Drama as Therapy

Drama as Therapy: Theatre as Living presents an integrated theory of Dramatherapy, focusing on how and why it can offer the opportunity for change. With a unique combination of practical guidance, clinical examples and theory, the author shows how Dramatherapy can be used with a wide range of clients and applied to their individual needs.

At the heart of the book is a definition of the nine core processes involved in Dramatherapy. Practical advice is given on how to structure sessions and the various techniques available to the therapist. The author draws on a variety of case studies taken from clinical practice; ranging from an autistic adolescent who enacts his life through a story about a prince locked in a tower to a woman who deals with her physical and sexual abuse by working with mask.

The author retraces the origins and development of Dramatherapy, taking into account the contribution of therapists throughout the world. He profiles the work of international innovators in the field such as Evreinov and Iljine and includes interviews with key figures Peter Slade, Sue Jennings and Billy Lindkvist.

Drama as Therapy will be an indispensable text for Dramatherapy students internationally and those working with drama therapeutically.

Phil Jones is Principal Lecturer and Course Leader of the Postgraduate Diploma in Dramatherapy, University of Hertfordshire. He also edits *Dramatherapy*, the journal of the British Association of Dramatherapy.

'A thoughtful and scholarly work! This book will be a key text in Dramatherapy for years to come.'

Alida Gersie, Director of Studies,
Graduate Arts Therapies Programme, University of Hertfordshire

'This remarkable book is essential for all Dramatherapy reading. Not only is it the first book to thoroughly research the European history of Dramatherapy, it also provides an illuminating, integrated model of practice.'

Sue Jennings, Senior Research Fellow, Royal London Hospital
Medical College, University of London and Honorary Fellow of the
Shakespeare Institute, University of Birmingham

'Phil Jones takes us on a journey through Dramatherapy – its history, processes, healing factors, theory and practice. When I started to read, I found it difficult to put the book down. Each chapter impelled me to read on. He has the ability to both describe and analyse Dramatherapy whilst firmly linking it with practice. This book cannot fail to stimulate the reader. It is a valuable resource for students, a useful review for practitioners and of interest to all who are involved in drama, theatre and therapy.'

Dorothy Langley, Lecturer in Dramatherapy and
Psychodrama, South Devon College of Technology

'A valuable and greatly needed resource for all Dramatherapists.'

Professor Robert Landy, Associate Professor and Director
of Dramatherapy Programme, New York University

'*Drama as Therapy* is an impressive book, meticulously researched. In it Jones covers Dramatherapy from early times to its emergence in the twentieth century.

He uses a broad brush to describe Greek and Roman theatre and more unusually, that of the Seneca Indians and the mask carving of the "False Face Society" of the Iroquois Confederacy. Shamans powerful for centuries, masks, puppets, all are there reinforcing our knowledge that, however much some of us would like to think so, nothing is new in this world!

Imperceptibly the brush strokes narrow until by the end of the book everything or nearly everything seems to be there as Jones probes deeper and deeper into the various modes, shapes, structures and methods used in the twentieth century.

Jones details the emergence of what he calls Dramatherapy in the Western World. He describes nine core processes and and theatrical core processes which he considers crucial to its effectiveness, with illustrations from his clinical practice.

In a word, Jones seems to have come a long way towards overcoming what he calls the "struggle to find clear concepts, working methodologies and language" to explain why and how it is that "drama is a therapy in its own right".'

Marian R. Lindkvist, Founder and Director of
the Sesame Institute, London

'Reading this mighty work has been a fascinating experience. This book describes all that Dramatherapy is, what people think it is and contains a mass of information based on wide research. This basic and most valuable book distinguishes between theatre and drama-the-doing-of-life.

It is a treasure chest of detailed information that no student or interested person should miss.'

Peter Slade, pioneer in Dramatherapy

Drama as Therapy:
Theatre as Living

Phil Jones

London and New York

First published 1996
by Routledge
11 New Fetter Lane, London EC4P 4EE

Simultaneously published in the USA and Canada
by Routledge
29 West 35th Street, New York, NY 10001

Typeset in Times by
Florencetype Ltd, Stoodleigh, Nr. Tiverton, Devon
Printed and bound in Great Britain by
Biddles Ltd, Guildford and King's Lynn

British Library Cataloguing in Publication Data
A catalogue record for this book is available from
the British Library

Library of Congress Cataloguing in Publication Data
A catalogue record for this book has been requested

ISBN 0–415–09969–2
    0–415–09970–6 (pbk)

This book is dedicated to my parents,
Esther and William Jones

I have in mind the instinct of transformation, the instinct of opposing from without images arbitrarily created from within, the instinct of transmuting appearances found in nature into something else, an instinct which clearly reveals its essential character in the conception of what I call theatricality.

Evreinov, *The Theatre in Life*

Contents

x   *Contents*

Plates

Figures

Boxes

Tables

Case studies

Don Quixote and the magic of action

'Pray look better, sir,' quoth Sancho: 'Those things yonder are no great giants, but windmills; and the arms you fancy are but their sails . . .'

'Tis a sign,' cried Don Quixote, 'that thou art but little acquainted with adventure! I tell thee they are giants; and, therefore, if thou art afraid, go aside . . . for I am resolved to engage in dreadful, unequal combat against them all.'

Cervantes, The History of Don Quixote

Cervantes takes pleasure in confusing the objective and the subjective, the world of the reader and the world of the book.

Borges, Partial Magic in the Quixote

In his travels and adventures Cervantes' Don Quixote (1898) suffuses reality with fantasy. His personally created world becomes confused with the world as experienced and lived in by others. The act of using the dramatic state and the creation of fictive, theatre worlds in a therapeutic context might be seen to encourage a similarly unhelpful confusion. Participation in dramatic activities has been seen as encouraging a removal from reality – as an escapist way of being, of relating to others and to the world.

Some have argued that theatre and life are separate states. If drama and life do connect it is only within the strict confines of a theatre with its formal demarcation of performance and audience areas.

Within the tradition of psychoanalysis enactment has often been viewed with suspicion. Fenichel's (1945) language reflects this in his essay 'Neurotic Acting Out'. When discussing the ways in which clients unconsciously avoid material within therapy he speaks of some clients having a 'bent for dramatisation' (1945, 198). A significant part of Fenichel's notion of avoidance through dramatisation relates to a 'Don Quixote' way of being – of wanting to satisfy a need within a fantasy which cannot be dealt with in reality. He speaks of this difficulty in terms of the client having a 'largely unconscious belief in the magic of action' (1945, 99). The argument is that adult dramatisation is a regression, an attempt to return to the experience of the child in play. The child is seen to believe that they can have magical effects upon the world through playing, creating a playful reality.

This book will argue against both the notion that acting or dramatised reality are not helpful in therapy and that life and theatre are essentially separate. It will argue that drama and living are vitally connected. Drama as a therapy asserts that human beings need enactment and theatre. As Evreinov (1927) wrote, theatre is a human impulse necessary to healthy living. Dramatherapy recognises that a part of this need and impulse can be used in the maintenance of health and in dealing with emotional and psychological problems. The creation of fictive worlds, of play states, the creative process itself, need not be seen only in terms of an unhelpful retreat from reality. The playful 'magic of action' need not result in Don Quixote's severance from the real world, rather it can be seen to be an important part of living in the world. Müller-Thalheim has spoken of this healing, life-affirming aspect of creativity: 'We know the fantasies and the artistic daydreams which help to conquer the painful limits of existence and lead through play to art. They also help us to manage our basic conflicts' (1975, 166).

There now exists a substantial body of theoretical knowledge and a range of specific practical approaches which relate to Dramatherapy. This book will consider specific techniques which have been devised during the twentieth century alongside the theoretical basis for linking drama, theatre and therapy. It aims to describe what Dramatherapy is whilst indicating why and how it is effective. A crucial part of this efficacy concerns the ways in which the creative and the fictive can be vital to living and to health.

Acknowledgements

I would like to thank Neil Walters for his support, editing skills and insight. Without his assistance this book would not exist.

This book was written in London, and during a sabbatical in Xania and Athens. I would like to thank my friends in Greece for their support whilst I lived there. This book owes a debt to Annie and Frank Nowak, Nicos Marinos and Giorgos Simou, Manolis Filipakis, Jannis and Gogo Bolaraki.

A number of people have helped in the research and writing through interviews and commentaries on my work. I would especially like to thank Peter Slade, Sue Jennings and Billy Lindkvist – both for the interviews they offered and for the documentation they have provided from their personal collections. Alida Gersie, Robert Landy, Ditty Dokter and Rea Karagiourgiou-Short have given me valuable assistance by their comments on my developing text. Alida Gersie, Hank Guilickx, Ana Palma and Cristina Calheiros assisted with the writing of the history section. Ann Cattanach and Dorothy Langley also must be mentioned in terms of their contributions to the field and to the development of my ideas within *Drama as Therapy*. Helena Ivins, Margaret Walters, Deborah Loveridge and John Convey have all assisted in the preparation of the book. Similarly I must thank the many students whose views have helped hone my ideas and research – from the Division of Arts and Psychology through to the Postgraduate Arts Therapies programme at the University of Hertfordshire. Penny Dade and the School of Art and Design's Library services have also greatly assisted my research. Many thanks also to Edwina Welham, Alison Poyner and Nikky Twyman.

The practice described in this book has been supported by a number of organisations and funders. I would like to give special thanks to the creative and financial input of Mike Sparks and the Sir John Cass Foundation. The Calouste Gulbenkian Foundation, the European Community's Horizon Programme and Greater London Arts also supported some of the work. I would also like to thank my co-workers Lesley Kerr Edwards, Pat Place, Ayad Chebib and Rosemary Sanctuary.

How to use this book

Drama as Therapy is divided into four parts. The first gives an overview of the definition of Dramatherapy and reviews Dramatherapy's main forms and formats. Included in this is a guide to the structure of Dramatherapy processes and sessions. Part II describes the history of Dramatherapy. The third part of the book is formed by a definition of the core processes which are at the heart of Dramatherapy's efficacy and the fourth considers the main areas of theory and practice. Each area is given a specific chapter which includes a theoretical background, an illustrated guide to practice with clinical examples, along with a summary or definition of the area.

Part I

Chapter 1
What is Dramatherapy? An introd

> Drama is mimetic action, action in imitation or representation of human behaviour.
>
> Esslin, *An Anatomy of Drama*

There are two perceptions at the heart of this book. The first is that drama and theatre are ways of actively participating in the world and are *not* merely an imitation of it. The second is that within drama there is a powerful potential for healing.

The term 'Dramatherapy' refers to drama as a form of therapy. During the twentieth century developments in a number of different fields such as experimental theatre and psychology have resulted in new insights into the ways in which drama and theatre can be effective in bringing about change in people: emotional, political and spiritual change.

The way in which Dramatherapy relates to dramatic and theatre processes is of a particular nature. 'Two Masks' illustrates one way in which a form from theatre, the mask, changes when worked with in Dramatherapy.

Case study 1.1 Two Masks

The Noh mask (Plate 1.1) is a theatre product. Its use and purpose originate from a tradition of acting. The mask covers the actor's face in order to depict a specific role; when wearing it the actor moves in a particular way. The portrayal of character is linked to a script which is performed for an audience's enjoyment. The actor is a paid employee; the mask is made by skilled specialist artisans.

The second mask (Plate 1.2) is also worn over the face and in this way is similar to the first, but it is a product of a therapy session. It was not produced primarily for the performance of a script to entertain an audience, nor was it produced by skilled artisans.

It was created by a client attending a Dramatherapy group. She was trying to deal both with her relationship with her father and with an aspect of herself. The mask was made as an image of a part of herself which she felt was caught in a web of her father's deceit. She was

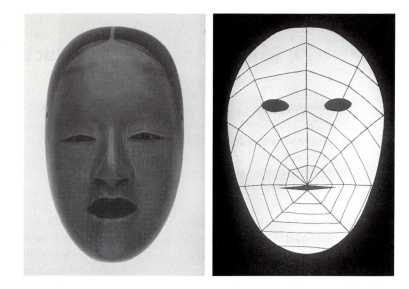

Plate 1.1 Image of Noh mask
Copyright British Museum

Plate 1.2 Image of client's web mask

physically and sexually abused as a child. The mask, for her, represented an internal role: a part she felt was stuck to her, that she kept a secret. She said that the centre of the web was over her mouth to stop her speaking.

The mask was important in three ways:

- The creation of the mask was a means of communicating to people in a powerful way what had happened to her. *It provided a concrete way of putting her internalised feelings outside herself.* Once outside they could be worked with rather than remaining locked inside. The mask provided a new language for her to work with the problem and trauma.

- Previously, the web around her had felt 'sticky' and 'trapping'. She said 'I couldn't get it off me'. The mask reflected this quality in that it was worn close to her face. But unlike the web, the mask could be taken off. This meant that after expressing the feelings of being trapped within the web mask she could experience taking the mask off – being released from the web. The physical expression through the mask changed her experience of the internalised role. *She could work dramatically with the mask and use it to try to find a new relationship to the trauma.*

- The work with the mask achieved change in the way the client felt about herself. It also *resulted in action in her life outside the therapy*. She began to consider ways in which she could be freed of the 'mask' in her life. One way she chose was to confront her family. She refused 'to wear the mask for them any longer', as she put it.

The mask was used over a period of time in different ways whilst she worked through the processes of revealing and dealing with the secret. She considered both what actions she wanted to take, along with the feelings that had been 'masked' for so long. The paradox of the mask in Dramatherapy is that the *concealing* of the face often *reveals* a great deal of personal material.

The comparison of the masks illustrates some of the key ways in which Dramatherapy relates to drama and theatre processes. The Noh mask is primarily a part of a theatrical product and the actor uses it to work creatively, portraying a fictional role in a religious or entertainment context. For the client in Dramatherapy the primary use of the mask was in expressing and working through personal issues and trying to resolve her distress.

Drama as necessary to living

In the past 100 years the theme of drama and theatre as 'necessary' to healthy societies and to healthy individuals has re-emerged. Evreinov says that theatre is 'infinitely wider than the stage', and is not just for entertainment or instruction; it is, 'something as essentially necessary to man as air, food and sexual intercourse' (1927, 6).

This phrase is echoed across the century. Forty years later Peter Brook seeks a theatre that is as 'necessary as eating or sex' in *The Empty Space* (1968). Schechner says of the special world created in performance, 'no society, no individual can do without it' (1988, 11). But *why* should theatre be so essential? *How* can theatre be necessary?

The general theme is not a new one. However, Western society in the twentieth century understands its implications in particular ways.

This understanding considers that participating in drama and theatre allows connections to unconscious and emotional processes to be made. Participation is seen to satisfy human needs to play and to create. The festive act of people coming together through drama and theatre is seen to have social and psychological importance. Theatre is both an activity set apart from everyday reality, which at the same time has a vital function in reflecting upon and reacting to that reality.

A theatre has been sought by practitioners such as Grotowski, Brook and Boal which can bring people together and can comment upon and deeply affect their feelings, their politics and their ways of living.

I consider that Dramatherapy originates from these beliefs which see theatre as being necessary to living. This book will explore one particular way in which drama and theatre processes are essential, a part of the maintenance of well-being or a return to health.

At the beginning of the twentieth century drama was used as a recreation, as an adjunct to the main therapeutic ways of working with people in care or health settings. The key aspects of the therapy remained outside the clients' experience of drama. Drama was seen only as a way of making stays in hospital more enjoyable, or sometimes as an opportunity to raise emotional material which would be dealt with later in the hands of the psychologist or psychiatrist. In this there was a gender issue: that, whilst a large number of practitioners using drama were women, the 'main treatment' modalities were practised by male psychiatrists and psychologists (Barham, 1994).

Over the past two decades a change has come to be fully acknowledged: that the drama itself is the therapy. This change marks the emergence of Dramatherapy as it is currently practised. There are two main aspects to this change or development. One is that the Dramatherapy session can deal with primary processes involved in the client's change rather than being an adjunct to other ways of working, such as psychotherapy. The other is that the root of this process is in the drama. Dramatherapy is not a psychotherapy group or behavioural therapy programme which has some dramatic activities added to it. The drama does not serve the therapy. The drama process contains the therapy.

The drama is the therapy

Oatley's analysis of healing and therapy adds to the understanding of the general notion of 'therapeutic change' in Dramatherapy. He connects the term and concept 'to heal' to its etymological origin: 'hale' meaning 'whole'. He defines therapy as becoming involved in a relationship which might become healing: 'It can allow the self and relationships to become more whole, less a set of fragments . . .' (Oatley, 1984, 2). He rightly acknowledges that 'wholeness' as a concept is culture-specific in its meaning.

Here therapy is seen to involve change towards a greater integration where there is currently fragmentation. Irwin also defines therapy in terms of change and relationship but within the context of Dramatherapy. The relation becomes the planned application of drama/theatre techniques 'to aid in remedition, rehabilitation, or personal or social adjustment' and 'a specific form of intervention to bring about intrapsychic, interpersonal, or behavioural changes' (Irwin, 1979, 23). A piece of research published in 1993 has indicated that the concepts of Carl Jung are seen by British Dramatherapists as being the most relevant to Dramatherapy (Valente and Fontana, 1993, 64). It is safe to suggest that many Dramatherapists would echo Jung's definition of therapy, as less 'a question of treatment than of developing the creative possibilities latent in the patient himself' (Jung, 1983, 211).

In Dramatherapy it is the client's creativity as developed, expressed and explored within the therapeutic framework, and the focused dramatic processes, which provide the opportunity for health and for the kinds of change which Irwin describes.

Dramatic processes are worked with in ways which facilitate therapeutic change. These ways are inherent in drama and theatre forms. Dramatherapy focuses and emphasises these healing aspects of drama and theatre. In terms of historic process, as Chapters 3 and 4 will show, Dramatherapy marks the connection between two main areas. One area is the discoveries and understanding of therapeutic processes developed over the past century. The other is the experiments and work which have taken place regarding the potentials of dramatic processes to achieve personal change.

As this book will demonstrate, any area of drama or theatre such as the taking on of an alternative identity through drama, may have a therapeutic element to it.

Case study 1.2 Gertrude and *Hamlet*

Clare Higgins, in talking about the Royal Shakespeare Company's rehearsal of *Hamlet*, describes how a painful personal memory was suddenly triggered within improvisations around the script.

> Mark took the knife out and threatened me, a lot of things clicked . . . I was not expecting it . . . It triggered something that had actually happened to me in my life, which he could not possibly have known.
> (Cox, 1992, 66)

The distress of the memory was used within the rehearsal and the creation of the role of Gertrude which Higgins was developing. The personal connection and distress was mostly channelled into the creativity rather than in looking to engage directly with the memory and the experience of being attacked. The 'therapeutic' aspect of this lay in the way in which the drama evoked a powerful personal issue or trauma from the past. Even within the theatre context Higgins says that she found the expression of the memory and working it into the role 'freeing' and cathartic.

In Dramatherapy itself the therapeutic aspects of drama are foregrounded, developed to their fullest potential. They are utilised within a clear framework of a therapeutic relationship.

The premise of Dramatherapy is *not* that all art is therapy. It does not preclude art made primarily for creative, political or financial purposes. It does not seek to pathologise the artist or artistic activity. It does, however, recognise that artistic processes and products have healing potentials and that, if worked with in particular ways in specific contexts, drama can be a therapy.

Basic tenets of Dramatherapy

Definition of Dramatherapy

Dramatherapy is involvement in drama with a healing intention.

Dramatherapy facilitates change through drama processes. It uses the potential of drama to reflect and transform life experiences to enable clients to express and work through problems they are encountering or to maintain a client's well-being and health.

Clients make use of the *content* of drama activities, the *process* of creating enactments, and the *relationships* formed between those taking part in the work within a *therapeutic* framework.

A connection is created between the client's inner world, problematic situation or life experience and the activity in the Dramatherapy session. The client seeks to achieve a new relationship towards the problems or life experiences they bring to therapy. The aim is to find in this new relationship resolution, relief, a new understanding or changed ways of functioning.

Who is Dramatherapy for?

Dramatherapy is practised with groups and individuals in care settings such as clinics, hospitals and specialist centres such as adolescent units. It is also offered as an individual or group therapy available outside institutions. Work is undertaken with both adults and children.

Dramatherapists are employed in family centres, prisons and borstals, special schools and educational units, centres for young adults with behavioural problems, in mental health and rehabilitation settings, community centres and within alcohol or substance abuse programmes. Individual or group Dramatherapy is offered to people in the community who are dealing with emotional difficulties through GP, social worker or self-referral.

Settings employ Dramatherapists on a full-time or part-time basis. Dramatherapy is often offered alongside other arts therapies, as part of a multidisciplinary approach. Prior to the establishment of training courses and the professional registration of Dramatherapists it was more usual for individuals occupying posts in other fields such as occupational therapy or social work, to use part of their time to run Dramatherapy groups and to have 'Dramatherapist' as part of their professional identity. Whilst this is still so in many cases there are an increasing number of specialist Dramatherapy posts.

What happens in Dramatherapy?

A facilitator, the Dramatherapist, works with groups or individuals over a number of weeks for sessions lasting between forty minutes and one and a half hours. Each session usually consists of a warm up phase which develops into an active exploration of areas which are problematic for clients, followed by a closure. The kind of problems which can be dealt with and the form of the sessions are extremely varied. The main process involves the client engaging with a problematic area through dramatic form and work with the group and/or therapist. Closure often takes the form of discussion and reflection upon the work undertaken within the session. Dramatherapy takes place within clear boundaries which protect the therapeutic space.

The basic processes of Dramatherapy

A number of key processes lie at the heart of Dramatherapy and they are the main ways in which therapeutic change occurs. These are described in detail in Chapter 5; important amongst them are 'dramatic projection' and 'transformation'.

Through *dramatic projection* the client becomes emotionally and intellectually involved in encountering the problems in dramatic forms such as characters, play materials or puppets.

Transformation describes the ways in which the client's experience of the expressed problems changes during Dramatherapy work. This change is due to the use of dramatic processes to express and explore (to transform) the client's material. It is also due to the experience of the relationships formed in the Dramatherapy, both with the therapist and with other clients if the work is in a group.

This process can open up a number of creative, altered ways of dealing with and experiencing the problem.

The expressive forms of Dramatherapy

Dramatherapy sessions include a wide repertoire of dramatic expressive forms. These have different therapeutic potentials as is described in Chapter 3. They include:

- the use of created or scripted roles and characters, or playing oneself in a fictional reality, in order to explore life experiences
- the use of materials such as objects, small toys and puppets to play out and work with problematic feelings, relationships or experiences
- the use of the body in dramatic form through disguise, masking, mime or performance art to explore the self, image, relationship
- the use of scripts, stories and myths to evoke and act out themes, personal issues or archetypal material with a view to the exploration of problems
- the creation of dramatic rituals to work through areas of life experience
- moving through different developmental stages in drama to assist in the development of new ways of relating to oneself and to others

Basic ideas underpinning Dramatherapy

Building blocks: creativity, play, drama and healing

Dramatherapy builds upon the healing aspects which are present in dramatic and theatrical activities. Generally speaking these healing aspects are based in the processes of creativity, playing and acting. Klaesi (1922) and Müller-Thalheim (1975) have put forward the idea that creativity has within it inherent self-healing processes. Müller-Thalheim discusses this specifically in relation to people in psychotic states, but considers some general implications. These include the Freudian notion that creative products are formed from elementary impulses from the unconscious, rather like dreams. However, he goes further than framing creative expressions as symptoms, which Freud seems to consider as the main quality of art. Müller-Thalheim sees 'inspiration, change, new combinations, new actions' (1975, 164) as inherent to much creativity, and claims that these are central to health and to development from ill-health or problematic conditions. He indicates a natural healing process involved in art making. As an example he discusses Ernst Josephson's use of a few symbols in painting: 'His paintings seemed not only to reproduce his difficulties, but also to free him from them' (1975, 165).

His faith here is in the natural healing potential within the artistic medium and process. This lies in the healing value of creative expression and the value of playfulness as a way of creating new insights. In addition he suggests that expressing problematic material and emotions through the arts changes the relationship to the problems or feelings. For example, 'Real fear is being converted into fictional fear' (1975, 166) and is therefore more able to be faced, talked about and dealt with. He believes in the arts as a counterbalance of 'sense and order' against the 'nonsense and disorder' (1975, 166) which many people experience in distress or illness.

Whilst his notions of artistic activity and experience are romantic and culture-specific, there are a number of points here which have been developed by empirical research and which are pertinent to Dramatherapy. These are: the emphasis upon the healing potential inherent in creative processes, the notion of playfulness, and the creation of fictive representations of emotions as being useful in the healing process of therapy.

Drama and therapy have been linked by a number of people from different disciplines. Peter Elsass, for example, notes an 'apparent similarity' between the work of the actor and that of the psychotherapist. He identifies this connection as the aim of creating new insights or making implicit knowledge explicit for audience or for patient (Elsass, 1992). Antinucci-Mark notes that theatre and psychotherapy are 'from similar roots and meet similar needs' (1986, 15). She notes that both involve an interplay between fantasy and reality, the manipulation of internal objects and images and the creation of an 'as if' scenario in terms of time and place (1986, 15).

However, such connections do not usually go beyond acknowledging a parallel in order to understand aspects of theatre or psychotherapy. For example, Antinucci-Mark does not take her exploration beyond noting the parallel. Elsass uses it as a point to begin a consideration of shamanism – indeed, he says in his conclusion that theatre 'is not like therapy' but that it is a useful analogy to make (1992, 342).

Dramatherapy is more than an acknowledgement of the connections between therapy and theatre. It takes the parallels or similarities and actively seeks to bring about a new form of therapy which builds on the relationship. In addition to recognising similarities it also seeks to acknowledge the differences and to use these effectively, as this book will show.

Fantasy and reality: a paradox for change

Drama and theatre have always dealt with the interface between reality and fantasy. Mast has said that the actor participates simultaneously on 'everyday' and 'dramatic' levels of reality (Mast, 1986, 79). Drama as a therapy seeks to work with the connection – the relationship between reality and fantasy – in a particularly intense way.

Dramatherapy uses the connection between fantasy and reality to intervene in the way people live. A boundary is made between being inside the therapy group and the world outside. However, the theatre of Dramatherapy is life. By this I mean that the theatre created by clients in Dramatherapy deals with, and is a part of, their own lives.

Schechner has summarised the space in theatre as a special world where people can make the rules, rearrange time, assign special values to things and work for pleasure (1988, 11).

Dramatherapy often creates a paradoxical state. It has the safety of the above qualities described as inherent in a special theatre world by Schechner. Yet . . . it creates a state which is very much to do with reality.

Clients may create roles where they encounter actual feeling states. They cry, feel anger, hope – these are not experienced as fictional. Real tears are wept. Real anger is vented. But at the same time it is within a fictional construct, they may be doing so whilst playing a role or handling a play object. The most fantastically unreal tale of jinn and sea demon, of castle and warrior maiden will be at the same time fictional yet to do with the innermost realities of the individual's psyche.

In Dramatherapy the paradox that 'what is fictional is also real' is crucial to its efficacy as a therapy. The enactment in the therapy group is a part of the client's reality. The dramatic experience is focused upon the client and their life. It is different from everyday living, but it is an equally valid way for the client to experience the different facets of who they are and how they are.

Dramatherapy does not seek to create the high level of distance between stage and life, between being involved in performance and being involved in life outside the drama, which many theatre forms aim for. This is not to say that Dramatherapy confuses the client's experience of life and theatre: this is often very clear. However, there is great intimacy between the two, the interface between life outside the drama and life inside the drama is extremely close and vital. It is a form of theatre as living rather than theatre as an escape from life.

The creation of fictive, dramatic worlds aims to challenge, to alter and directly bring about change for the client, both within the time of the Dramatherapy and in the client's life outside therapy. This book will give example after example of people living and changing their lives within the enactments of a Dramatherapy session.

Therapeutic change and Dramatherapy: how psychological disturbance is construed

One of the simplest definitions of therapy is that it is a form of intervention aiming to bring about personal change.

The nature of this change within Dramatherapy practice in part reflects the setting of the work and the orientation of the Dramatherapist.

In recent research the major influences cited by Dramatherapists reflected the variety of ways in which Dramatherapy is practised. Dramatherapists cited group dynamics theory, psychotherapy, theories of play, the work of Jung, Winnicott, Rogers, Freud and Klein, for example. Psychodrama is cited as an influence 'which many Dramatherapists now see as a sub-division of Dramatherapy' (Valente and Fontana, 1993, 63).

This diversity is also noted by Dokter. She asserts that differing cultural notions of drama and healing result in different treatment orientations based on culturally specific concepts of illness. In Spain and Portugal, for example, she says that, 'Given the different concept of drama, the acceptance of drama as therapy would be problematic' (1993, 85). In developing a critique of Dramatherapy in different contexts she describes a tendency to see Dramatherapy within an 'either/or' framework. This sees it either as 'a form of psychotherapy' or 'a creative healing art form in itself' (1993, 89). I do not see the division as necessarily present in the way that Dramatherapy is practised. Currently Dramatherapy functions within a number of theoretical and therapeutic paradigms. As the book will demonstrate, it serves within behavioural frameworks as successfully as it does within family therapy, or within dynamic psychotherapy contexts.

The ways in which psychological disturbances are construed vary widely. It could be that at some point in the future Dramatherapy theory and practice might develop or work with one particular model of the mind, or become attached to one particular school of thought concerning the ways in which the individual or group experiences psychological distress. This is not the case at the moment.

Authors such as Ciornai (1983) and Canda (1990) have stressed the importance of cultural and socio-economic factors in considering change within the arts therapies. Ciornai places emphasis upon the need to orientate work within the cultural and social background of the client. She notes the possibility of areas such as oppression, discrimination and poverty being overlooked in therapeutic approaches which focus exclusively on intrapsychic factors. The need is to balance internal and external factors affecting the clients' life (1983, 64). Both authors emphasise the necessity for therapists to be conscious of their own cultural assumptions about the expressive forms used within the arts therapies. Clients' expressions and intentions through dramatic form may operate within cultural traditions which differ from those of the therapist. Ciornai and Canda both advocate the necessity for arts therapists to 'provide service in a manner that is accessible and meaningful to the client' (Canda, 1990, 58). This entails the need for the therapist to be 'culturally literate', contextualising the work within accurate cultural knowledge, positive regard for cultural diversity, practical cross-cultural communication skills and familiarity with relevant artistic expressive forms and traditions (Canda, 1990, 58; Ciornai, 1983, 65).

As Chapter 5 will illustrate, key processes in Dramatherapy are constant and there are basic assumptions about how Dramatherapy can facilitate change. The task of the Dramatherapist is to comprehend how these basic processes and expressive forms connect with the context of the work. The context is the way in which the client presents a difficulty and the philosophy or ethos of the setting or framework in which the therapy will be undertaken.

Drama and theatre

Often the terms 'theatre' and 'drama' are used interchangeably. Dramatherapy conceptually and practically includes aspects of both theatre and drama processes. As Chapter 3 will show, some of its antecedents, such as Evreinov's 'Theatrotherapy', have used the term 'theatre' rather than 'drama'. It could be that the exclusion of 'theatre' from 'Dramatherapy' is due to the comparative lack of traditional performative processes such as staging a scripted play within Dramatherapy.

There are many different models and definitions of 'theatre' and 'drama'. Barrault echoes many when he defines theatre as follows: 'A theatrical representation is a meeting of two human groups. First, the audience. Second, the players' (Barrault, 1972, 24). Southern arrives at the same conclusion: it is 'the act . . . of performing something before a group of other people' (Southern, 1962, 21). Drama is defined by Landy as 'a separation of self and non-self . . . a separation of realities' (Landy, 1986, 5). Within the context of discussing Dramatherapy I have taken the following as my basic definitions based on Barrault, Southern and Landy. Theatre is the production of a performance, and drama is the entry into a special state where individuals, the space they use and the things they do, exist in a pretended reality.

Dramatherapy and meaning

Drama and theatre are social activities. As O'Neill and Lambert have said, an important facet of drama is social and involves 'contact, communication and the negotiation of meaning' (1982, 13). The discovery and communication of meaning in Dramatherapy is a key concept within my discussion of how Dramatherapy is effective for clients. Important aspects of the relationship between Dramatherapy, meaning and the client include the ways in which:

- life experiences are given *added validity* by depicting them dramatically with and in front of others.
- an individual's dramatic work is *recognised and understood* by others. The feelings and experiences they depict are empathised with and responded to by others.
- the process of dealing with life problems through enactment leads to the creation of a *vital relationship between the client's life experiences outside the Dramatherapy and the enactments they take part in within the therapy.*

By establishing a link between the client's life experiences and the Dramatherapy group the possibility of finding new meanings in their life through the playful, experimental space of Dramatherapy is created. Laurel of the Japanese Atari Research Division, has documented the positive potentials of virtual reality through computer graphics. She sees this in terms of the relationship between the process of finding meaning and the creation of dramatic worlds. Laurel argues that virtual reality creates access to areas of

> Meanings that are only rarely afforded by the real world. Dramatically constructed worlds are controlled experiments, where the bare bones of human choice and situation are revealed . . . If we can make such worlds interactive, where a user's choices and actions can flow through the dramatic lens, then we will enable an

exercise of the imagination, intellect and spirit of an entirely new order.

(Laurel, 1991, 14)

This aspect of constructing dramatic therapeutic 'controlled experiments' is an important way for the client to find meaning in their world and to deal with problems they are encountering.

Past and current models of Dramatherapy

As Chapters 4 and 5 will show, the way in which drama has been perceived in terms of therapy has changed radically. Courtney has described the current variety of models within the arts therapies as a whole, and says of Dramatherapy, 'Even within the one form . . . there are major differences of approach' (1988, 192). The definition of Dramatherapy is especially problematic. As Landy has pointed out, 'because both drama and therapy are conceptually complex terms, confusions are inevitable' (1982, 135).

Previous definitions have often tried to divide the functions of Dramatherapy into different types or models of therapy. One way of doing this has been to try to divide Dramatherapy into various levels of practice with different kinds of drama attached to each level (Langley, 1993). In this way, for example, one approach defined Dramatherapy as having three 'models': a creative/expressive model, a tasks and skills model and a psychotherapy model (Jennings, 1987). This is unsatisfactory in that it tries to separate out aspects which do not actually exist as clearly defined entities within Dramatherapy. Creativity is not separate from psychotherapy, skill cannot be separated from expression. In recent years the proliferation of definitions has reached epidemic proportions – with anthropological models, paratheatrical models, shamanistic models, role-theory models, etc. (Jennings, 1987; Mitchell, 1992; Landy, 1994). These seem to try to meet the need to define Dramatherapy and its efficacy by hiving off a particular element and calling it a model. I find this unsatisfactory and incomplete.

This book will define Dramatherapy in its entirety. It does not seek to separate out different aspects into models. Rather it will define the key processes which operate within Dramatherapy and show how they can be used in different ways according to the needs of the client group or context. Hence *the basic processes are constant*, and are utilised in different ways according to specific client need. The processes are defined initially in Chapter 5, but the understanding of how they operate underpins the whole book. By working in this way I aim to provide a substantial base to all Dramatherapy practice and the theory which facilitates work with clients.

Chapter 2
Forms and formats
Dramatherapy practice

Introduction: form for feelings

Dramatherapy is practised in a series of sessions. The aim of the shape
of the Dramatherapy session is to find a form for feelings to be explored
with the intention of achieving personal change.

This chapter considers the basic format or shape of a Dramatherapy
session, and it will also look at the different elements which are part of
this shape. Dramatherapy uses a wide range of expressive forms – from
playing a role to creating environments. The chapter will examine the
ways that these forms relate to the basic shape.

The basic shape

The session – introduction

The content of a Dramatherapy session usually happens within a basic
shape or form. In any session it is necessary to find a way in which the
therapeutic needs and creative potentials of the group or individual can
connect with the expressive forms and processes of Dramatherapy.

Some work is highly structured. Aims will be set and the Drama-
therapy session, content and process will be agreed with the group.
The case study 'Leaving Home' (see pp. 36–37), illustrates this approach.
It is more usual for the content and process to relate to the material
brought to the session by the group or individual. The case studies
'Villa Grumpyview' pp. 37–39), 'Creature in a Box' (pp. 20–31) and
'Role Play' (pp. 20–31) all illustrate this approach. However, as
Schattner points out, a Dramatherapist will often have some prepared
ideas based around the work the group or individual has done to
date – it is important is to remain sensitive to the group's needs and
situation.

We might start with a very structured session which we might have
to change on the spur of the moment, because we have to work
according to the needs of the special populations. There are patients

who want to perform; there are patients who want to sit and do nothing.

(Schattner and Courtney, 1981, 144)

A usual form for Dramatherapy is a basic shape which divides into five sections or elements as Box 2.1 illustrates.

Box 2.1 **Dramatherapy – the basic shape**

- Warm Up
- Focusing
- Main Activity
- Closure and de-roling
- Completion

The length of each of these sections varies according to the way a group uses Dramatherapy. Each section has a different function within the therapeutic work. Usually a Dramatherapy session will include all the sections. In many cases the warm up and focusing will take up a third of the time, the main activity another third, and closure, de-roling and completion the last third. However, as is discussed below, as a group develops the warming up time may be reduced.

The basic shape illustrated

The next section will discuss the parts of this basic shape. Two sessions from two very different kinds of Dramatherapy work will be described section by section to illustrate the five elements of the shape. One concerns a Dramatherapy group using role in a psychiatric day centre, the other group involves puppetry with a group of children with severe learning disabilities.

Warm up

Often the warm up phase can be divided into two – a general warm up time followed by a focusing.

The warm up is an activity which helps an individual or group prepare for dramatherapeutic work. It usually takes the form of a variety of exercises which concern the emotions of the group and/or the group's use of dramatic processes or language.

With the increase in the use of improvisation in rehearsal processes over the past century, many theatre practitioners use exercises to prepare actors. The warm up in Dramatherapy is analogous to this in that part of its function is to begin to help the group to prepare for dramatic activity. However, it has an additional function in that the Dramatherapy warm up also seeks to help individuals begin to consider the area of content they might work with in the therapy. Unlike a conventional theatre warm up or improvisation, which aims to rehearse a specific text, there is often no set agenda or script to be worked with.

The warm up often helps to mark the start of the creation of a special Dramatherapy space. This will be discussed in detail later in the book. The basis of this can be a specific pattern which is followed at the start of each session – the rolling out of a carpet, the completion of a name game. It can also consist of exercises which mark entry into dramatic work – a role-based game or activity, the bringing out of play materials or the building of an environment.

It has been argued that an individual using drama does so more effectively if they are physically, emotionally and mentally prepared. This can be true of Dramatherapy. An individual's use of dramatic media within the therapy session can be enhanced by warm up. In addition, the warm up can help individual, group and therapist orientate and focus themselves towards the therapeutic material with which they will work. This can be described as part of the 'need-identifying' period within a session.

Figure 2.1 sets out some of the key areas with which warm up activities engage.

Some have questioned the notion of the warm up in Dramatherapy. Often the therapist will suggest a warm up based on what they perceive to be happening in a group or for an individual. Some have argued that this seeks to avoid resistances and that the resistance to the work needs to be acknowledged rather than diverted by a warm up. For example a group of adolescents might present as being resistant to doing anything in the group. The Dramatherapist has to decide whether the group will stay with the resistance to any active work – experiencing its state – or whether the therapist will create a warm up activity to help the group to overcome its resistance and engage in active work.

Why does Dramatherapy need a warm up? It might be argued, for example, that verbal psychotherapy does not use a formal 'warm up'. A psychotherapist does not directly ask the client to play with language, practising the voice, preparing to lie on a couch prior to a session. However, Dramatherapy uses dramatic languages, not just speech.

Body/Mind
- physical co-ordination
- concentration
- physical expression

Working with others
- engaging in physical activity with others
- engaging in imaginative activity with others
- working on emotions with others

Use of materials
- using objects physically
- using objects imaginatively
- projecting feeling into material

Issues
- group or individual emotional material

Figure 2.1 Key warm up areas

Whereas most people use verbal language as the main mode of communication in their daily lives, they do not tend to act or create a fictive world.

The warm up need not be confined to the start of a session. It can be used in terms of a particular activity. For example, during the later stages of a session a group might be involved in role work. To use role effectively the therapist may ask the group to engage in warm ups specifically connected to the building up of roles.

A warm up might help to achieve a level of focus for a group or individual too excited to work, or too 'over-aroused'. It has been said that to engage in dramatic activity it is necessary to be in a state of balance in terms of over- or under-engagement. For some groups and activities it is true that, should the aim be to engage in ongoing enactment or focused work, a group may be too aroused or distressed to do this. However, the therapist needs to be clear that he or she is not imposing a form upon a group. For example, a group may naturally have a short focus or attention span – the therapist needs to think whose needs are being truly met if he or she wants to work towards a longer form of concentrated work. Usually the therapist aims to find a balance between the emotional needs and capabilities of a group or individual and identifying the appropriate vehicle to explore and work with the material.

Case study 2.1 Role Play in Dramatherapy (context, aims and warm up)

The group was ongoing, weekly, and was part of a psychodynamic therapeutic programme in a psychiatric day centre. Each week the group would bring issues they wanted to explore. The main focus had been upon individuals working on particular problems and the relationships between group members. Often themes would emerge which would be dealt with on both a group and individual basis. There was a general feeling of low self-esteem, and the previous week a woman, Annie, had taken part in a role play depicting her mother's response to her attending the day centre and her breakdown. Her mother saw the 'whole thing' as a 'terrible let down'.

Warm up
The group began with a silence which lasted for just under five minutes. One person began to talk about a theme which had emerged at the close of the previous session and which had been touched on briefly a number of times within individual and group work. This concerned 'how other people see us'. The theme became how other people's expectations were 'the worst thing to deal with' and how 'impossible' it was when other people's opinions were so damning and so low. This extended to family, friends and the staff at the centre. This verbal warm up carried on for ten minutes or so.

Case study 2.2 Creature in a Box (context, aims and warm up)

The work was with a group of 12–13-year-olds in a special school for children with severe learning difficulties. The children were considered to have problems with social contact, and often were unsure of how to engage in establishing relationships. The twelve-week group was aiming to help the group to acquire social skills in establishing relationships and to help them deal with shyness and lack of self-esteem. The group did not have a complex verbal vocabulary able to deal directly with this material. Their self-consciousness had been perceived during the assessment period to indicate that to try to deal directly with first-hand experience would be less valuable than a more oblique way of letting the group work with the material. The group had shown a high level of interest and creativity in working symbolically with objects and could use objects to represent a fictional persona.

Working with the teacher it was decided to create a shadow puppet which would hold the personality of an extremely shy socially naive creature. The puppet would then be used to help the group to develop a social vocabulary and to enable them to explore their feelings of shyness and self-consciousness. Other puppets were created with different personalities. Some of these were given characteristics which would encourage the creature, other puppets would be discouraging or difficult.

Each session was to have a particular goal in developing a particular skill. We would both deal with the skill and explore some of the feelings around the topic. These included: Feelings when meeting a stranger, What to say, What is a friend?, What to do if you don't want to be a friend, What is the difference between wanting to know someone and not wanting to know someone, Strangers and friends – different ways of behaving and feeling when someone isn't friendly.

Warm up

Third session: In the second session the shadow puppet creatures had been created by the group. The pupils had worked together using thin card and pens to create shadow puppets which were then used on a large screen. The small creature had been introduced. Staff and students had manipulated the puppet and the group had given it particularly shy and 'naive' qualities. The group had made the creature rather small and furry with two large eyes. It lived in a box with a lid it could bring up or down.

The intention had been to warm up straight into using the puppets. However, a fight had occurred in the playground prior to the session and one of the group had been marginally involved, though, as the school was small, all the group had witnessed what had occurred. Hence the energy and concentration level of the group was dispersed and distracted. As the aims of the group were to work with the puppet I decided to try to work with the themes that seemed to be around ('aggression', 'unfriendly' and 'friendly'). However, the group were not in a state to be able to concentrate on using the puppet. They were distracted, there was much cross-group shouting, looking out of the window and running around the room.

I used warm ups to try to help the group to focus and work together. An example of this was to bring the group in a circle sitting in chairs, and to work physically with stretching and shaking. This tried to focus the wild energy which was within the room, not suppressing it but channelling it into patterned activity. Initially the group focused upon myself, the therapist, as a pattern of movement was introduced. This then shifted to the group imitating each other in turn. This aimed to bring the group together – moving in parallel with each other. It also aimed to help the group to inhabit their own bodies in a way that was more focused than the distracted running around. A small bean bag was then passed around the group; each member said what the bean bag could be. This aimed to help the group to focus and to engage imaginatively with an object. The bag then had to become an animal experiencing different feelings. Many of the themes which had seemed to be around the previous week, and feelings which seemed to be in response to the playground incident, were present: 'sad', 'shy', 'cross', 'smelly'.

The group were making a song as a way of memorising the development of the work and to demarcate the start and close of the activity. At the end of each session a new line was devised by the group and added to the song. At this point the therapist reminded the group that they'd made the first line of the song the previous week. With a little help the group managed to remember the line and sang it. Though some of the group had remembered the puppet and had asked straight away, for others the song activated their memories of the puppet; on singing the song their attention went to the screen and the puppet box.

Focusing

Focusing is a period when the group or individual engages more directly with the area or areas to be worked on – the subject or content of the work. Whereas the warm up section may be general, this section usually involves a move towards more specific areas. Blatner (1973) has referred to an aspect of this as 'Act Hunger'. In Chapter 5 of this book, along with the warm up, focusing is described as being part of the 'need identifying' period in a Dramatherapy session. Focusing can be said to be the way in which clients arrive at a state where they are ready to explore an issue in some depth and with involvement.

This section often includes negotiation as to the work which can be included within the session. It may include specific warm up activities or preparations linked to the development of a main activity. This might include: building roles for a specific role play, creating a focused improvisation, an intensifying of playing, or a particular way of engaging with material brought up in the first, warm up stage.

A session may have more than one period of focusing – it might shift after the completion of a main activity to move into another theme or another piece of work.

This phase is often not structured by the therapist, but occurs spontaneously in the session. For example, an individual might offer to begin to work dramatically. A specific theme might emerge from the warm up which the group naturally develops into deepening, exploratory enactment.

As a group becomes more used to working within Dramatherapy, there can be periods when the warm up stages diminish. The entrance might be straight into a brief focusing followed by a main activity.

Case study 2.3 Role Play in Dramatherapy (focusing)

The group was ranging far and wide in its discussion of other people's power to disempower and destroy self-image, and to leave people with a sense of no worth. I perceived that another of the group's themes was not present – a sense of despair at never being 'well' again, and that they were powerless. I noted to the group that it seemed that they were leaving themselves out of the discussion except as victims and wondered how they felt about this role? The discussion was broadened into a sense of 'What on earth would anyone want to know me for?', as one member put it. This became a new focus for the depressed feelings of isolation, despair and disconnection; they did not know what they could offer to people. I felt that this could be explored using enactment.

The task was to try to provide a way of relating the material to an enactment. This would enable group members to feel more activated and empower them to confront and work through the issues rather than to remain solely in victim roles. The suggested activity was to sit on two chairs which illustrated their dilemma. One chair could represent facets of themselves with which they felt people might want to connect. The other would represent a different experience of themselves. Examples of this other chair included the following: one person said how 'ill and frightening' they were, another said 'diffident' and 'difficult to talk to'. Clients took it in turn to sit in each chair and to speak briefly about themselves.

Case study 2.4 Creature in a Box (focusing)

The shadow puppet creature was brought out and looked at by the group – the qualities of the creature were remembered and spoken of. The puppet was then put on to the screen inside a shadow puppet box. The group greeted the creature and the creature, operated by a staff member, lifted the lid of the box and waved an arm out.

Following the warm up, the focus of the session – the screen and the puppet – was introduced. The simple production of the puppet and the screen was a way of establishing the concentration and engagement of the group.

Main activity

Within most Dramatherapy sessions there is a period of time which marks an intensity of involvement. This can take many forms and the ways in which the intensity is shown varies between groups. For a group of people with severe learning difficulties it might be marked by an increased concentration in their work with an object – from a lack of interest to a three-minute period of focus. For another group it might be a period of sustained improvisation.

The main activity might take the form of (a) one or more individuals dealing with an issue, (b) a group as a whole working together with a specific theme or focus, or (c) all members of a group working on their own material with each other in small groups, pairs or in the large group.

Examples of these three main forms are as follows:

- One person portrays a problem they are encountering in their life. If this takes place in a group other clients are involved in creating this scenario and in being audience members.
- The group deal with an issue within the group – concerning the dynamics or relationships within the group.
- Individuals create stories – time is given in small groups for all the stories to be performed. Individuals then share personal issues relating to the stories created.

The range of main activities within Dramatherapy sessions (e.g. play, role work) is described in the later chapters in this book. The following gives a representative sample of the kinds of ways the main activity period is used:

- improvising a traumatic, real-life event
- physical depiction of a symbol from a dream
- using objects to play, to see what unconscious material emerges
- creating a sculpt to illustrate a problematic relationship
- making and using masks to depict split parts of the self
- enacting a fantasy story to reflect personal events causing difficulties
- developing an environment to explore a troubling theme

- physical activity with the body to deal with relationship problems with a significant other

It should be noted that catharsis is not necessarily a part of this phase.

Case study 2.5 Role Play in Dramatherapy (main activity)

After group discussion an individual, Mark, said that he felt the chair representing 'what other people might want to connect with' to be entirely empty. I asked him if he wanted to explore that feeling further. He acknowledged that he did, saying that it was a situation he often experienced. He doubled the chair and then sat in it. Doubling involved placing his hand on the chair, imagining that it represented himself, and saying aloud what he might feel or think in that position. He said, 'I have nothing to offer. There is nothing there.' He was asked who he might be saying this to. At first he said it could be anyone; when asked if anybody in particular came to mind he identified his wife, his son and his father. I invited him to sculpt the other presences. Sculpting involved creating a physical sculpture of his wife, child and father by using other group members to represent his family. He placed his wife and child closest to him and his father behind the wife so that she blocked the line of sight between him and his father.

He sat in the chair and began to cry. After some moments I asked him to try to speak to those he'd placed around him. He addressed his wife first: 'Why do you stay with me? I'm just a burden. Why don't you go away?' To his child: 'I love you so much but I feel a failure to you. How can you face me when I've behaved the way I have?' He said there was nothing he could say to his father.

At this point in the session the material presented here could have gone in several directions. He could have focused on his relationship with his wife, son or father, or the sense of 'nothing'.

In order to animate the sculpt Mark was asked to take on the role of the wife, son and father. In each role he could try to speak to the chair representing himself about how they felt about his feelings of being 'nothing'. He left his chair and took up the positions of each family member in turn. He spoke for a couple of minutes from the viewpoint of his wife, then his son, and finally as his father. The people portraying his family listened to the way he acted each role and then the therapist asked them to use the material as a prompt to their playing of the characters.

The sculpt was improvised with for a brief period of time. The father, wife and son all interacted with Mark. This time was largely spent in

Mark saying how depressed and worthless he felt. He seemed hardly to acknowledge their presence – only speaking about his 'terrible life' and how awful he felt. I intervened to ask Mark if there was anything he felt like saying directly to any or all of the three. He said to his wife and son that they should leave him. His 'wife' asked him 'Why?', and he again cried, saying that he couldn't understand why they stayed with him through 'it all'. I asked him if he had ever asked either of them why they stayed. Mark replied, 'Of course not. We don't talk like that. I couldn't.' It was suggested that he try it out here. After a pause he nodded and then worked with each in turn.

Mark directed the question to his wife, Jane. I suggested that he reverse roles – to take up the role of his wife whilst the person playing Jane took up the role of Mark. I asked the person playing Mark to repeat the question to Jane. It was suggested to Mark that he should reply as his wife, but to give the reply he considered what she might actually feel rather than what she might actually say to him. The question was again asked and Mark, in the role of his wife, replied, 'You know that I stay with you because I love you. I want you to be well, but I don't know what to do. I can't help you.' I asked Mark to return to playing himself again and asked him to reply to her as himself. He said, 'The most important thing is that you stay there for me, and I know I can pull through this if you're there. I'm frightened I'll get lost.'

This dialogue continued for a while and the structure was used with both the son and the father. I asked Mark to step out of the enactment and to give advice to each of the protagonists. To his wife he said, 'I want you to know that I can pull through this, only I can do it, but I need you to be there like a lighthouse.' To his son he said, 'I know you don't understand this. Maybe I should talk to you about what's happening rather than thinking it'll make things worse.' To his father he said, 'I feel cut off from you.' He was asked to try to find advice, but he said that he couldn't find anything. To himself he said, 'There might be light at the end of the tunnel. Try not to forget that you're not alone.' Then he cried again. He was asked if there was anything he wanted to do with the sculpt. He said that he wanted to hear his wife and son say that he wasn't alone. He sat in the chair once more and Jane and his son both said simply, 'You're not alone,' and 'You're not alone, Dad.' He was asked if there was anything else to say at this point, and he said there wasn't.

Case study 2.6 Creature in a Box (main activity)

The group discussed ways in which the behaviour of the other puppets might make the puppet come out of its box or go in. Other puppets were used to demonstrate these kinds of behaviour. The students took it in turns to manipulate the boxed puppet. Staff manipulated the other puppets, who behaved in 'friendly' and 'unfriendly' ways – some were angry strangers, others were friends and the students decided what the creature in the box would do.

The group were then asked to help the puppet in the box come out. What might help? The group discussed what might work – offers of food, being nice, singing, were elicited. Then each member came up and sat near to and in front of the screen and worked with the puppet in turn; trying to tempt it out of its box with offers of sweets, singing or treats such as television programmes.

After each student had interacted with the puppet, the group gave feedback on what they had done to help the creature come out of the box.

Closure and de-roling

This phase marks the closure of active work involving dramatic forms. It is usual for there to be a clear point at which individuals leave or disengage from the dramatic space or activities and the ending of any audience/performer divisions. This closure period includes 'de-roling' exercises if character, role or improvisation are used. If materials such as play objects are used, this phase includes an opportunity for individuals to shift their engagement with the materials – to leave the direct, dramatic involvement. If group activities have taken place then 'closure' is a time for group dramatic relationships to be ended.

This phase differs from both verbal therapy and from theatre practice. It is usual for a theatre play or rehearsal to end and the actor is assumed to be able to leave the activity. Applause has been described as a way of helping the cast of a play to disengage with the play reality and their roles and to re-engage with their everyday selves, and for the audience to mark the ending of their witnessing roles by clapping (Jones, 1993). In forms of analytic therapy the end of the session may be marked only by the therapist verbally acknowledging time. For Dramatherapy neither of these states is usually desirable.

To leave a client in role or suddenly to close the dramatic activity can be highly problematic. It can result in role confusion or in an individual or group leaving in a state of high identity confusion. Some sort of disengagement is usual within a Dramatherapy session.

De-roling

De-roling involves an activity which assists all those involved in enactment to move out of the dramatic engagement in which they have been involved. It also helps those watching to leave their roles as audience members. For Dramatherapy, de-roling does not refer only to leaving a character or role which has been played during the session. It has a much broader meaning. It describes the process of leaving any enactment or dramatic process. This could include playing, work with objects, mime activities or physical-theatre-based work.

In Dramatherapy it is usual for the de-roling to consist of two phases. The first involves specific exercises designed to help the move out of roles to occur. The second phase involves both those who have been engaged in enactment, and, if people have been watching, audience members gathering together to reflect and absorb what has happened.

The first phase might, for example, include an exercise which directly requests the actor to leave their role and state their usual identity. A typical exercise involves moving the client out of the dramatic space and emphasising the return to the non-acting arena of the group. One approach uses chairs. The client sits in a chair within the dramatic space or 'stage' area in role. They might briefly summarise the dramatic persona they have played: 'I am Murray's father.' The Dramatherapist then asks them to move from the stage area to another chair placed by the audience area, verbally acknowledging that, as they leave one chair and move to the next, they leave the role and return to being their usual identity.

When on the second chair the therapist will invite clients to speak as themselves in order to reinforce the change. This might be a request to say their own name and to talk to the group about one or two simple things about their life: where they live, what they had for lunch, their favourite activities. Another way of working is to ask the client to comment upon the role they played. This could include their opinions about the role, their personal response, something they would have liked to say to the role, what it was like to play the role. The client can be asked what they consider to be similarities or differences between the role and themselves.

The activity is important in any Dramatherapy work in order to start to help the client to begin to have a new relationship to the enactment. It gives the opportunity to look at the role or enactment rather than to be in the enactment. De-roling is not just about separating from the enactment. It can mark a distancing from the playing. It can also mark an important shift which involves the change from being in the dramatic activity to digesting or absorbing the enactment. Quite often the significance of a piece of work will only begin to emerge once this digestion or absorption has begun. De-roling is often associated with a 'cooling off' from the heat of dramatic work. In many cases this is so. The move from action to quieter reflection can be a part of de-roling. This need not be a time when the client disengages with their personal material. In de-roling, the client can often make painful and important connections between the enactment and the issues they have brought to therapy. This might be verbal and occur in discussion, or it might emerge as a feeling which is encountered when the client begins to connect the experience of the role to their own identity. On occasion the process of reflecting on the activity which has taken place can mark the emergence of material which needs to be further worked with.

It is, therefore, important that the therapist leaves an adequate amount of time for de-roling. If this time is not left then much of the potential of the work can be left undeveloped. This way of looking at de-roling also makes clear the importance of a completion phase to follow on from de-roling. During completion there is time and space to absorb the process of de-roling itself!

Case study 2.7 Role Play in Dramatherapy (closure and de-roling)

All those involved in taking on roles sat on chairs in the 'stage' area. I confirmed that the enactment was over and that they were leaving the roles they'd taken on. They moved from the area where the acting had taken place into the 'off stage' area and sat on another set of chairs. Each person who had played a role was asked to state their own name and to talk about any similarities and differences between themselves and the role. Mark was asked to de-role in a different way. I requested that Mark say something about himself in the role play he had shown the group. Then the group as a whole, audience and players alike, returned to a circle of chairs.

The client who had played the father identified a similarity in his relationship to his own father. It, too, contained many things that were unsaid. The client who played Mark's wife said that one difference was that she did not have a son. Mark said that he was pleased that in the role play he had been able to express his feelings and hoped that he could do so to his wife and son in real life.

Case study 2.8 Creature in a Box (closure and de-roling)

The previous week the group had been asked how they wanted to stop the work with the puppets and they had said that saying goodbye to each puppet was the best way. This was established as a way of de-roling the puppets. The group said 'Goodbye' to each of the puppets. The puppets were brought round from behind the screen. The group briefly recollected what had helped the creature come out of its box. This was a way of reinforcing the process of the work. The group put the puppets away into the puppet box. The screen was then taken down.

In some work, closure is a pause rather than a completion. There is no expectation that an issue should have reached a full conclusion. The main activity might have taken the form of 'work in progress', with the client or clients aiming to return to the content or the issue. There is a danger that an illusion of completing the drama means that the client expects that the issue is closed – solved. But the closure in these cases marks an ending with a particular scene or act rather than the whole play.

Completion

This is a crucial aspect of Dramatherapy. It is an activity which is separate from the immediate disengagement from the drama which constitutes the closure stage; it is also separate from de-roling. Completion has two main components. The first is a space for further integration of the material dealt with during the main activity. The second is the preparation for leaving the Dramatherapy space.

Integration can take a purely verbal or a dramatic form. In some cases it might involve discussion of the work: the making of personal connections and sharing of perceptions and feelings. In others it might take the form of active exploration of integrating or responding to the main activity. For some groups this might be a time of internal reflection, so the time might be spent partly or wholly in silence.

Case study 2.9 Role Play in Dramatherapy (completion)

There was room for individuals, including Mark, to reflect on the enactment. The group were given alternatives. They could discuss what had happened or choose to take up a physical position indicating an important moment, reaction or interaction within the enactment. Those playing roles could talk about how they felt in role and about what it felt like for them to play the roles. Mark could talk about how he felt in the role and the audience could talk about the feelings the enactment raised in them. This took approximately twenty minutes.

The group finished with each person making a statement about what they would take away to consider or think about until the next group.

The preparation for leaving the Dramatherapy group also takes place during completion. This can be a ritualised activity to mark the ending, or might be a structured time for individual endings through statements. For some groups and in some work a formal closure is helpful to mark the end of a particular way of relating which is different from the usual rules and boundaries.

Completion can often reflect the initial warm up stage – e.g. an exercise – such as a name game, or a pulse game whereby a squeeze is passed round the group, which has started a session – might be repeated to demarcate the ending.

Case study 2.10 Creature in a Box (completion)

As described earlier, the group had a song which added a line each week about the creature.

The opening line had been made the previous week:

He is small and can't be seen
Hiding in his box

This week they added:

But if you're kind and say nice things
He might come out

The song was sung five times. The group enjoyed singing, and though some individuals could remember the song after one repeat, for others it took a while.

This section has described the basic shape of many Dramatherapy sessions. It has discussed each of five stages within this shape and given illustrations of these stages. As said earlier, not all Dramatherapy groups follow this process – some work may not contain any warm up activities, at other times the session may not reach a main activity but involve being 'formless', without any focus. The Dramatherapist attempts to reflect the issues and processes at work within the Dramatherapy in the shape and form of the session.

Beginning and closing Dramatherapy

In some ways the pattern of an individual session is reflected in ongoing Dramatherapy work. The first few sessions, the initial phase, for example, can often involve a general warm-up to the work. The focus of this phase involves finding out what issues might be worked with, what dramatic language can be used and what the boundaries and aims of the work might be. The following briefly summarises this starting process.

Starting Dramatherapy groups

It is usual for the initial stages of Dramatherapy groups to contain:

• referral
• diagnosis and assessment
• aims setting
• the creation of boundaries

Referral involves the ways in which clients arrive at Dramatherapy. There are three main routes. One involves self-referral – the client deciding that they want to come. This might be in response to an advert, a poster, a verbal invitation or description, or a sample session. A second involves referral by a professional such as a general practitioner, a social worker, or a department such as Occupational Therapy within a particular setting. The third involves the Dramatherapist assessing someone's suitability for Dramatherapy. This might involve considering file material, taking part in a case conference, meeting and talking with potential clients or running a referral session which has a clear selection agenda. A referral session is often a two-way process – the Dramatherapist and client or clients considering individuals' participation in a group. If, for example, a Dramatherapy group is being offered to deal with bereavement, then referral might look at whether a client is concerned with this issue, or whether enactment in a Dramatherapy context might be the most effective way for them to work with this material. A client might decide that they would prefer to work with art-making processes in an art therapy group, or to talk in counselling.

Diagnosis, assessment and aims setting are dealt with in Chapter 12. In these areas the focus is upon identifying what the presenting problems or issues are, what the possible work might be, and what kinds of dramatic language can be used.

The assessment period is important in terms of the language chosen to deal with the presenting problems or issues. The therapist, as will be discussed in detail in Chapter 12, considers the issues which are to be the content of the therapeutic process, but also the language in which the group can find meaning and can best explore and deal with the material.

In much Dramatherapy, boundaries are important. The way boundaries are dealt with varies according to context and approach. For certain clients, such as for some people with severe learning difficulties, verbal negotiation may be impossible. In this kind of situation boundaries may involve non-verbal negotiations or maintenance. For some work, boundaries may be formally provided by the setting, for others they may emerge as part of the work. Boundaries often concern:

- *time* (e.g. how frequently the sessions occur, whether people can come late)
- *space* (e.g. location, making sure that the sessions are not interrupted)
- *behaviour* (e.g. issues such as no physical violence, damage to materials, smoking, drinking, eating)
- *equal opportunities* (e.g. rules or guidelines on expressed racism, sexism, homophobia, able-bodiedism)
- *confidentiality* (e.g. whether material expressed within the session can be spoken of by Dramatherapist or by other clients outside of the Dramatherapy group)

For some work issues such as the amount or nature of contact between clients, or between client and therapist outside of the Dramatherapy group, need to be dealt with. In some contexts it may be important for clients not to meet socially outside of the group, or to discuss their material with the Dramatherapist outside of the Dramatherapy group.

Ending Dramatherapy groups

It is usual for the ending of Dramatherapy groups to contain:

- reflection
- evaluation
- acknowledgement of closure

Reflection and evaluation of the work at the close of the individual or group Dramatherapy can use enactment, verbal discussion or a mixture of the two. In some sessions this will be formal – with each client evaluating their experience of the Dramatherapy according to previously agreed criteria. A client may have formed individual aims to be achieved within the work. At the close of the sessions these aims would be evaluated in the light of what had occurred during the time of the Dramatherapy sessions. In other work the process of looking back, looking towards the future and looking at how the ending of the work is experienced might be more unstructured. Here themes and issues might emerge during enactments or during reflection on the Dramatherapy.

Issues relating to the basic shape

Entry into drama: using dramatic language in Dramatherapy

The way a group or individual uses the shape of the session and the language of drama can help to understand what is happening in the Dramatherapy. Often groups will develop particular speeds of entry into material. The therapist will need to be sensitive to this and to understand the ways in which the group dynamic or relationship is reflected in this. For example, a lack of engagement in role playing might be due to a lack of adequate warming up; a lack of clarity might be due to the lack of adequate focusing.

However, other factors may also be present; the way a group engages with the Dramatherapy activity may reflect its response to the content of a session. For example, a lack of engagement in playing might be to do with inadequate warm up or might be to do with a lack of interest or a fear of dealing with the material. This might be a necessary stage. It should not always be assumed that an apparent lack of engagement is somehow a 'failure'. Often this can be a protection or a way of responding that avoids a feeling of being overwhelmed.

It is important to note that some main activities need a specific level of dramatic skill. The warm up and focusing periods of sessions can also be places to develop the skills of participants pertaining to the main activity. With some groups a long period of time is spent in basic work developing dramatic skills.

A group might need to develop role playing skills prior to running role plays. Inadequate skills might mean that the force of the therapeutic work might be muted. Similarly the capability to create stories to be enacted might need to be built up.

In some situations the kinds of relationships present between group members will affect the dramatic content of the work. In order to develop enactment it is necessary for clients to be able to work together dramatically. Factors such as trust and being confident enough to enact personal material with others are important in this.

To an extent warm ups can be used to create and develop dramatic skills and capabilities in working together. However, the work undertaken in the main activity may also need to develop in dramatic complexity over time. For example, a group may initially only be able to hold roles in relation to each other for brief periods of time. This will mean that only short dramatic engagements can take place. More sustained exploration and development of role work may be possible once skills have been developed by familiarising a group with role work skills and practising these skills in subsequent warm ups.

It is important that the group can develop some sense of congruent meaning in work. This means that during an enactment the group can understand each other and be congruent in the reality created in the drama. If this does not occur then the work can be too fragmented for people to participate together.

For others it may be important to develop a clarity that acting is different from being. For some individuals it can be confusing to play a role – they might become confused about whether the role is them or a fictive creation. Mast, in her study of actors, has highlighted this issue. She says that the trainee actor must learn where identification of self with role is called for and where separation of self from role is called for (Mast, 1986, 41). She notes that one individual she observed in her research 'was clearly embarrassed by acting as though *she* was seductive' (41). This may be especially true for clients who are engaged in therapeutic work where personal involvement in created roles is encouraged, or where their identity is confused due to their condition or illness. Hence training in the dramatic processes and skills of moving in and out of role is important for some. The therapist must not assume that a group can naturally and easily move into the expressive forms of Dramatherapy.

Dramatherapy and therapeutic paradigms

As described in Chapter 1, Dramatherapy is practised within a wide range of therapeutic contexts and its aims respond to these contexts. Its development has been in a number of fields and settings. It has, to date, developed as a therapy which can be utilised within a number of frameworks. Its basic therapeutic assumptions as described in the last chapter are able to be applied within a broad range of therapeutic paradigms. And, although, Valente and Fontana's research has shown that Dramatherapy 'looks more to psychodynamic psychology than to either cognitive or behavioural psychology in its search for appropriate psychological models' (Valente and Fontana, 1993, 65), the practice of Dramatherapy takes place within behavioural, psychodynamic, cognitive and systemic contexts.

The context and paradigm in which a Dramatherapist works need to be considered in the forming of the aims and in the way the sessions are structured or shaped. For example, working within a behavioural framework might entail having a clear focus and structured content designed with a group.

The following two case studies, 'Leaving Home' and 'Villa Grumpyview', give examples of Dramatherapy as practised within different paradigms. One is a behavioural framework and one takes place within a systemic, psychodynamic framework.

Case study 2.11 Leaving Home

A group of eight people met once a week for fifteen weeks in a psychiatric day centre to develop members' assertiveness skills. At the first session a methodology and a series of topics were agreed. These included: being more effective both in decision-making and inter-personal relationships, and dealing with aggression. Each member, in consultation with the group and therapist, decided on a small number of personal goals in terms of the group and their lives outside the group. Improvisation and role playing were agreed as the main ways of working. At the start of the group the individual goals were shared with the group; midway through the series of sessions and at the end each member evaluated themselves in terms of the work they had done in the group and in terms of their lives. Group members gave feedback on their development in the group. An example of a personal aim was 'To be able to decide what I want and don't want to do each day'. Participants were encouraged as the group developed to consider whether in choosing their goals they had set themselves up for failure.

Sessions included – practising using the voice, role playing situations in which they had wished themselves to be more assertive, handling fantasy situations in assertive ways and preparing for real life situations by role playing them in advance.

Ben, for example, a 22-year-old man diagnosed as schizophrenic and as having moderate learning difficulties, was preparing to confront his parents with the fact that he wanted to leave home to stay in sheltered accommodation. He experienced his parents as being over-protective and wanting to keep him as an adolescent or a child. He felt overwhelmed by his mother, who was often aggressive, and by his father's indecision. He had already tried to deal with it, but his mother had forbidden him to leave home. The situation was role played with group members as his mother and father. Ben was able to rehearse telling his mother and sticking with his decision. He tried it four times, each time handling the situation differently. The group gave him feedback after each attempt – pointing out his language, the way he introduced the situation, the way he used his posture, eye contact. Small changes were discussed, such as making statements rather than asking permission, saying that he understood her point of view but that this was a decision he had to make for himself. To an extent Ben was able to rehearse and script the situation.

At a later session he came back to report how things had gone. It had not gone according to the script he had prepared, as this seemed to be, in part, a wish-fulfilment. His mother had become furious and had walked out of the room, refusing to speak to Ben. However, the role playing had prepared him: he had made her listen and had the confidence and capabilities to 'stick to his guns'. Eventually Ben did leave home. He said that the confrontation with his parents in the Dramatherapy and in his life outside the group were pivotal in the process.

In the above case the Dramatherapy sought to find a structure and language to achieve aims of changing behavioural patterns and to learn new ways of relating. Here the projection of personal material into roles, the use of enactment to create a transformed, changed perspective on a life situation, and the group working together in witnessing and improvising with the client combined to produce change. The processes of the Dramatherapy were all centred around the achievement of change within a behavioural framework.

Case study 2.12 Villa Grumpyview

Working within a psychodynamic context entails an approach which attempts to follow the form of the group's or individual's dynamics.

This example of Dramatherapy involves a family described by Leguijt and van der Wiel (1989). The parents had registered with RIAGG, an institute for out-patient mental health care. The presenting problem involved Jacqueline (9), one of three children, Mirjam (6) and Jan Jaap (3½).

There were initial meetings and an assessment prior to a decision about the method of treatment being made. Dramatherapy was felt to be a useful treatment mode as it would help the family to express and work with material without having to depend upon verbal communication. Dramatherapy also allowed play and experimentation with 'as if' situations to consider threatened or denied aspects of their relationships.

Leguijt and van der Wiel add that the children were too young for verbal therapy. Twenty-six sessions over a one-year period were run. Areas of potential therapeutic focus were decided. These included – the relationship between Jacqueline and the parents' problems, Jacqueline's denial of negative feelings, along with problems in verbally expressing and communicating needs.

The initial phase involved an introduction to Dramatherapy with an emphasis upon playing.

The first session included an offer of clothes to dress up in and a potential scenario of shopping. The family and therapists put on costumes and improvised a story about an ambush on a train. The children held up the train and killed the inhabitants – the parents and therapists.

At times the therapy took the form of free improvisation and play with adults and children alike taking on roles and dressing up. At other times roles and scenarios were suggested by the therapists.

Through playing and using materials such as costumes the clients made clear what they would like to do, what they feared, and what they 'cannot (yet) accept from others or oneself in play' (1989, 19). Post-activity discussion attempted to help the family to perceive that the play was experienced by each other in a different way.

Events such as the death of the mother's father and her pregnancy are reflected in the sessions. For example, it is planned that Jacqueline will play a baby. In addition to responding to events as they occur, underlying themes as described in the aims of the work were explored. In part they emerged spontaneously, in part the therapists suggest structures to explore themes.

An example of this is in the creation of a building. The dynamics of the family are played out through fantasy stories in a hotel, 'Villa Grumpyview' (1989, 21–22).

Change is noted in individuals' role flexibility, in the way the family relate to each other in the play, and in the way that they use the content of the Dramatherapy to reflect and resolve familial tensions or difficulties. In improvisations the family as a whole began to recognise family and individual needs through acknowledgement rather than destructiveness. For example, an improvisation creating a war is developed. The mother wants peace and quiet and takes the role of someone writing their memoirs. A fight ensues and a child playing a 'landowner' protects his mother and negotiates in the war. The situation is resolved and the action has a sense of unity and co-operation, 'the roles relate logically to each other' (1989, 29) and do not destroy or negate.

Jacqueline, after a series of tough, aggressive roles allowed herself to be sung to sleep. At another point the family play out a fantasy of being challenged by a government official with eviction plans. Mirjam is able to indicate what displeases her without withdrawing – a change in the way of relating to her family.

Here the same Dramatherapeutic processes as discussed within the previous example are utilised but within different aims. Personal and family issues are projected into the roles and characters created, enactment helps to look at situations and transforms the way the family experience each other, the family as a group witness each other's work and improvise together. The piece aims to enable a psychodynamic exploration of material presented by the family. The playing and enactments result in the family working with and through unconscious desires and issues; family dynamics are reflected and resolved through the play and the involvement of the therapists.

Summary: forms and formats

These two examples illustrate how the same basic processes – such as dramatic projection, the transformative potential of enactment, the ways in which participating with others and witnessing others in improvisation – can create change. The examples also show that, though processes are parallel, the way the change is understood and undertaken can differ in Dramatherapy. One example operates within a behavioural framework, the other works along systemic and psychodynamic lines.

As will be seen, the basic processes at work within Dramatherapy are constant, even though the specific context, paradigm and aims of the practice vary. The therapist and group seek to identify and work within the processes as best suited to these aims and the paradigm. These basic processes will be described in detail in Chapter 5.

This chapter has also shown that much Dramatherapy can be seen to operate within a basic five-step shape or format: that of warm up, focus, main activity, closure/de-roling and completion.

The descriptions of the forms of the sessions in this chapter have also tried to illustrate that variety is at the heart of Dramatherapy. Though the chapter has defined some of the shapes which Dramatherapy work often takes, it has also stressed that these vary greatly. The idea of this chapter has been to offer a shape to work *from* rather than to define a shape which must always be worked *within*.

Part II

Chapter 3
From amphitheatre to operating theatre?
Drama, theatre and therapy – a history

Introduction: three histories

How has Dramatherapy come into being? This chapter will describe the background to the emergence of the intentional use of drama as a therapy. Chapter 4 will describe the evolution of the term, practice and profession of the Dramatherapist.

There are three kinds of history relating to drama as therapy.

Healing, drama, theatre

The first involves the general, historical uses of theatre and drama in ways which we would now interpret as being to do with healing, or as having a healing function. This history has importances in the examination of the roots of the twentieth century development of Dramatherapy.

A twentieth-century context

The second involves the evolution of new attitudes towards therapy and theatre which created the environment to make it possible for Dramatherapy to exist. This could be described as the 'immediate prehistory' of the emergence of drama as a specific therapy within twentieth century Europe and the United States. The increasing awareness of, and contact between, other cultures and different models of health and 'drama' add to this 'new attitude'. It is, therefore, also important to examine the way the potentials seen and used in theatre during this period are viewed by non-Western or non-European cultures.

The emergence of Dramatherapy

The third involves the specific emergence of the term 'Dramatherapy' and the practice of Dramatherapy which occurs mainly in postwar Western Europe and in the United States. This history will be discussed in Chapter 4.

Healing, drama, theatre

The earliest documented use of the term 'Dramatherapy' in the United Kingdom occurs in Peter Slade's 1939 lecture to the British Medical Association (see Chapter 4 for details). In the United States one of the earliest recorded uses of the term in reference to contemporary practice is by Florsheim in a paper, 'Drama Therapy' (1946), delivered at the American Occupational Therapy Association. However, the notion of the intentional therapeutic use of drama and theatre is much older than this, both within the UK and in Western culture as a whole.

Aristotle proposed that the function of tragedy was to induce the emotional and spiritual state of catharsis – a release of deep feelings that originally had a connotation of purification of the senses and the soul. The method by which the emotions of pity and terror are evoked is 'mimesis' – a combination of vicarious participation and suspension of disbelief (Aristotle, 1961).

His work formally established a theme which recurs throughout the history of writing about theatre and one which is relevant to the relationship which drama as therapy has to theatre.

The theme can be characterised as drama having a unique and direct relationship with human feelings, and as being able to produce change in people's lives. At different times in history different kinds of change have been emphasised – from religious to political change, from an individual's psychological make-up to mass societal change.

One contemporary way of understanding the processes which Aristotle discussed is to see this 'change' in terms of healing. Goodman summarises this approach: he says that tragedy is said to have the effect of purging us of pent up and hidden negative emotions, or of 'administering measured doses of the killed virus to prevent or mitigate the ravages of actual attack' (1981, 246).

Traditions such as the medieval Feast of Fools, the Roman Saturnalia and survivals of ancient customs, such as the Padstow Horse or the 'Reign of the Wild Men' on the eve of St Nicholas' Day in the Bavarian mountains, are often considered within a framework of catharsis – of a healthy psychological and emotional 'release' for individuals, groups and communities (Landy, 1986; Jennings, 1987; Turner, 1974; Southern, 1962). The past history of other cultures is often considered within a similar framework – of looking at ritual and rite as a form of drama concerned with healing (Turner, 1974, 37). An example of this is Fryrear and Fleshman's consideration of the Seneca Indians and the Iroquois Confederacy's 'False Face Society' curing and carving masks as elements of treatment or therapy with drama as a primary means of change. The radical innovations in experimental theatre, educational drama, psychotherapy, the study of play, anthropological study of ritual, cross cultural contact and the development of the field of dramaturgy in sociology all made important connections between the potentials of drama and direct change in people's lives.

This section documents some of the ways in which this contact between drama and therapy began to emerge; the way a 'twentieth-century context' formed. A series of different contexts will be described: hospital theatre, twentieth-century theatre, early pioneers – Evreinov, Iljine and Moreno – and developments in therapy and education.

Context – hospital theatre

There is evidence that some of the early European asylums had theatre facilities, though this was by no means the norm. In the eighteenth century a move towards reforming attitudes and treatment of people with mental health problems resulted in 'Moral Therapy' which involved occupational and some artistic activity for patients (Fryrear and Fleshman, 1981, 13). Many patients were still locked in prisons or work houses, especially the poor. The majority of asylums in nineteenth century Britain, for example, were places with very few facilities. There were exceptions. Ticehurst Asylum, founded in eighteenth century England and 'favoured with the aristocracy' had fortnightly concerts with as many as thirty-six patients taking part. Also 'an excellent theatre with scenery' was constructed for the use of patients in an environment 'to restore health to diseased minds' (Souall, 1981, 207). Coulmier, director of the asylum of Charenton, outside Paris, worked with his patients using theatre productions between 1797 and 1811. De Sade was an inmate of Charenton and wrote and directed a number of these productions.

Reil, a German author, wrote about the uses of theatre in psychiatric hospitals in 1803. He wanted special theatres in hospitals where patients would be urged to portray scenes of their 'former life' by 'acting them out'. The therapeutic advantages, however, were seen in the following dubious way: 'through the proper assignment of roles other advantages could be gained such as ridiculing the follies of each patient' (in Zilboorg, 1976, 287).

By the mid-nineteenth century a number of the large asylums were being built with theatres as part of the main structure. Broadmoor, for example, has a stage (Cox, 1992, 116). In Italy the psychiatric hospitals in Aversa, Naples and Palermo built at the same time (1813) have theatres.

Alexandre Dumas in 1863 describes a theatre performance directed by Dr Biagio Miraglia in Aversa. Miraglia notes his intention as keeping patients occupied and 'to lead them to the exercise of the intact functions, relaxing in the meantime the impaired functions' (Mora, 1957, 268). Scripted plays were worked with, and rehearsals used in preparation for performances, though only male patients were allowed to take part. Dumas noted that patients were 'considerably better on the stage while still in hospital' (Mora, 1957, 268).

Fryrear and Fleshman say that most psychiatric institutions were at best involved in caretaking and that this situation was the prevailing one well into the 1940s in many countries. They suggest that the groundwork for the arts therapies lies in the arts and crafts movement in hospitals as part of occupational therapy. These were introduced after the First World War in parts of Europe and the US. This period also marked the beginnings of 'recreational therapy' (Fryrear and Fleshman, 1981, 14).

This emphasis upon the recreational or occupational aspects of drama and theatre activities is evident in much work in hospitals during the mid-twentieth century. Examples of this include the annual theatrical reviews in New York Creedmore State Hospital and the Menninger Clinic in 1942. However Mazor (1966) notes that some of those involved in hospital theatre in the 1930s and 1940s saw a more exciting potential for these productions. Reider, Olinger and Lyle (1939), for example, stressing amateur dramatics as 'outlets for . . . unconscious strivings', and Price and Nagle note that theatre performance 'unconsciously brings about a socialising effect in both hospital personnel and patients' (1943). Insights such as these mark the beginnings of significant changes in the understanding of the potentials of drama.

A history of a hospital theatre – Julio de Matos, Lisbon

As described above, the tradition of theatres in psychiatric hospitals existed in many parts of Europe. The history of the theatre at Hospital Julio de Matos in Lisbon from the 1930s is not untypical in terms of its structure and usage. Initially built as a part of the recreational services of the hospital, the idea was to create a self-sufficient community according to notions of asylum, whereby the hospital had within its walls a bakery, a tannery, and fields in which to grow its own crops. The theatre was part of this process – a centre for entertainment within the life of the hospital. As such it was used for concerts and folk-dancing exhibitions with the occasional outside company coming in.

Though the evidence is sparse from the early years of the theatre, it also seems that staff may have been involved in performances.

Later, in 1968, theatre activity involving patients in performances was initiated. A theatre director, João Silva, was invited in by a group of psychiatrists motivated and influenced in part by the writings of Foulkes and Moreno. Initially the director worked with clients with a mainly recreational purpose – staff and patients participating together. The initiative was integrated into a 'cultural group' and club within Julio de Matos. A play script was chosen by staff for the group to work with, *O Oleo (Oil)* by Eugene O'Neill. Fifteen patients took part. Some of these patients were diagnosed as schizophrenic, most were psychotic, though some had depressive or hysteric illnesses. The performance was internal within the hospital. In 1969 Pirandello's *O Torno* was chosen. Both were seen as being mainly recreational in purpose. Hospital psychiatrists worked with the director to support and inform the way he worked.

In 1970, however, a change occurred and the play performed was written by one of the patients – *Caleidocopio* by Eduardo Gama. The play dealt with his own experiences as a patient and the problems he had encountered with his family, with the hospital and Portuguese society. The client's play was critical of his experience of the hospital, the professionals there and the military government of this time. The play text was registered with the Portuguese author's society. It was performed twice and was open to the general public.

At this time, however, Portugal was ruled by a military junta and artistic expression, along with many other forms of social and political activity, were governed by censorship and strong repression. There was no formal complaint from the censors. However, communication was sent through the Ministry of Health to the Hospital Administration indicating that such work should not be allowed. The existence of the group was called into question and the theatre activity threatened with closure. Plays were to be sent to the Censorship Commission for approval prior to performance. In 1971, in response to the threats, the staff chose to confront the censors by choosing Bernardo Santereno's *A Traição do Padre Martinho* (*The Treason of Father Martinho*) and the censors forbade the performance.

The role of drama and theatre has expanded within the hospital. Since the mid-1970s there has been the development of psychodrama, playback theatre and Dramatherapy. As well as dramatic productions, patients are regularly involved in psychodrama and the occupational therapy department is involved in providing Dramatherapy for patients. Individuals had contact with Moreno's ideas and practices and with Dramatherapy work in England. This contact has helped to encourage ideas and develop the hospital's provision.

In the history of Julio de Matos, then, the initial use of the theatre is for recreational purposes. This is followed by the involvement of patients in performance and writing processes. More recently this had been added to by the uses of drama as a direct therapy in the forms of Dramatherapy and psychodrama. This is the shift many hospitals and institutions have seen: a gradual development in the range of drama and theatre processes involved in work with clients. The range includes the move from drama as recreation alone to drama having a primary role in the therapeutic programme.

Mazor, a consultant in the American Occupational Therapy Association, wrote in 1966 of a historical shift in the United States in the treatment of people with mental health problems. This shift involved viewing 'All the patient's activities in the hospital [as being] potentially therapeutic' (1966, 8). Mazor goes on to say: 'An activity such as play production can be therapeutic if it provides the patient with an opportunity to recognize and utilize his capacities more fully, both in the activity and his relationship with other people' (1966, 10). This attitude is reflected in the work of João Silva in the hospital of Julio de Matos.

The tradition of performance was widespread. Examples include the community theatre which was begun in 1943 by Gibson, the Riggs Theatre, at Austen Riggs psychiatric centre, Stockbridge, Massachusetts. Later Brookes produced *The Persecution and Assassination of Jean-Paul Marat as Performed by the Inmates of the Asylum of Charenton Under the Direction of the Marquis de Sade* in Austen Riggs psychiatric centre (Brookes, 1975). Chase, working with women in the St Elizabeth's Hospital, in the United States producing 'Hotel Saint Elizabeth', about their lives in the hospital, is another example.

The practice of creating performances within health settings is still extant. As the next chapter will show, this area of cultural activity has an important place in the development of Dramatherapy. For example, professionals and patients alike were able to discover, in working with this area of theatre and drama, potentials and effects which were wider than those of recreation or artistic expression. These discoveries related to therapeutic change, and would lead to some individuals attempting to find ways to hone the therapeutic possibilities of drama.

Context – twentieth-century theatre and therapy

The tradition of experimentation in theatre and drama during the twentieth century is relevant to the development of drama as a therapy. The most important facet of this tradition is the establishment of certain themes in experimental theatre. This made it possible to view theatre and dramatic processes in a way which helped to open up the possibility that they could be powerfully therapeutic. Another important aspect is the development of certain methodologies, approaches and techniques in theatre training, rehearsal, research and performance out of which the language and techniques of Dramatherapy have developed.

The key schools and approaches include the psychological approach to character construction and performance developed by people such as Stanislavski; the emphasis upon political change and representational theatre and *Verfremdungseffekt* of the Brechtian approach to theatre; the theories of Artaud; along with the experiments of Brook and Grotowski.

Later on, the new political theatre born in the 1960s and Boal's work are also important. Their relevance lies in the emphasis they laid upon the role and potential of drama to change society and people's lives as seen by the achievements of feminist, black, lesbian, gay and disability theatre.

This section briefly outlines three themes in experimental theatre relevant to the development of the notion of a form of drama which can result in personal change. It also touches on the development of particular acting techniques related to Dramatherapy's way of using drama and theatre.

Memory, the unconscious, empathy and character

The work of Stanislavski at the Moscow Arts Theatre initiated an approach to creating theatrical roles which stressed the ways in which memory, the actor's individual unconscious and the portrayal of feeling could effectively connect. One of the cornerstones of acting described in 'Building a Character' concerns the 'psycho-technique'. The actor creates a physical and emotional state in themselves in order for inner feelings to emerge from the 'subconscious' into the portrayal of the role (Magarschack, 1950, 274). The importance lies in a chain of empathy. An actress sees or experiences someone encountering a particular feeling or encounters something in her own life. In creating a role she tries to enter into a state where she can re-create this feeling. The technique involves a series of exercises to create an emotional state whereby an unconscious memory or feeling can enter back into her. In turn the idea is that the accurate re-creation of this feeling will enable the audience to connect through empathy with her, and be involved and moved by the drama. These themes are reflected in Dramatherapy's work linking character and life experiences, as Chapter 9 will describe.

An important link in Stanislavski's work is formed between the actress or actor's life, the individual's experience of it, the storage of unconscious material, and the creation on stage and in rehearsal of a system by which the actor or actress enters into an emotional state based in their own life experiences. Stanislavski's stress upon rehearsal and the development of character through improvisation was also innovatory and influential.

Transgression and change

Another strand of experimental theatre has concerned itself with different kinds of transgression. Theatre is seen as violating and transforming everyday reality. Theoreticians and practitioners of this form of theatre often claim that they are returning to the origins of drama by rediscovering its religious and mystic roots. Its forms and inspiration are found in carnival, ritual, rite and subversion. This movement can be seen in the late nineteenth century symbolist movement with their attempts to create an unconscious dream world upon the stage. An example of this is seen in Symons's description of pantomime as a form of inspiration:

> Pantomime is thinking overheard. It begins and ends before words have formed themselves, in a deeper consciousness than speech . . .
> And pantomime has that mystery which is one of the requirements of true art. To watch it is like dreaming.
>
> (Symons in Gerould, 1985, 12)

This is echoed by Artaud in *The Theatre and Its Double*, in his search for a 'universal language that unites the total . . . space . . . to the hidden interior life' (Artaud, 1958, 65).

This search and approach can be traced through many of the experimental theatre companies and projects in the twentieth century – it is present in Brook's travels in Africa in the 1970s and in both Grotowski's 'Poor Theatre' of the 1960s and his Paratheatrical activities in the 1970s and 1980s. Barrault's practical experiments (1974), performance art and Barba's Odin Theatre (Barba and Savarese, 1991) are other notable examples.

In these approaches ritual forms of expression and working are stressed. There is a move away from narrative, character and script to an approach which looks at the creation of a situation where 'the stage ceases to be a physical representation of the world and becomes a projection of myth or the . . . inner self' (Innes, 1993, 36).

Theatre, distance, disturbance, revolution

Political theatre, in particular the methodologies of Brecht and Boal, has been important in the development of connections between theatre and change. In the 1930s Brecht formulated an approach and a set of theories of performance. These advocate theatre's potential to create direct political change in society and in the life of individuals attending performances. A series of techniques such as *Verfremdungseffekt* and the ideas of Epic Theatre were devised to effect this change. The *Verfremdungseffekt* is central to Brecht's work and can be characterised in the following way: the actor does not enter into an empathic relationship with character and audience, rather they seek to remain a reader, making personal political judgements and comments on the action and text of a play. This process also seeks to encourage the audience to remain alert, critical, thoughtful.

These techniques have been widely used in subsequent theatre of the political left. The idea that a political theatre can achieve direct change in the lives of its performers and audience has been taken up by the left in a number of countries, particularly in the 1960s and 1970s. Groups based on this belief include: 7:84 (formed in 1971), the Welfare State (1968), Feminist Theatre such as the Monstrous Regiment (1976) or the Women's Theatre Group (1974), Lesbian and Gay Theatre such as Gay Sweatshop (1975), Black Theatre such as the Black Theatre of Brixton and Temba, and Disability Theatre groups such as Graeae. These and other groups have tackled direct political, social and personal issues and thus attempted to create change and social revolution.

Since the 1970s Boal (1979) has developed a political theatre methodology which seeks to assist individuals in changing their lives. Boal's Theatre of the Oppressed and Forum Theatre see drama as a way of achieving direct change in people's lives. Methods are devised to enable this to occur, and performance is used as a tool to work towards personal and social revolution.

As this and the next chapter will demonstrate, the emergence of Dramatherapy can be said to have a clear relationship with hospital theatre and with educational drama. From the interviews conducted for this book and from existing documentation it cannot be concluded that the field of experimental theatre has the same direct relationship with the early manifestations of Dramatherapy. Several practitioners, for example, say that they had not heard of the work of Stanislavski, Brecht or Artaud during the initial stages of their work.

However, it is possible to say that the above areas contributed to a climate of experimentation, of pushing the boundaries of theatre and drama. It is in the later developments of Dramatherapy, from the 1970s onwards, that these influences become more direct.

On the one hand the theories of the unconscious and drama, the notions of transformation, areas such as distancing and emotional sincerity in acting have contributed to Dramatherapy theory (Landy, 1986; Jennings, 1987). In addition, during the 1970s and 1980s the development and refinement of specific techniques such as distancing or enrolement have been influenced by the work of Stanislavski, Brecht and Boal. These areas will be discussed in more detail in Chapters 9 and 11. In the late 1980s and 1990s specific ways of working in Dramatherapy have been linked to the innovators described above. Jennings (1994) has written about work related to Artaud, Jones in relation to Grotowski and experimental theatre (1991) and Mitchell on the theatre of Peter Brook as a 'model' for Dramatherapy (1990).

Context – Early pioneers: Evreinov, Iljine, Moreno

Evreinov and Theatrotherapy

In revolutionary Russia a number of new theories and experiments in theatre emerged at the beginning of the twentieth century. Many of these have relevance to Dramatherapy in that they helped create ways of understanding and approaching theatre and dramatic practices which re-frame the purpose and technique of theatre.

One of the innovators working in the Soviet theatre at this time was one of the first to articulate a formal connection between theatre and therapy in the modern era by his description of 'Theatrotherapy' as Nazaroff translates it. This innovator was the director and author, Nikolai Evreinov (1879–1953) who produced a series of pamphlets and monographs between 1915 and 1924. These included 'The Theatre for Oneself' in St Petersburg (in three parts 1915–1917), 'Theatrical Innovations' (1922) and 'The Theatre in the Animal Kingdom' (1924). A collection of his works was translated and published in the US in 1927 as *The Theatre In Life*. This collection includes a description of his key concept of 'Monodrama' (1927, 187) and of 'Theatrotherapy' (1927, 122). Golub has described him as 'One of the first and most insistent modern exponents of the will to play as an instinct basic to mankind, and therefore the theatre as not a pastime but a necessity' (1984, 212).

Evreinov's ideas are very similar to most of the current basic tenets of Dramatherapy. Unlike most theatre practitioners both before and since his time, he did not put too much emphasis on the creation of theatrical products. Instead he focused upon internal and psychological processes involved in acting. The key ideas outlined in his work in terms of drama as therapy are:

- theatre as a therapy for actors and audience
- theatre as an instinct
- theatre and play linked as necessary to the development of intelligence
- the stage management of life

Evreinov characterised theatre as entertainment, instruction and aesthetic enjoyment, the theatre of public spectacles such as military and state functions and even the ritual of the operating theatre as examples of 'a commercial exploitation of my instinctive liking for theatre' (1927, 6). He puts forward the idea that our relationship to theatre is in many important ways 'pre-aesthetic'. By this he means that it 'is something as essentially necessary to man as air, food, and sexual intercourse' (1927, 6). He links the play of the child, acting and the viewing of theatre with the play of animals. The basic psychological foundation is described by him as a series of instinctual drives:

> The instinct of transformation, the instinct of opposing images received from without to images arbitrarily created from within, the instinct of transforming appearances found in nature into something else, an instinct which clearly reveals its essential character in the conception of what I call theatricality.
>
> (Evreinov, 1927, 22)

Theatre is seen as being the desire to imagine and to be different. This is an instinct – not something entered into for its effect or outcome. The experience of transformation is a need. He sees the self as a dramatic dialectic – of the ego and 'another ego'. The second ego 'can leave this world of realities and wander in some other world which it has itself created' (1927, 29). This second ego can 'theatricalise'; in other words it can imagine, it can imitate reality and by imitation master reality. Following on from mastery it can transfigure reality by imagining difference. By this process an individual gives the world 'a new meaning, it becomes his life. . he has transformed the life that was into a life that is different' (1927, 27). This is to 'imagine himself' different from that which he really is: 'he selects, so to speak, a part for himself. And then he begins to play this part' (1927, 27).

Life is seen as being theatrical. In 'The Stage Management of Life' (1927, 105) he analyses everyday interaction, politics and the military in terms of theatre. Evreinov describes the transgressive elements of life in terms of theatre; the violation of norms set by 'nature, by the state, by the public' is seen as the 'essence' of theatre (1927, 116).

Evreinov's Theatrotherapy is based upon these notions. In his writing about this area he does not propose a specific methodology, but rather seeks to demonstrate a facet of the way in which this instinct can have beneficial effects. Theatrotherapy concerns the ways in which engagement in dramatic or theatrical activity connects to healing, alleviation of illness and the creation of well-being: 'The theatre cures the actors. It can also cure the audience' (1927, 126).

He speaks of health on several different levels. On the general level of society he claims that theatre is one of the strongest weapons for safeguarding the health of mankind (1927, 127). On an individual level he considers a number of the ways in which theatre can heal – from clowns working in children's hospitals to the alleviation of toothache.

Evreinov describes theatre as a stimulant: an actor's ailment is overcome by the 'transfigurative energy' of the role he enacts (1927, 125). He cites the example of a performer who is suffering from an illness prior to taking on a role. When on the stage the symptoms may disappear. He says that the actor, when engaged in theatre, enters into an energised state and this helps to alleviate illness – mental or physical. He writes of the reworking and reforming of unhealthy roles in life and the changing of patterns of living which cause distress or illness through theatre. The actor can create roles anew as a way of engaging with their life differently. Here re-playing roles is linked to auto-suggestion and behavioural relearning: 'Play a role well, and you will live up to it' (1927, 125). The ability to utilise the skills of drama is seen to be helpful. The capability to transform the self and the ensuing potential reworking of difficult life situations is enhanced by the development of the abilities to act: 'The theatre "cures" an actor skilful in the art of self transformation' (1927, 125). Theatre can also enable a change in the framework within which someone sees their life. This change can help to alter and reframe difficulties: 'you were induced to leave the place where you had so adapted yourself to things occupying your attention that you could no longer maintain a contemplative attitude to them' (1927, 122).

In formalising these elements of Theatrotherapy Evreinov anticipated many of the writings and workings on theatre, drama and therapy of the later twentieth century. In Revolutionary Russia his ideas were partly realised in theatre events in the early 1920s. He then emigrated to the

United States. His ideas were not to bear direct fruit there. However, the basic ideas of much of his writings are similar to those formulated in Europe and America after the Second World War which underlie the basic tenets of Dramatherapy.

Nilli, in an article referring to Evreinov, 'On the Theatre of the Future' ('O teatre buduscego'), saw theatre as a way of living life: of the connection of fiction and reality. This future theatre extends Evreinov's ideas of theatre in life:

> a group of actors performing a single play and each actor [takes] a single role for an entire season. At the conclusion of the season, the actor would take this role into life and play it among the people, modifying the role according to his observations of the people.
>
> (Nilli in Golub, 1984, 74)

The neglected writings and theories of Evreinov as set out here give a historic example of one of the early experiments in formalising the uses of theatre in relation to personal change. Though his writings have been all but forgotten, 'Theatrotherapy' and the related ideas and notions deserve to be restored to the history of the interplay between life and theatre and to drama as a therapy.

Iljine

During the early twentieth century Vladimir Iljine developed a way of working in the Soviet Union called Therapeutic Theatre. Petzold (1973) indicates the main years of this work as being between 1908 and 1917. During this time Iljine was developing his techniques through activities with psychiatric patients in hospitals, with students who had emotional problems, and in the theatre. His work brings together theatre and therapy in the form of a particular methodology.

After being made a Professor at the University of Kiev he had to leave Russia for political reasons – he travelled widely, settling eventually in Paris in the late 1920s. His travels took him to Hungary where he came into contact with Sandor Ferenczi and his 'Active Techniques' in psycho-analysis which included role playing.

Iljine describes Therapeutic Theatre as trying to combine sciences such as biology and medicine with the humanities, music and theatre.

Like Evreinov his methods were connected to the turn-of-the-century experiments in theatre taking place in Russia. Three key areas which formed the basis of his methods were improvisation training, instant or impromptu performances and the forming of scenarios around which improvisations could occur.

Work could be undertaken with individuals or with groups. A group would usually consist of between ten and fifteen people, though with more therapists a group of thirty could be created. Iljine says that there should be a minimum of thirty sessions, with meetings occurring twice a week. Sessions could last as long as between three and five hours. Within the two weekly meetings one would focus upon improvisation training, the other would work with Therapeutic Theatre performances. The idea behind this combination was that one area would enhance the clients work in the other.

Improvisation training

Improvisation training is an essential element of Iljine's methodology. This sought to develop clients' creativity through drama games and exercises. The training encouraged spontaneity, flexibility, expressivity, sensitivity and the ability to communicate. Iljine saw these attributes as qualities which people in general neglected, and said that this phenomenon was especially prevalent in people with emotional or mental health problems. He viewed the loss of these qualities as a distinctive part of their illness. He would analyse clients' presenting problems in terms of deficiencies or problems in these areas. Therapeutic Theatre had as its main aim the bringing about of change for participants so that they could have access to them once more.

Within the improvisation training emphasis was put upon the clients' use of their body and voices. The idea was that the body is essential to the expression and exploration of emotion. By training clients in using their bodies and voices in drama, the aim was to enhance their ability to express and explore emotions in the Therapeutic Theatre sessions and in their lives in general.

To overcome any blocks against playing and creativity Iljine developed the idea and practice of warm up techniques such as sensitivity and the ability to communicate.

One warm up used the qualities of animal and bird movements, such as the jumping and falling of cats or the motions of snakes. Iljine observed animals and used them as a basis for exercises concerning self-expression. Clients would use the movements of puppies at play, birds of prey, reptiles, big cats. He used a wide variety of such drama games, developing them over the years. Yoga-based activities were often included within warm up activities.

Therapeutic theatre

Therapeutic Theatre consists of a series of stages: theme identification, a reflection on themes, scenario design, scenario realisation and reflection/ feedback.

Theme identification

At the beginning of a piece of work a relevant theme would be established. This theme needed to have the potential to be improvised with. In working with an individual it could be identified by consideration of the client's case history, through the recounting of autobiographical details. Diagnostic techniques such as the Rorschach test could be used to assist this process. The aim was that the raw material gathered in these tests and explorations would be developed into dramatic material. In a group context the theme could also arise out of group discussion. Individuals would discuss the details of their lives and situations and from this a theme would be identified. In this way material from clients' lives was gathered together.

A collection of ideas for dramatisation would then be brought together and selected from. Some of the forms for playing out and exploring the theme mentioned by Iljine include fantasy games, the enactment of incidents, folk-tale based performances, specific situations such as problems at work, hospital scenes and political themes. A theme and format would be chosen which the majority of the group felt to be the most relevant to their current needs.

This process of choosing themes was seen as giving diagnostic information to the therapist(s). This concerned the identification of issues which troubled clients, but could also involve the interpersonal dynamics which emerged during the negotiations. The therapist(s) could give interpretations or make interventions which aimed to stimulate the selection process. Iljine says that this would usually take the form of asking questions, or interpreting what was happening within the group or the decision-making process.

Reflection on themes

Once the theme had been established it was thoroughly examined and debated. In relation to individual therapy this means that the therapist and client discussed the choice of theme, its relevance, the key areas of conflict contained within it, and the ways in which it might be expressed and explored through drama. Within the group a general discussion of the theme would occur. Therapists and clients alike discussed and explored the key aspects of the theme. Other means of reflection could be used in addition to verbal discussion; for example, group members might paint or draw a picture in relation to the theme.

Scenario design

The next task involved the creation of a scenario, which entails a structure giving a shape to the theme. A scene is established, though this does not involve a specific script. It takes the form of a brief outline to act as a focus and springboard for improvisation.

In individual therapy the therapist and client would work together to arrive at the scenario. In a group everyone took part in the design.

The selection and distribution of roles followed. Within a group this occurred by considering the needs of each role in relation to the needs and potentials of the participants. This process involved a high degree of self- and peer assessment, and discussion. Within individual therapy both client and therapist would be involved in enactment. In group situations Iljine says that, depending upon the size of the group, there can be four or five staff who can also take an active part. The role of staff is to assist or stimulate the realisation of the enactments.

A scenario design would include: the theme, key words, details about roles and the characteristic behaviours attached to the roles, a short series of basic situations or scenes to be focused upon, and the location or locations.

Scenario realisation

Within the realisation stage the actual improvisation is practically prepared for and enacted. A stage and materials such as masks and costumes can be used, or the work can take place with a defined space in a room using only some chairs to sit in. If no stage is to be used, Iljine recommends that participants close their eyes and imagine the details of the location. A series of improvisation training exercises could be used prior to the enactment, aiming to warm up the participants to the situations and characters they were to portray. As with Stanislavski's approach to preparation for performance, emphasis is placed upon the use of the five senses in developing an imaginative context for the playing.

The scenario is then enacted. Iljine places emphasis upon the importance of a high level of emotional and imaginative involvement for those taking part.

If a number of basic situations or scenes are included then the group pause after each one to reflect and discuss it before moving on. The idea was that the discussions would deepen the exploration and portrayals in the following scene. A key character might form the centre of a scenario and be at the centre of three or four scenes or situations.

Reflection/feedback

The aim of the reflection section was to help each player discuss their whole emotional experience during the work. Each person discussed how they felt whilst in role. Particular attention was paid to the levels of emotion and the behaviours manifested by individuals within each scene. The belief was that issues from the life of the player could become connected to the enactment they were making. The reflection time offered the opportunity for clients to make spontaneous connections between the scenario and their own lives. The idea was that memories would emerge and the therapist could assist this process by interpretation and comment.

As reflection periods followed each situation or scene, Iljine intended that the emerging issues and memories could be worked on and resolved through the ongoing alternation of the enactment of the scenes followed by reflection times. Emerging emotions or ideas could be pursued, deepened and resolved. The client could gain insight into themselves and personal issues through the combination of the enactments, connections to their own life, their own reflections and the interpretation of the therapists or group members. Emotional material which might be repressed could be expressed and examined during the scenarios and discussions. The scenes within the scenario were seen to be flexible, enabling the emerging material to be followed.

Iljine says that the length of time taken by these different stages varies. As an example he states that the consideration, identification and reflection on a key theme or themes might take between three and five sessions. The scenario design might take a further one or two sessions. The realisation and reflection might take another three to five sessions. These weekly sessions would be running alongside the weekly improvisation training sessions.

Although Iljine's ideas have not been influential in Dramatherapy in the UK and US until recently, they have been used in Dramatherapy training in Germany and in the Netherlands. This difference can largely be accounted for by the unavailability of any English language translation of his ideas and work.

Moreno

Moreno created his first psychodrama theatre at the Beacon, New York in 1936. In the 1920s he had developed the theatre of spontaneity at the

Viennese Komodienhaus (Marineau, 1989). In 1924 he published *Das Stegreiftheater*, or *The Theatre of Spontaneity* (published in translated form in the US in 1947). This form of theatre aimed 'to bring about a revolution' (Moreno, 1983). The theories employed in the Komodienhaus emphasised the elimination of the playwright and written play; everyone was seen to be both actor and audience; improvisation was the main medium of expression. However, these theories met with 'great resistance' (1983, 38) and the Komodienhaus had to close due to lack of public interest and financial problems.

In the 1947 American edition of *The Theatre of Spontaneity,* Moreno divides his ideas into three parts – the spontaneous theatre, the living theatre and 'the therapeutic theatre or theatre of catharsis' (Moreno, 1983, 38). The Therapeutic Theatre 'uses the vehicle of the spontaneity theatre for therapeutic ends . . . The fictitious character of the dramatist's world is replaced by the actual structure of the patient's world, real or imaginary' (1983, 38).

Moreno published a plan for a new form of theatre at the International Exhibition of New Theatre techniques in Vienna in 1921 (Marineau, 1989, 83). When he moved to the US he started working with children at the Hudson School for Girls and also at Sing Sing Prison. Later he began a series of experimental activities – including work with the Living Newspaper – a group improvising and dramatising aspects of current news to an audience. The *New York Morning Telegraph* of 7 April 1931 noted how 'all the members of the impromptu came up on the stage and the doctor told them off for parts' (Moreno, 1983). Moreno eventually opened the first psychodrama theatre in 1936 at the Beacon Hill Sanatorium. The first public hospital to build a theatre of psychodrama was in June 1941. This was followed the next year by the first official position for a psychodramatist, Frances Herriott. In 1942 the Socio-dramatic and Psychodramatic Institutes were opened by Moreno in New York. In this year he also published a paper on the subject of psychodrama. This paper outlined the principle of three parts to a session: warm up, action and sharing; it also described the key aspects of the process, such as the protagonist, auxiliary ego, director and audience, doubling and role reversal. Psychodrama training was established by Moreno at the Beacon, New York.

The therapist is termed 'director' and groups meet for between one and a half and two hours. In classic psychodrama a protagonist emerges within each session, and this individual is the focus of the work. Their problems are depicted and worked with using role improvisations. During the enactment of a situation or issue other clients or staff take on the roles of people relevant to the portrayal of the problem. Specific techniques are used to explore and deal with the protagonist's material. In 'role reversal', for example, players swap the role they are playing to take on a different persona within the action. The psychodrama is divided into different parts. The warm up stage aims to select a protagonist and to help the group to prepare for dramatic activity. The main action consists of role work. In classic psychodrama a catharsis is aimed for. After this a period of reflection, discussion or sharing occurs.

A more detailed discussion of psychodrama in relation to Dramatherapy can be found in Chapter 9. Moreno's work has been influential in a number of spheres, from psychotherapy and family therapy (Brown and Pedder, 1979), to the study of social organisation in girls' schools (Jennings, H.H., 1943)! In the field of psychiatry many early occurrences involving drama as a therapy took the form of psychodrama. The field of Dramatherapy has emerged as separate from psychodrama, as the next chapter will discuss. However, there can be no doubt that the structure of much Dramatherapy has been influenced by the warm up/action/sharing pattern. Specific techniques such as role reversal are used and adapted within Dramatherapy. The relationship between the two is still in flux and papers are still attempting to clarify elements of this relationship (Landy, 1986; Langley, 1989, 1993; Chesner, 1994).

Context – the drama in therapy

Authors such as Bentley (1977), Elsass (1992) and Antinucci-Mark (1986) have indicated parallels between the theatre space and the therapeutic space.

In some forms of therapy, such as play therapy or Gestalt, the language of enactment or drama is used. The development of these forms by Melanie Klein (1932) and Fritz Perls (Perls, Hefferline and Goodman, 1951) acknowledged that the processes of enactment, of action and representation using dramatic form had therapeutic uses and importance. In Gestalt, dramatisation is used to explore the self in the 'here and now'. In a 'Dialogue', for example, the patient might act out a split or division within themselves. This is done through the use of two empty chairs. Each chair represents a part of the split and the client takes on the role of each part of the split by sitting in the chair. In play therapy, as described in Chapter 8, toys are used in dramatic play to express and explore problems.

In other forms of therapy, such as psychoanalysis, some have argued that the process itself is inherently dramatic, or that the form could be understood through analogy with theatre. Antinucci-Mark has drawn parallels between the way in which psychoanalysis creates a fictional space where the client and therapist take part in an 'interplay of fantasy and reality, past, present and future thoughts, feeling and emotions' (Antinucci-Mark, 1986).

In this way key aspects of the analytic or psychotherapeutic work such as the transference relationship can be seen within a dramatising framework. The analyst Casement has spoken of the 'as if' nature of the analytic relationship. Within the therapy an 'illusion' is created. The patient re-experiences in the transference aspects of earlier relationships 'as if' the analyst were the original person. The transference is seen to be a crucial element in psychoanalysis, and it is interesting to note the way Casement describes the potency of the process: '. . . when trauma is brought into the transference, it is the illusion of realness that accounts for the transference experience being so immediate' (Casement, 1990, 82).

The process is couched in theatrical terms – the creation of a fictive reality, the substitution of a fictional identity on to the therapist by the client, the encountering of this situation 'as if' it were real. A core concept in Stanislavski's system of psycho-technique is the 'magic if'. In this lies the key to the efficacy of acting as Stanislavski saw it. The actor believes in the actions on stage – as Magarshack says, 'the actor . . was able to believe in it . . as sincerely, if not with even greater enthusiasm, as real truth' (Bentley, 1977, 227). Seen in this way the process which the client goes through is akin to that which an actor can go through in an enactment – the encountering of a fictive reality which is accompanied by feelings which are experienced as 'real' not as purely pretended or as 'fictive'.

Bentley (1977) has pointed out that psychoanalytic therapy is dramatic. An early traumatic scene, for example, is 're-enacted with the patient playing his childhood self and the analyst the hated father' (1977, 41). He criticises the analytic tradition, however, for failing to fully realise the dramatic potential of such a situation. The analysis stays with the client lying upon the couch, the analyst in a chair. Bentley understands this 'restriction' in terms of Freudianism being part of a Judeo-Christian tradition of a hatred of the body – overemphasising the mental aspects of the therapeutic process to the exclusion of the physical.

This way of seeing analysis and therapy implies the presence of latent dramatic and theatrical processes in areas such as psychoanalysis and psychotherapy. In Dramatherapy the latency was to be realised by the actualising of the inherent drama in the therapeutic encounter.

Context – dramaturgy: doing is being is acting

An important parallel development which has influenced thinking in Dramatherapy was the emergence of symbolic interactionism and dramaturgy or dramaturgical thinking in social psychology. Dramaturgical social psychology is usually traced to the writings of Kenneth Burke in the 1930s and the development of a dramatistic model of human behaviour. The emphasis was upon interaction as opposed to the analysis of individuals in terms of a 'psychobiological entity consisting of conscious and unconscious elements' (1975, 55). Individuality was understood as a social and not a psychological phenomenon. Within this understanding emphasis was placed upon the ways in which people were subject to external conditioning by their environment.

The writings of Mead (1934), for example, advocate the view that it is only through interaction with others that we learn to identify, recognise and value objects. One of these objects is the 'self' – the 'me' as seen by other people. The individual can have multiple selves resulting from different interactions with others. A 'social self' is developed and defined by interaction:

> Certain interactions will lead us to label ourselves as male or female, mother or daughter, clerk or customer, and will lead us to learn sets of behaviours associated with these and complementary labels.
>
> (Knowles, 1982, 6)

Burke put forward the idea that human action and interaction was best described and analysed in terms of drama. This was developed by Peter Berger, Hugh Duncan and Erving Goffman.

Drama is used as a way of understanding the nature of the self. Individuals are termed as actors in everyday life and the way people relate to each other is described dramatistically; that is, in dramatic terms. For example, people in life are said to play different roles, they use props to portray and arrive at their identity. The self is arrived at through interaction with other 'actors'. Society assigns us no permanent identity while at the same time 'exposing us to many alternative universes of discourse' (Travisano, 1975, 92).

Life and humankind are seen as inherently theatrical. In a way the approach assumes that living is a form of theatre. For example, Goffman takes the notion of theatrical performance and uses it to understand the way an individual relates to another: 'A "performance" may be defined as all the activity of a given participant on a given occasion which serves to influence in any way any of the other participants' (Goffman, 1975, 75).

Brissett and Edgeley (1975) in *Life as Theatre* describe dramaturgy as the study of meaningful behaviour. A person builds up meaning through day-to-day activities with other people, 'the meaning of the human organism is established by its activity and the activity of others towards it' (1975, 3). Individuals are provided with basic resources that enable them to act meaningfully, not in narrow proscribed ways, but in terms of the whole range of human possibilities. The individual is viewed as 'one who creates new meanings' (1975, 3). As Turner (1974) states, roles are not necessarily fixed. He says that role making is as important as role taking. 'Role making' as a term denotes the way an individual creates and modifies their roles.

Crucial to this area of thought is the notion described by Berger as 'Ecstasy'. He uses this not in terms of a heightening of consciousness through trance but as

The act of standing or stepping outside (literally ekstasis) the taken-for-granted routines of society.

(Berger, 1975, 14)

The player becomes conscious of the play. Rather than being in a state of constant submersion in the roles they take on, the individual enters a state of awareness that roles and role playing involve choices, decisions, 'The actor has established an inner distance between his consciousness and his role-playing' (1975, 14).

Dramaturgy also becomes connected to a way of understanding forms of illness and distress. Illness is seen as an inability to play roles. Change is a consensual affair between actor and audience: 'Change in identity is ... in the eye of the beholder. But who is the beholder? He is the self-reflexive other, the actor's others, the generalised others, the sociological observer' (Travisano, 1975, 91). Problems arise for individuals who cannot follow social ritual rules, the sustenances of the 'social fiction of shared meaning' (Becker, 1975, 299).

Dramaturgy creates a way of connecting the worlds of drama and of real life. On one level, by drawing an analogy between theatre and living, a conceptual link is made. On another level the individual is seen to function through the creation and negotiation of roles. This way of functioning assumes a level of consciousness – actors can work and rework their roles. Hence who they are and who they become is linked to an ability to be effective actors in life. This way of perceiving individuals has been influential in the use of role playing, and has affected the way a number of Dramatherapists see their work. Dramatherapy has been understood as an arena for the client to experience the kind of 'ecstasy' Berger talks about. Roles can be looked at, examined and reworked. The relationship between one's own roles, other roles and society can be examined.

As Chapter 9 discusses, certain forms of role play work in the social sciences have been strongly influenced by this school of thought. In recent years a number of Dramatherapists have also been influenced by dramaturgy. Meldrum has gone so far as to say:

Although most Dramatherapists use role and characterisation in sessions with their client group, it is the American School of Dramatherapists, led by Robert Landy, who base their theories in role theory as such and on Erving Goffman's dramaturgical model in particular.

(Meldrum, 1994, 75)

Context – play and drama in education

The late nineteenth century and twentieth century have seen the emergence of the use of drama and theatre in education. Caldwell Cook's *The Play Way* (1917) developed a way of using drama for learning. A special room was built in Perse School, where he was head of English, called 'The Mummery', and was described as the first purpose-built drama room. Part of this approach asserted that dramatic literature was better understood through enactment rather than formal learning. Drama was also given a wider significance in the education of a child:

The natural means of study in youth is play . . . A natural education is by practice . . . It would not be wise to send a child innocent into the big world; and talking is of poor avail. But it is possible to hold rehearsals, to try our strength in a make-believe big world. And that is Play.

(Caldwell Cook, 1917)

Hornbrook links the development of drama as an acceptable part of the curriculum and of learning with the development of theories of play and playing within the field of psychology. These developments, as described in Chapter 8, in part concerned the ways in which play related to learning processes. He demonstrates how drama was seen to be allied to this new way of seeing play, quoting a Board of Education Report on primary education from 1931 which states,

> Drama . . . for which children . . . display such remarkable gifts, offers further good opportunities of developing that power of expression in movement which, if psychologists are right, is so closely correlated with the development of perception and feeling.
>
> (Hornbrook, 1989, 9)

In the US, John Dewey refocused education by advocating children's natural 'learning by doing'. Neva Boyd formed the Chicago Training School for Playground Workers and in 1911 and 1921 the Recreational Training School in Chicago. This included work with drama, games and story-telling to develop creativity in children and adults. In 1945 she wrote that games have therapeutic value for hospitalised children, the efficacy in the treatment of 'mental patients' and in corrective work with the re-education of 'problem youth'.

In the US in 1925 Winifred Ward began a drama department and the community at North Western University – this included the development of 'creative dramatics' and the move into special education. In 1930 she published *Creative Dramatics*. By 1975 this field, of Creative Dramatics, was defined by the Children's Theater Association of America (CTAA) as an

> Improvizational, non-exhibitional process-centred form of drama in which participants are guided by a leader to imagine, enact and reflect upon human experience . . . the process is appropriate to all ages.
>
> (in McCaslin, 1981, 7)

The development of the use of dramatics in educational and community settings was widespread, another example being Viola Spolin's work in teaching improvisation for use in community work.

Peter Slade (1954) also reflects the shift in the ways drama is used. From a perspective of Dramatherapy certain significant areas of thought and practice can be highlighted. His aims for Child Drama, for example (1954, 106) include the following benefits for the child: emotional and physical control, confidence, ability to observe, tolerate and consider others. Another later example is the way in which Heathcote emphasised drama as a way of enabling the child to develop insight and understanding. In the late 1960s she saw the important potential of drama in – 'putting yourself into other people's shoes' and in 'using personal experience to help you understand their point of view'. The emphasis was upon discovery and enabling the child to develop personal capabilities through drama.

In Germany, between 1880 and 1940, a number of publications and articles were written on the function and uses of play in 'personality development', in the enhancing of personality characteristics and the development of the individual's social awareness. This area was called *Spielpedagogik*. After the war, in the 1940s and 1950s the Kultur Muhle initiated a number of training programmes which looked at the role of drama in the context of personal change. Germany also saw the development of *Spieltherapie* involving the use of dramatic play and games in therapeutic contexts. Courses in *Spieltherapie* began to be offered in some teacher training colleges.

The emergence of drama in education involved an increase in the understanding of the ways drama could function in personal development. Drama was seen as a way of helping children to learn about the world and its relationship to them, and as a way of developing empathy, insight and interpersonal skills. As such it can be seen to help the movement towards seeing drama as being connected to personal processes and as a way of apprehending and developing a relationship with the world. As the next chapter will show, this field was to be important in the emergence of Dramatherapy.

Summary

This chapter has described the variety of ways in which connections between theatre, drama and therapeutic change began to form. New theories such as those of playing and psychoanalysis, dramaturgy and psychodrama, experiments by people such as Evreinov and Stanislavski, the new uses of the arts in areas such as hospitals and schools all made different but important connections between forms of enactment and the creation of change.

Key areas include:

- the development of psychotherapy and uses of playing made by psychoanalysis
- the work of Evreinov, Iljine and Moreno in formalising the connections between therapy, theatre and drama
- the introduction of drama as an educational force

- the experiments of theatre practitioners and theoreticians in developing new insights and methodologies concerning the processes of acting and performance
- the development of theatre in hospitals and of drama as part of the recreational and occupational services in psychiatric hospitals
- the emergence of group therapy and action-based therapies such as Gestalt

The importances for the emergence of Dramatherapy lie in the fact:

- that dramatic processes can be connected to contemporary forms and notions of healing
- that drama as a process, rather than as a product, has value
- that playing out problems is a natural way in which children deal with difficulties
- that working in groups can be therapeutic
- that the reworking of experiences in psychotherapy can help change

As I have described, these importances were already utilised in part in areas such as the recreational use of drama or theatre and in psychodrama's uses of enactment. However, the potentials which were being discovered in all the areas above created a context of thought, a background of experimentation and recorded practice, and created opportunities for individuals and groups to begin to make discoveries as to the depth and breadth of drama's potential for healing. As the next chapter will show, the emergence of Dramatherapy as a discipline and specific area of professional practice and expertise followed on from the wider discoveries, developments and connections described in this chapter.

Chapter 4
The emergence of Dramatherapy

Introduction

The emergence of Dramatherapy as a specific discipline and as a profession has taken place since the 1930s. There is documented evidence of the use of drama as a therapy from a wide range of countries: from Bellevue Hospital's work in Jamaica in the 1970s (Hickling, 1989) to the development of the Greek Society of Theatre and Therapy in the 1980s (Robertson, 1990). The nature of Dramatherapy's emergence can be said to be parallel in countries such as the United States, the Netherlands and Great Britain: the main countries which mark its origin as a distinct field and profession. This chapter will trace Dramatherapy's development thematically, focusing upon material from these three key countries.

The emergence is marked by a number of phenomena:

- Dramatherapy's development of a *separate identity from other main therapeutic and educational uses of drama and theatre*. This includes a separation from psychodrama's use of theatre processes and from the uses of theatre and drama in educational drama, child drama and what was known as 'remedial drama'.
- *A movement away from dramatic processes being used as an adjunct to other therapies or treatment processes* into Dramatherapy being a therapy in its own right.
- Dramatherapy, along with the other arts therapies, achieving *an identity distinct from arts in hospital settings* or other care settings – such as theatre performances in hospitals or drama projects in day centres.

The process occurs in stages. As discussed in the last chapter, unlike psychodrama or psychoanalysis, there has been no one individual who developed the field in such a way that their name can be uniquely linked with the 'birth' of Dramatherapy. The process seems to have involved the gradual evolution of a form, with a number of pioneers contributing to its development in a number of different settings and countries.

In the introduction to *Dramatherapy, Theory and Practice* (1987), Jennings states that 'current Dramatherapeutic practice as we now accept

it began in the UK in the early 1960s' and that this is discussed within
a context of a 'development in the remedial application of drama within
the educational framework [beginning] to direct itself towards work in
clinical areas' (1987, xiii). The history of Dramatherapy is often viewed
in this way. This chapter will show, to the contrary, that the term and
concepts were in use by clinicians well before that date. The emergence
of Dramatherapy 'as we now accept it', occurred in a number of countries
and is much more complex than is suggested by the notion that it started
in the United Kingdom in the 1960s. Dr Alfred Solomon's extensive
work 'Drama Therapy', for example, published in the USA in 1950 refers
to a wealth of practice already in existence.

From the 1930s onwards, and in the postwar period especially, there is
a marked increase in the exploration of the uses of drama in health and
special educational settings and the growth of interest in its application.
This usually involved individuals with an interest in drama who were
employed as occupational therapists, teachers, psychiatrists or drama
specialists being brought into care settings from other fields such as
theatre. There was little or no co-ordination of this work – it happened
in relative isolation.

The next stage is marked by the coming together of these individuals
to form groupings of people who developed ideas and ways of working.
This is accompanied by the emergence of specific concepts and ways of
working concerning drama in therapy or drama as a therapy.

This is followed by the development of specialist trainings, associations and professional negotiations to establish a specific identity and
form of practice. During this stage there is an increase in the amount of
material documenting Dramatherapy practice and theory.

The pattern in all three countries follows that described above: firstly,
individuals from various professions begin to see how drama could be
used in therapy and in the context of personal change, then groupings
of these individuals form, followed by the formalisation of the parameters
of drama as a therapy.

The Netherlands, for example, follows this pattern. There are records
of artists of varying sorts working in settings such as psychiatric hospitals
and centres for people with learning difficulties from the 1920s and 1930s.
Especially after the 1939–1945 war there is an increase in drama and
theatre activities undertaken with psychiatric clients, for example in the
late 1950s in the 'Festival Room' of the Rotterdam Hospital. Then, by
the 1960s, groups come together, with the formation of trainings and a
professional association following in the 1970s.

Why did Dramatherapy evolve?

In relation to Dramatherapy's emergence Fleshman and Fryrear point to the influx of returning disabled soldiers from the war and the devising of 'new therapeutic techniques' to deal with the 'tremendous demands' (Fryrear and Fleshman, 1981, 14) including some art approaches. Examples of such practice can be found: these include Solomon and Fentress' work with the Veterans' Rehabilitation Center, Illinois (1947), and Cohen's work with puppets in the treatment of 'psychoneurotic soldiers' at the Marine Corps, Army Services Center (Cohen, 1944). However, as pointed out earlier in this book, there are numerous and complex factors relating to the development of 'Dramatherapy'.

Though Iljine and Evreinov had pioneered the use of drama in therapy, there is not a traceable line from their work through to the postwar emergence of Dramatherapy in the United States and United Kingdom. Iljine's ideas have been more influential in the Netherlands. Moreno's work in psychodrama has had a significant effect on the use of drama in health settings, especially in the United States. However, Dramatherapy's use of drama in therapy is seen to differ from psychodrama. Dramatherapy *has* been influenced by Moreno: however, it cannot be assumed that the early development of Dramatherapy owes anything to psychodrama. For example, British pioneers Slade, Lindkvist and Jennings in their interviews for this book claim not to have known about psychodrama at the time of their early work. Though key ideas and ways of working were initiated early in the twentieth century, it is not possible to say that they played any significant part in the later emergence of Dramatherapy as a profession and a discrete field of therapy.

As described in the last chapter changes and developments in a number of areas created a context which made it possible for drama to be seen differently – in terms of personal, therapeutic change. The developments in educational drama, with its emphasis upon process rather than product, created opportunities for people to work with drama in a new way. Not only did it allow for the development of new ideas and kinds of practice, but, perhaps more importantly, it allowed these individuals to witness, encounter and be part of the benefits of drama – not just in terms of education but in terms of personal growth. It is interesting to note how many of the individuals involved in the early use of drama as a therapy comment upon the importance and influence of children's play or educational drama in their early thinking (Horwitz 1945; Moreno, 1983; see interviews with Jennings, Lindkvist and Slade later in the book).

As also described in the last chapter, changes in the care of people in institutions, in psychiatry and psychotherapy, in the development of group work and the use of the arts in health settings created an environment and interest base for Dramatherapy's development. Sue Jennings, an innovator of Dramatherapy in the United Kingdom, in her interview (see pp. 89–92) summarises this phenomenon based on first-hand experience. She remarks on the relationship between the emergence of Dramatherapy and the early use of drama and theatre in psychiatry,

> Because play reading and drama activities were seen as 'a good thing' in the nineteen thirties and forties it was easier for the likes of us to take it a stage further in the fifties and sixties. It wasn't virgin territory.

What can be concluded is that changes within health services, therapy, education and in the way drama and theatre were used and understood created opportunities for individuals to see the potentials for drama and therapy to connect. These changes also resulted in the creation of contexts for Dramatherapy to be practised in. As Sue Jennings remarks indicate, notions that clients could 'benefit' in some way from arts experiences were becoming more widespread. This liberalisation of treatment programmes away from, for example, a complete orientation in drug treatment or mere containment of 'inmates' meant that there were opportunities for new ideas and practices to emerge.

The emergence of Dramatherapy: an overview of documented practice from 1939

Work written about in the 1940s, 1950s, 1960s and early 1970s tends to be in three areas. One area concerns dramatic events or activities taking place in health settings. Another concerns the ways in which drama can be an adjunct to other therapeutic or rehabilitative work. The third begins to concern itself primarily with the therapeutic nature and effects of drama and theatre processes – drama as the main agent of change in Dramatherapy.

In the 1930s and 1940s much of the work recorded is based on Moreno's ideas and psychodramatic practice. Some *individual* pieces of work do deal with drama in a wider sense and the use of the term 'Dramatherapy' does occur. However, there is no *widespread* notion of a separate field called Dramatherapy. In 1939, for example, E. Davidoff and colleagues write in the 'Reaction of a Juvenile Delinquent Group to Story and Drama Techniques' (Davidoff, 1939). This, like many pieces, describes a particular technique rather than advocating a whole approach or new form of therapy. Practitioners struggle to define what they are doing – this can be seen in the strangulated language which is often used! A fine illustration of this is Solomon and Fentress' title of their 1944–1946 work: 'A Critical Study of Analytically Orientated Group Psychotherapy Utilizing the Technique of Dramatization of the Psychodynamics' (Solomon and Fentress, 1947).

An increase occurs in the frequency of the third area of work in the 1970s. However, it is not really possible to divide the three kinds of writings and practice into neat time periods. As this chapter will show, practitioners such as Slade, Horwitz and Florsheim were writing about and using drama as the main agent of change, or using the term 'Dramatherapy' in the late 1930s and 1940s. This lack of a neat, uniform process of development can, in part, be explained by the fact that much early work was being undertaken in isolation. Hence individuals were making discoveries and developing their work at different times without coming into contact with each other. During the late 1960s and 1970s, as organised groupings became common, more coherence began to evolve under the banner of 'Dramatherapy'. The interviews later in this chapter, which focus on early developments in the United Kingdom, for example, bear witness to this process.

The following sections give examples of the three areas of documented practice described above: drama events or activities taking place in health settings, drama as an 'adjunct' to therapy and drama as the main agent of change in Dramatherapy. All contribute to the emergence of Dramatherapy from the 1930s to the present day.

Drama and theatre: arts in hospitals

Examples of theatre and drama in health settings from the 1930s to the present day occur widely. In the *Nursing Times* of 1956, for example, there is a 'Christmas Story Presented by Patients at a Mental Hospital'. Mazor's 'Producing Plays in Psychiatric Settings' (1966) and Green's 'Play Production in a Mental Hospital Setting' (1966) both describe the creation and performance of theatrical productions. Here the emphasis is upon creativity, performance and the special circumstances of a mental health setting.

In the late 1950s Steger and Coggins' work in Tampa General Hospital, Davis Island, Florida is an example of this area of practice considered from the point of view of therapy rather than purely as performance. In an article titled 'Theatre Therapy' they describe the formation of a performance group meeting on a weekly basis. Its primary objective is described as 'entertainment' of patients with an additional by-product of 'the betterment of personnel relations' (1960, 127). 'Gifted' staff were selected by department heads and invitations sent out to patients on Thursday evenings on their supper trays. An audience of 160 patients are recorded as attending the staff performances. The work is firmly set within the context of rehabilitation processes:

> Attending patients are heartened in many ways, both as individuals and in general. For the long stay patients, from the rehabilitation and convalescent departments, the show brings welcome relief from the tedium . . . Patients from the psychiatric department . . . discover in being members of a theatre audience that their return to reality is a smoother path than it might otherwise be.
>
> (Steger and Collins, 1960, 127–128)

This example of 'Theatre Therapy' with its' 'gifted staff' performing represents one strand of this area of work. Contemporary attitudes have become more critical of staff being the performers and patients as audience saying that it reinforces the notion that staff are capable and patients able only to receive. More work has involved patients themselves becoming involved in the creation of productions as writers, directors and performers. In some settings this is clearly part of a therapeutic programme. Others see theatre work in this context purely in terms of its artistic value, with no therapeutic function attached (Pickard, 1989). Some work tends to be undertaken for social reasons or to create access to theatre and drama in the special circumstance of a hospital or health setting (Green, 1966; Brookes, 1975).

In this area of practice the emphasis is upon the performative process with therapeutic benefits arising from the creation and showing of the work. More recent examples include the accounts of the Royal Shakespeare Company's theatre performances and workshops at Broadmoor Special Hospital (Cox, 1992) and Emunah and Read Johnson's research into the ways in which participation in performance work can positively affect the self-images of clients in community and residential mental health care contexts (Emunah and Read Johnson, 1983). Other work, such as that at Tampa General Hospital described above, hints at potential therapeutic benefits from participating in or watching theatre or drama events. Some work considers the direct therapeutic value of theatre form and describes it as a part of Dramatherapy (Read Johnson, 1980, Read Johnson and Munich, 1975; Mazor, 1966).

Handmaid and adjunct

In 1947 Lassner writes in the *Journal of Clinical Psychology* of 'Play Writing and Acting as Diagnostic-therapeutic Techniques with Delinquents': dramatic techniques are used to aid assessment for a verbal therapy programme. Similarly Ellis's 'The Use of Dramatic Play for Diagnosis and Therapy' (1954) and Gunn's 'The Live Presentation of Dramatic Scenes as a Stimulus to Patient Interaction in Group Psychotherapy' (1963) use dramatic techniques in assessment and as a way of assisting verbal therapy. These, along with many other examples, form a second common strand of work with drama in therapy. Here the emphasis is upon drama as an adjunct to therapeutic processes, or to other areas of therapy such as assessment prior to treatment, group psychotherapy or rehabilitation and recreation.

This approach is best summed up by Dr Alfred Solomon in his extensive work, 'Drama Therapy' (1950) when he says that drama can be used with a therapeutic intent: 'This therapeutic intent, however, cannot be accomplished by the use of drama alone, but drama used in conjunction with the technique of psychiatry and psychoanalysis in a group psychotherapy setting' (Solomon, 1950, 247).

Frank Curran's work in 1939 is an example of this phenomenon. Adolescent boys, in therapy due to behavioural problems, write and perform plays such as *Framed* and *How Gangsters Are Formed* (Curran, 1939, 215). Costumes, scenery and performance were involved, but this is seen as a way of creating material for smaller verbal group work and individual therapy 'where deeper probing took place' (1939, 269).

In this strand of work drama is seen to be useful in therapy, but it needs the context of another 'accepted' form of therapy to be effective or safe. Drama can be a servant or handmaid to help elicit material to be dealt with elsewhere, or can assist change for clients as part of something else – a brief enactment during ongoing verbal psychotherapy, for example. It is an adjunct or subordinate to an established therapy.

Drama as the therapy?

From the late 1930s to the early 1970s there is an increasing emphasis upon the drama as the primary medium of change and as a therapy in its own right. Usually, though, the concepts, terms and forms are still confused with those of other areas.

The phase is typified by the struggle to find clear concepts, working methodologies and languages and to establish whether the use of drama is effective as a therapy. The work is often marked by the attempt to describe a specific piece of work and to extrapolate a method or general set of statements or hypothesis. These characteristics of the work can be explained by the fact that the notion of drama as a therapy is emergent. It is beginning to leave behind the notion of an adjunct or handmaid, but does not yet have a full identity or sense of what it is doing. Much of the work is still taking place in relative isolation. A number of individuals are working in parallel directions, or start to come together into groups from similar backgrounds such as education or occupational therapy.

Examples of the third area include Lefevre's 'A Theoretical Basis for Dramatic Production as a Technique of Psychotherapy' (1948), McMillen's 'Acting the Activity for Chronic Regressed Patients' (1956) or Kors' 'Unstructured Puppet Shows as Group Procedure in Therapy with Children' (1964).

Cerf's practice in 1968 is typical of this phase. He takes a particular way of working based in his approach with one group and starts to generalise about it as a broader methodology. 'Drama therapy' is used as a term and drama is the main means of working. However, it is seen as involving taking methods from education/training into a care setting and not as a special, different type of practice.

In 1968 Cerf was working with young adults at the Children's Treatment Center at Central State Hospital in Louisville, Kentucky. Cerf at this time was director of a children's theatre and ran ongoing workshops. The Department of Mental Health permitted a trial run of six weeks and later funded a regular programme. Cerf describes his work as drama therapy. Sessions were weekly and again ongoing and there is an emphasis on skills learning for the 'students'. He describes his work as follows:

> Drama experiences can enhance personality development in the disturbed young person. Both role playing as well as functional technique exercises can be valuable aids in realization of self and in making contact with others. I use the same exercises with mental patients that I employ in the training of actors.
>
> (Cerf, 1972, 112)

He stresses creativity – when discussing objectives they consist of areas such as creative imagination, voice work and the ability to concentrate. The main aims of his drama therapy focus upon process rather than theatre product (1972, 117). Cerf contrasts psychodrama with drama therapy: psychodrama is identified as being more 'confrontative'; this route to dealing with patients' problems is seen as too direct. In drama therapy the patient resolves emotional problems 'while he is comfortably hiding behind his face-saving shield' (1972, 123).

A pamphlet produced by the Educational Drama Association, *Drama with Subnormal Adults*, describes Dramatherapy as 'working through drama in a constructive way' (Slade, Lafitte and Stanley, 1975, 3) and shares some of the traits of Cerf's writing. The practitioners whose work is documented in the pamphlet had been trained on the United Kingdom's Slade-influenced Child Drama Certificate Course. The work is described as Dramatherapy and is seen as 'child drama' used with adults: 'Child Drama adapted with care and really only a part of a much larger total form of Dramatherapy . . . which [can] include a high level of social training and understanding of various grades of ability' (1975, 4).

The work, documented by Eileen Lafitte, was described to patients and staff as 'Creative movement' in order not to 'make claims' that it was Dramatherapy 'before its value as therapy had been assessed by the hospital doctor' (1975, 5). The pamphlet states that the practice's aims were to assist participants' personal space awareness, to increase language flow and to communicate through fantasy in order to redress isolation. Half-hour sessions were held five days a week for four weeks. The practice is a mix of Laban-influenced movement work and Child Drama techniques including improvisation, 'imaginative play' and 'individual movement play'. Each day had different themes and structures designed by staff.

In their pamphlet a number of the ambiguities and difficulties in this area of emergent Dramatherapy practice are illustrated. There is a hesitancy to call drama a therapy, for example. Clients are given one frame of reference whilst the staff have a different framework. There is a shifting between educational and therapeutic terminologies and ways of describing the processes at work. Child Drama, for example, is an approach firmly rooted in educational ideas and practice. From a historical point of view the piece is fascinating as it is a picture of Dramatherapy emerging – its birth struggle. The sense that drama can be used thera-peutically is there, along with a desire to validate this notion by empirical testing, combined with a hesitancy and a need to be approved of by a recognised authority – the hospital doctor.

Some very early work places drama at the heart of therapeutic change, and uses the term 'Dramatherapy'. Slade's practice, as described later (see pp. 83–86), is one example from the late 1930s. Two excellent examples from the same period are found in the work of Florsheim and Horwitz.

Florsheim, in her paper 'Drama Therapy' (1946), brings the drama process to the fore in her work. She utilises the enactment of plays as the therapy. Using texts as varied as A.A. Milne's 'A Boy Comes Home' and a marionette show 'Marmaduke and the Red Bananas', she describes the therapeutic value for clients as being in the identification with the played role, the awareness and benefits of being part of a group creative process, and that unconscious, repressed forces (hostility being given as an example) can find needed release and expression in a socially acceptable form.

Case study 4.1 Sylvester's Dream

One of the most interesting early examples of this third area of practice is undertaken in the early 1940s by a group working with Selma Horwitz. She describes 'spontaneous drama' in group therapy as a technique to be used with children. Dramas are created by the whole group, incorporating the fantasies and providing the therapist with what she describes as 'a medium of operation' (Horwitz, 1945, 252). The aims of this therapeutic drama are summarised by her as follows:

> The implications of the drama for child and group are often far reaching and the therapeutic task, as we see it, lies not only in bringing about the invention of the drama and the production of fantasies, but also in the handling of the material that grows out of the drama.
>
> (1945, 252)

In 'The Spontaneous Drama as a Technic in Group Therapy' she illustrates the dangers involved in allowing clients to act out personal material without the therapist engaging in the issues arising from the drama.

Each child communicated their problem to the group by acting in the group. A specific example describes how a 'group drama' was employed to bring out 'problems that were inaccessible to the therapist yet urgently required handling' (1945, 259). Nine boys, aged 9–11, were in a group together and described themselves as 'The Hawks'.

In the eighteenth session Horwitz notes new tensions in the group. It was revealed that four of the boys were in trouble at home and school. Bill and Danny were threatened with expulsion from school, Tom had been told his parents were to divorce and Eddie had learned that he was to be placed in a foster home. These things had already been communicated to Horwitz by colleagues outside the group. She says that they had not told her of these things previously – 'perhaps because of their urgent need at this time to be good children and because of their fear of losing the therapist's love' (1945, 260). She arrives with costumes and encourages the development of 'spontaneous drama'.

The group do not, in this instance, perform, but instead write a play together containing 'Sylvester's Dream',

The idea was taken up enthusiastically by the group, and the resulting play was 'about two brothers who fight'. The boys propose that Horwitz play the mother, who is very angry when her two boys fight. The boys are sent to bed for being naughty, and then Sylvester, the 'big brother', has dreams. Each of the boys then contributes a dream within the drama.

The dreams include Sylvester robbing the bank, the teller is his 'little brother', who is in school with a 'mean teacher'.

> And then all the kids are sitting around with rubber balls that look like apples. And the teacher thinks that they have apples for her ... And the minute she gets up to talk all the kids start singing 'An apple for the teacher' and every kid throws the ball he's got at the teacher.
>
> (1945, 263)

Horwitz notes that within the different dreams several themes are interwoven – sibling rivalry, aggression against the mother, stealing, class aggression against teachers. She also notes a slip when 'therapy group' is briefly referred to instead of 'class' during the drama. Within the enactments the role of the therapist is seen as thinly disguised in the parts of mother and teacher.

The rehearsals start. Horwitz uses both the process of creating and working together and the content or subject matter of the enactment therapeutically. She says that, whilst playing Sylvester, Bill is 'carried away' by the role, he becomes wild and noisy, curses the little brother and pummels him with 'joyous hate' on the floor. She was instructed to be 'a real mean mother' (1945, 265).

Bill becomes 'irate' as director and 'tyrannical' as Sylvester and the group refuse to work with him. He storms at the others for deserting him. This whole process is described by her as 'for the first time ... Bill bring[ing] out, in relation to the other children and the therapist, his problems as he acted them out at home and school' (1945, 265). This pattern follows on during subsequent groups.

Horwitz considers that the group drama allows Bill to transfer the full impact of his feelings from his mother and sibling to the group therapist and the therapy group. She says that the acting out of his problems within the group made accessible to therapy a whole area of conflict of which Bill had permitted expression elsewhere but until then not in the group (1945, 267). He is then able to work with this material within the enactments and in discussion afterwards.

Horwitz sees the enactments and the creation of the dramas in the context of 'content and transference implications' (1945, 273). She works with the process in the group to an extent, but also in individual verbal sessions with Bill. Though she attempts to help Bill gain insight into his work within the group, she does not do this fully in the presence of other children. She says that, as his 'rivals', they prevented discussion in the group.

Though the title of the piece places the drama in a context of group therapy, and though Horwitz partly moves outside the drama group to discuss material with the clients, she does work directly and deliberately with therapeutic change within the drama. The work uses drama substantially as a therapy – the clients express and explore their material using drama. It is clearly not play therapy, nor is it classic psychodrama.

Horwitz uses a variety of drama and theatre processes, including costume, scripting, improvisation, role work and rehearsal with a clear remit for therapy. There is no notion that drama is a handmaid for other therapies, it is the primary mode of working therapeutically. Horwitz has a laudable clarity about aims, purpose, the therapeutic value of drama, and her role within the dramatic therapy.

The term 'Dramatherapy', then, along with detailed recordings of practice and the formulation of theories and ideas to analyse and justify the work undertaken, was created by individuals well before the 1960s. The three areas described above, and the examples given, show how drama as a therapy was being explored in a variety of ways by a number of individuals.

From individuals to profession

Three interviews: Slade, Lindkvist, Jennings

Dramatherapy began to cohere and grow as individuals met up and started to form organisations, societies and trainings. As mentioned at the start of this chapter, the process is similar in the United States, the Netherlands and the United Kingdom. I will focus upon the developments in the UK as an example and describe the process in detail.

Interviews with Peter Slade, Billy Lindkvist and Sue Jennings follow. These three individuals were closely involved with the emergence of

Dramatherapy as a field and profession in the United Kingdom. Their work has spanned a wide period of time, but the following material concentrates on the early stages of Dramatherapy's development. Their accounts of this process reflect many of the aspects discussed so far. Within their descriptions the following can be found: the initial concepts of drama as a handmaid or adjunct to therapy; the move towards drama as a primary aspect of therapeutic change accompanied by the struggle to find a clear language, methodologies and to establish whether drama is effective as a therapy; and moving on to the creation of trainings and professional organisations.

Nearly thirty years after writing his seminal book on drama in education, *Child Drama* (1954), Slade described Dramatherapy as an attempt to explain a simple method 'of therapy for educational purposes' (Schattner and Courtney, 1981, 78). He contrasts psychodrama's 'imposed structure and symbols' with Dramatherapy's emphasis upon play-inspired activities and the way healing occurs through the drama experience rather than through a focus orientated by the facilitator. This is typical of Slade's perspective on Dramatherapy. As the interview shows he drew his inspiration for the use of drama as a therapy from the 'free play' of children.

There can be no doubt that Slade, in the United Kingdom, was one of the most important early developers of the field. As Billy Lindkvist says in her interview, his contribution has been continually underestimated. Slade is chiefly known for his work in Child Drama. His early work with Dramatherapy, as he has said, involved his exploration of taking Child Drama into work with adults. The following interview with Slade describes how, as early as 1939, he had used the term in a paper to the British Medical Association. He also describes his individual work in Dramatherapy alongside a Jungian analyst.

Interview with Peter Slade

My relationship with Dramatherapy started very much earlier than my discussion of it in *Child Drama* (1954). By the 1950s it was a culmination of a great many things: seeing a lot of children, seeing a lot of schools, my own experiences. I started to use drama as a child at school in the 1920s, because I wasn't happy at school. We would go up into the Downs and dance and improvise. We'd improvise about the masters we hated. The stage, the formal stage, was never enough for me. Later, when I was involved in theatre, looking at children gave me the feeling that a lot of what we were doing as professional actors was different from what children did. In fact they had a drama of their own.

Part of my early work involved starting an arts centre in Worcestershire. I developed my drama and Child Drama work during that time. There were people who came to me either as young actors or as older people who had not very much confidence, so I used to employ certain stage techniques that I used to train my actors on to build their confidence. That would be from 1935 onwards, in what was very elementary therapy.

Kraemer, a Jungian psychotherapist, and I went into a sort of partnership in London between 1937 and 1939. I was honoured by Doctor Kitchin who more or less started the Guild of Pastoral Psychology, a Jungian group, and Kramer and I were both made honorary foundation members of that society. Doctor Kitchin said, 'We think you will show us, and perhaps the world, what Jung means by the "active imagination" – to tell you the truth, we don't know.' It was such a wonderful thing to say! I don't know if I did, but I tried to!

In the late 1930s I was the first person to speak at the British Medical Association on Dramatherapy. It was one word from the start because I think it has more force that way. It was very tough-going then. Doctors thought it was ludicrous and they were all terrified of imagination. I used to say from the beginning, 'If your patients are going to do drama with me or with anyone else, and they're imagining a lot, then we start with the imagination because that's where they are.'

Kraemer didn't always understand what I meant because Jung means something slightly different than I do by projection. Though what Jungians mean by projection is involved in what I mean by it. I said projection involves playing with things which you project your drama into, on to and around – objects outside yourself. The Jungian and other concepts are that you project something unsatisfactory or unkind or full of animosity on to something or someone else so that the hate process is moved from one thing on to another.

In terms of my partnership with Kraemer, clients were referred to us through the Guild of Pastoral Psychology. I always held at the time that a Dramatherapist should not try to be clever and believe that he could do everything because psychotherapy itself was going through a bit of an early stage then and people would try to make more and more sure that you'd at least been through some of it yourself. I was saying 'I don't want to spend time on lone analysis and that's not my job. I'm not being a full psychotherapist in your sense. My job, until I know more, is to work with a doctor and to see how far my contribution can go towards what you people are not doing.'

Kraemer would reflect on and try to obtain dream sequences in Jungian therapy. They would come to me in another room and I would do improvised acting of situations and sometimes I would play through the dream with them if they liked me to or if they wanted me to. That would usually be a dream that Kraemer had been talking about in the other room. The work was one to one at that stage. I would get a tremendous breakthrough. By acting with me they got the breakthrough they hadn't got with Kraemer. They remembered something you know.

We'd work with whatever came to them. They could do whatever they or I felt would elucidate what we were after. But the great thing was that this was further proof of what I mean about projective and personal play, because Kraemer was doing projected activity, I was doing personal activity. What I've always been writing about since is that the balance of these things is so important. We need some of each at different times of our lives until ultimately we settle down into a personality that you know how much you need for the main part of your life. Then, of course, illness or inability to move comes in more and more, then the amount you choose of one or another of the activities changes again.

I remember a man who had some difficulty over getting into trains and he didn't quite know why it was and in his work with Kraemer this kept on coming up, this business of the train. He came to me and we were doing trains together. We would be sitting here and 'You're in a train and I'm in a train and perhaps we're having breakfast together.' I would say, 'Have you seen the paper today?' or something like that, and that would start him off. Then I would choose something that was in my pretend paper, probably trying to get closer to his mind, and so on and then something would come out of that. This man suddenly said, 'My God! The crash!' I said, 'no. I don't think we are in a crash. That's something that happened somewhere else.' 'My God, you're bloody right! Yes!' And he remembered the crash and that was why he was afraid to get into trains. It was somebody he had loved very much, they had died in a crash.

The breakthrough of memory is a very interesting thing. We don't always know why it comes, do we? I believe it's the mixture of personal play and projected activity. You're allowed to be like a child again and you can spit out what you want. At that time I would have said that drama is valuable both in education and in helping people to get better. I must have had the idea in my head for a long time because I wouldn't have used the word 'therapy' otherwise.

I read something by Moreno in the 1930s and wrote to him in New York. We met after the war. I sent him a copy of *Child Drama*. I was interested in a general way. I simply was interested that there was anybody doing psychodrama, when I was having such a tough time in this country persuading anybody that it was important or that drama would have a contribution to make. I think I would have to say that there aren't really any influences in my work. I came across Jung which enriched something in me. I'm often asked if I got my ideas about acting from the Russian gentleman, and I hadn't heard anything about Stanislavski and hadn't read anything until years later.

I believed that the inculcation of drama into people's minds in simple ways, and the use of it in a thousand different exercises, would enrich everything in life. Because drama in my sense is the doing of life.

In the 1960s and early 1970s a number of groupings began to form and these initiated training programmes and associations. At first the trainings were short courses in Dramatherapy or were part of other courses, such as community theatre, occupational therapy or performance.

The most important early training initiatives were the Sesame short courses and Kats programme. These were formed by Marian (Billy) Lindkvist and involved taking participatory activities to hospitals and care settings within the UK and abroad. Sesame was founded in 1964. Its early training consisted of brief intensives. The Principal of the Welsh School of Occupational Therapy, D.G. Connor, after attending the first courses, summarises a training workshop in 1966 as dealing with how

> Drama, mime, music and movement can be used with the mentally handicapped in the following ways: as a form of learning, for identification of body image, as a means of expression for those who cannot verbalise, for mentally ill patients. Drama gives confidence ... allows fantasies to be released in an acceptable form, and generally tones up both mental and physical faculties.
>
> (Lindkvist, 1966)

Sesame currently states its aims as the preparation of practitioners to work 'at a professional level through drama and movement in ... therapy' (Central Sesame Course Information, 1993). Its approach is now based in the work of Lindkvist and influenced by Laban, Slade and Jung. The first Sesame short training course was in 1964 at Guy's Hospital, London, with twenty-five occupational therapists. The identity of Sesame differs from all the other UK training courses in its orientation towards movement. In 1990 Lindkvist refers to the training as 'Drama Movement Therapists' for example (Lindkvist, 1990).

Interview with (Marian) Billy Lindkvist

What started me thinking and what motivated me in developing drama in what I though was a new way was a dream I had. I shall tell you the rationale about why I had this dream – but that's how it was! I had this dream! In a few words the dream was that I saw a hospital ward. Instead of the usual feeling of disintegration in hospital wards, especially psychiatric hospitals, everyone was coming together sharing movement and improvisation. There was an out-of-world feeling – a kind of transcendence – a merging. As I woke I knew what had to be done and I started doing it! So that is how it was – that is how it all started.

As to the rationale for the dream, I had an autistic daughter who was in hospital. I was visiting her all the time and having her home as well. It was about 1964 when I had the dream. I was visiting from 1954 and in 1964 they were still going on. Hospitals were anathema to me, I was terrified. All I could see was people who were not merging at all. I hated the atmosphere and I was terrifed as to what I might see and hear while I was there. At that time I was on the council of Radius, the Religious Drama Society. It was losing members and looking for a way to go. I was seeking a new path for them and the subject was on my mind when I went to bed on the night of the dream. So the dream seemed to be a culmination of the two – my hospital experiences and being involved in Radius. I'd also been training extramurally as part of the City Lit, London, for ten years – studying voice, improvisation, movement and straight play performing.

During the training I was noticing things that were happening to people as well as myself. One time, for example, we wore paper bags with holes in them over our heads and one particular person moved quite differently while she was in the bag. That was interesting to me. We played 'The Living Room' and I was Aunt Helen. The role of my sister in the play was played by someone with whom I had absolutely nothing in common. Yet when we were doing this play I got very close to her because we were sisters in the play. The closeness remained when the production was over. So I was noticing things. I was interested in how I changed according to the play I was in. All this was going on and I was agonising over the hospital situation as well.

I knew nothing at this time of Slade or Moreno. Nothing about any of these things. I knew nothing about Music Therapy or Art Therapy. To me it was absolutely fresh.

When I first put my ideas to the Radius Council, somebody said, 'Well, if the authorities had wanted to do this, don't you think they would have done something about it?' I replied that it was going to happen, going to be! We would run workshops, we would invite people to participate like occupational therapists and nurses, all the people in hospitals who were working with patients. We would teach them about drama and movement and they would take back what we'd taught them and use it with patients. This was a very naive concept. I didn't know about the psychological implications. I hadn't rationalised it or thought about it – I'd just had a dream!

Not long before the dream, I was listening to the radio and Sybil Thorndike, and she said, 'Drama is psychology' and that really hit me 'Bang!' I thought, 'She's absolutely right!' All these things happened.

I said, 'It's got to be everywhere.' One of the reasons I behind my statement was that Radius had performing groups all over the country in the churches and I thought they could take their latest play into places such as elderly people's homes. This was in addition to the training. It was going to be everything! So they were going to go and do plays, staff were going to come and train. I had the bit between my teeth. I was unstoppable!

One of my first contacts was Dr David Stafford Clark, psychiatrist at the York Clinic, Guy's Hospital, London. He said, 'Would you like to do a course at Guy's Hospital for occupational therapists?' I said, 'Yes I would, ' and that was the first course. My main job was to go all over the country to local authorities telling them about this idea and setting up workshops. I didn't really get any resistance. My colleagues, who were the first tutors and whose knowledge formed the basis of the early workshops, were actors and drama teachers.

We have never used the word 'Dramatherapy'. It did not come into existance for therapeutic work until the 1970s. We've always called ourselves Movement and Drama practitioners. We've always considered ourselves to be an adjunct to psychotherapy or part of a treatment team. I'm not sure if that's so much the case now. In the 1970s, twenty years ago, this was certainly the case. In 1972 we ran a day-release course at Casio College, Watford, for one year. In 1974 the Sesame one-year full time course started.

I suppose we talked about Drama and Movement in Therapy after we met Peter Slade in 1965. It was then that Peter said to a Sesame meeting,

'You know you're going to have to learn much more about psychology'. And we said, 'Stuff and Nonsense! We're the artists! The people we're working with know about the psychology. We have the pure art form. This is what we're using and this is what has the effects on people.' By effects we meant the psychological effects. We didn't know what we were talking about because we didn't really know this world and that language – we were artists. However, what Peter said made sense and so we did start to study.

Peter Slade worked with us and we read his books. I always feel he's never had the credit for what he gave to therapy through his philosophy of Child Drama. Of course it was we who set up the Sesame Organisation and it flourished. It has flourished for thirty years. Individuals may have done things that I don't know about, but bringing about a coherent picture of what Drama and Movement Therapy is, and staying with the same organisation for thirty years, being as well known as we are: it was the dream!

During the 1960s and 1970s Sue Jennings was involved in developing a number of important initiatives. These included the Prang project, the Remedial Drama Group and Centre, the Dramatherapy Centre, and the training programme in Dramatherapy at the St Albans College of Art and Design. She was also influential in setting up courses in England and abroad, and in the formation of the first professional association for Dramatherapists in the United Kingdom. In 1973 she published the influential *Remedial Drama* and has written extensively on the subject.

Interview with Sue Jennings

Looking back I don't actually think there's such a thing as 'began' for Dramatherapy anyway. Maybe I've used the phrase myself; if I did I retract it with later knowledge. It's an easy thing to say 'it began' . . . what I mean is this particular initiative, an impetus in relation to Dramatherapy, began. Maybe it had been fallow for a time and it began in a new way.

For me it goes back to a holiday job when I was 17 and at drama school and the supervisor at the local psychiatric hospital had heard about psychodrama, he didn't call it that, he'd heard about drama being done with patients. He knew I was at drama school and said would I come and do some drama. I had to put on a nurse's uniform and be called

Nurse Jennings. In addition, at some level for me, there was an understanding that in the early part of my theatre career drama was actually healing for me. It was mending me from a lot of early life trauma.

I worked closely with Gordon Wiseman. We were asking how one could take drama to unusual places, i.e. not just schools, but where else? For example children's homes, psychiatric hospitals, prisons and so on. The two words 'drama therapy' weren't used at all. The origins of the Remedial Drama Group were in the International Theatre Good Will project in the early 1960s. The sole aim was to take a theatre group across the Berlin Wall. Prang was a shorthand term for that project, it means a happening, a ritual, festival or event. As part of the tour we went to this hospital in Germany and none of the group had worked with people with severe learning difficulties before. Because the work there, the project, had gone so well we set up a programme to do that work. The Remedial Drama Group started in 1962 and went on to the end of the 1960s. The Remedial Drama Centre ran from 1967 or 1968 until 1971. Then Larry Butler started Playspace. In 1971 the Remedial Drama Centre moved to the Drama Centre and we took the plunge and put the two words together: Dramatherapy.

The Remedial Drama Group I started with Gordon Wiseman in the early 1960s. I was doing remedial drama in a special school in St Albans before the Remedial Drama Centre and at St George's Hospital, a psychiatric centre there, and also at the Marlborough, as an instructor explicitly to do drama. There was an interest in 'doing drama with special needs'. I was also employed by the London School of Occupational Therapy to teach OT students. I also worked at a Special Nursery in St Albans.

Drama and music were seen as ways of enabling children to do things that otherwise they couldn't have done. Quite a lot of work we were doing was helping maturation to happen. It was the same with the Remedial Drama Group and Centre – almost like a social education. Maturation steps were gained and retrieved through drama; steps that hadn't been there, or had been lost through institutionalisation, for example.

Moreno and psychodrama I didn't know about until the 1970s. Through Gordon Wiseman and his work with the Belgrade Theatre Group in Coventry I was aware of drama in education and Peter Slade. It was suggested that I contact the Religious Drama Society. They said, 'You should ring Sesame and Billy Lindkvist, she's doing similar things.' The Sesame Board and the Religious Drama Society of Great Britain wanted me to come to meet them, so I went but there wasn't much cross-fertilisation.

It was Peter Slade's pamphlet, that was what we all grabbed hold of: *Dramatherapy as an Aid To Becoming A Person* (1959). That was just like a beacon. The minute it came out in the mid-1960s we all got it. I remember the impact of that; the fact that somebody called this something.

I was very aware in the early 1960s of Occupational Therapy's use of drama for recreation. The problem with the emergence of the arts therapies is that they wanted to divorce themselves from anything the Occupational Therapists did, without acknowledging that this was where they'd actually come from, to an extent. In a sense, because play reading and drama activities were seen as 'a good thing' in the 1930s and 1940s, it was therefore easier for the likes of us to take it a stage further in the 1950s and 1960s. It wasn't virgin territory.

I hadn't heard of dramaturgy; that came later. I'd heard of Smalinsky's Sociodramatic Play – that influenced me. I found it in a shop. I took it to the special Nursery in St Albans and the Child Educational Psychologist there said, 'What will they think of next?' I was so excited – so many connections with my own work and how I was beginning to think! It was quite fortuitous. In terms of play therapy I'd never heard of it as such. To my regret I didn't know the work of Margaret Lowenfeld. In the 1960s I went into psychoanalysis and in my head I was making connections between drama and analysis – but it wasn't the right frame. I cast about, around 1969/1970 to find another frame for remedial drama or Dramatherapy to begin. At that time I felt it couldn't have a framework of its own, it had to be within something. It was anthropology, ritual, the anthropology of art.

Everything was ripe. Art Therapy started as Remedial Art. St Albans had a first course in Remedial Art before it became Art Therapy. We called our thing Remedial Drama and it was almost as if one had to make an enormous step to call something therapy. But it was about 1970 that the step from Remedial Drama to Dramatherapy was made. Dramatherapy – one word because psychotherapy was one word. Slade was anyway using the one word. We corresponded but we didn't meet up. He was patron of a lot of what we did. Veronica Sherborne was very formative by her presence, she came and did courses at the Remedial Drama Centre.

The Association for Dramatherapists started in 1976. There were early discussions that maybe there were to be two sorts of membership. One would be a drama type of membership. The other involved asking – should one indicate whether someone had had a psychotherapy training – nothing to do with their Dramatherapy training? People wanted to differentiate between people who had come through a psychology degree or psychotherapy training and had added on Dramatherapy, and those from drama or theatre backgrounds. This was so that the outside world would know they were psychotherapy or psychology trained. We dropped that pretty quickly. In the 1970s psychodrama and Dramatherapy started to develop more of a relationship. When we launched the Association in 1976 Zerka Moreno came along to the first Conference; I invited Marcia Karp to give the opening address to welcome Zerka to this country. A dialogue was set up between psychodrama and Dramatherapy.

Any decade brings people with energy, ideas and perhaps what people do is take the parts of a jigsaw and put them together in a new constellation that isn't unique. I don't think that anything can be unique. I think I've had the energy to move something forward in a postwar time.

I go back time and time again to the word transformation; that by having a structure like drama it was possible for people not to have something imposed on them but to actually have a way to transform energy.

Three individuals have described above aspects of their experience of the early stages of Dramatherapy. Though there was some contact between them, all arrived at their own position and developed their own perspective on Dramatherapy. Each person shows in the interviews how a mixture of personal circumstances and experiences, ideas, plans, opportunities and fortuitous events – such as hearing Dame Sybil Thorndyke on the radio, being asked to don a nurse's uniform and run drama activities at an early age or picking up a book by chance – all contributed to create unique combinations. However, the stages of development described earlier in this chapter are clearly demonstrated. Slade, Lindkvist and Jennings all progress from ideas and work as individuals, to coming into contact with others, through to the formation of groupings and organisations. The themes of drama as an adjunct, finding a language to describe drama in relation to therapy, attempts to prove efficacy through experimentation and the increasing emphasis upon drama as a therapy in its own right, all feature in the testimonies. The interviews also illustrate that Dramatherapy evolved gradually with a number of starting points which, to an extent, begin to converge, rather than being started in one place at one time by one person or group. What can be noted, though, is the importance of Slade in his being a touchstone for both Lindkvist and Jennings and the importance, historically, of his work and use of the term 'Dramatherapy'.

Training and associations

In the 1960s and early 1970s a number of groupings and training courses developed. These included the Child Drama Certificate Course, the Remedial Drama Centre, Dramatherapy Centre and Sesame in England, along with a course at Queen Margaret College, Edinburgh, in Scotland.

In the Netherlands the training and identity of arts therapists seems to be closely tied with the development of 'Activity Leader' training from the late 1940s. For example, in 1947 an educational programme for youth workers to apply art and play in work with war orphans was begun in Amersfoort. In Mikojel at the Middelau Kopsehof, a course trained workers in social welfare and youth care for settings such as community centres, youth psychiatry and residential care. Part of this training concerned therapy, and during the 1950s arts activities begin to be included as a part of this course. Drama as part of this approach was strongly influenced by Play Therapy. In the 1950s Lex Wils produced his book *Bij wijze van spelen* (*By Means of Playing*) and Jan Boomsluiter wrote a number of articles on drama as therapy. Both were influential in the development of drama as a therapy in the Netherlands. In the early 1960s the Nederlandse Vereniging voor Kreatieve Therapie (Netherlands Society for Creative Expressive Therapy) was formed along with the Netherlands Art Therapy Society. From 1974 Middelau offered a four-year Creative Therapy Diploma with specialisms such as drama; by 1978 the Hogeschool Nijmegen offered its four-year Arts Therapy course with a specialism in Dramatherapy. 1981 saw the formation of a branch of the Netherlands Society for Creative Expressive Therapy purely for Dramatherapists: the forming of a section needs 100 members.

In 1971, short courses in Drama Therapy had begun at Turtle Bay Music School in New York City. Gertrude Schattner was important in the development of these courses and of Drama Therapy in the United States. Her work had its origins in working with survivors of Nazi concentration camps. The group were involved in performing plays by the Jewish author Aleichen about life in a small Polish village community. She says that this process enabled the group 'to wake up, to enjoy themselves and to work together' (Schattner and Courtney, 1981, xxi). In turn she felt that the theatre work with the group enabled her to see 'drama as an instrument in the healing process' (1981, xxi). Like other initiators in the field she worked with children, at the Lincoln Square Neighborhood Center, New York and in the early 1970s was involved in the development of the Turtle Bay courses. The United States' National Association for Drama Therapy was established in 1979, and this period saw the founding of two Masters Programmes in the US: one was an MA in Psychology with a concentration in Drama Therapy at Antioch University in San Francisco, the other was an MA in Drama Therapy at New York University.

With the development of training programmes and associations, how did Dramatherapy change?

Writing in the early 1980s Fryrear and Fleshman (1981) note a shift involving a change in the primary modes of Dramatherapy practice. They describe a move away from performance, puppet shows and the presentation of formal dramas by clients, to spontaneous role-based work. It is interesting to consider some of the points which Davies makes in 1987 – he indicates a 'gradual shift into more specifically psycho-therapeutic areas', and from a general attempt to encourage spontaneity and creativity to a 'more intensively structured and carefully controlled system for exploring and solving important emotional issues through personalised dramatic action' (Davies, 1987, 120). This development would be acknowledged by many theorists and practitioners in the field.

Dramatherapy has established a clearer identity as a specific mode of therapy and as a profession, and, as described in this chapter, this is due to a number of factors. These include the increased contact between individuals involved in using drama as a therapy, the creation of professional associations and training programmes, and the increasing publication of material on Dramatherapy case material and theory. This has been accompanied by an increase in the attempts to evaluate the efficacy of the therapy which, in turn, has led to increased confidence in the potency and validity of drama as a therapy, to clear structures and standards in training and the organisation of professional validation.

Dramatherapy has developed within a number of countries during the postwar period, especially in the 1980s and 1990s. The work of the ECARTE (European Consortium of Arts Therapies Training and Education) formed in the 1980s has played an important role within the European Community in developing courses and contact between countries for example. Training and established practices now exist, or are being developed, in countries such as India, Israel, Portugal, Germany, Ireland, Jamaica and Norway.

Discussion and debate between the different arts therapies, (music, art and dance) has grown. An early forum for such debate was the British Institute for the Study of the Arts in Therapy (BISAT) formed in association with Sesame in 1977 and chaired by Dr Anthony Storr. Its stated aims were to 'co-ordinate and develop the work of healing through the practice of the arts' (Lindkvist, 1977). Some have argued for the main-tenance of separate professions and identities for the different arts therapies, whilst others have stressed their commonalities, pointing to the divisive nature of separation. McNiff, for example, argues that there is a clear, definitive and common identity for all the creative arts therapies that 'centres on the primary use of creativity as a process of therapeutic transformation'. He adds that the situation of the 1980s and 1990s, where professional identities exist 'through divisions of the media related parts of creativity' (McNiff, 1986, 15) is unjustifiable and unsound.

One of the struggles within Dramatherapy has concerned how to deal with its diversity. In Dramatherapy's early development, as this book has shown, a number of individuals and groups worked independently of each other. This resulted in a wide diversity of approaches and ways of working. Later developments have included the emergence of training programmes, the creation of professions governed by national associations along with state recognition and registration in some countries. This stage, of a coming-together through training, professionalisation and registration, has produced a desire for a more homogeneous, coherent form or model for Dramatherapy.

Summary

Mooli Lahad has said that 'We are moving towards that era where we have brilliant ideas, vast experience, and there is a need to conceptualise it into a more theoretical approach' (1994, 182). A number of practitioners have begun to call for work which tries to summarise from a theoretical viewpoint how Dramatherapy is effective. As noted in Chapter 1, much Dramatherapy writing tends to define Dramatherapy either by listing a series of techniques or by a seemingly endless series of models. As Lahad goes on to say, paralleling the comments made in Chapter 1 of this book, 'there is a need to move from experience and models to theory' (1994, 182). The next chapter considers this problematic area. It attempts to present a theory of Dramatherapy which summarises the core processes at work, which explains and accounts for Dramatherapy both theoretically and in practice.

Part III

Chapter 5
Dramatherapy: therapeutic factors
Nine core processes

Introduction

This chapter attempts to define how Dramatherapy is effective. It does so by identifying a number of different elements which combine in Dramatherapy work. These elements describe the ways in which drama and theatre forms and processes can be therapeutic. The factors or elements do not consist of specific techniques or methods. They concern fundamental processes within all Dramatherapy.

In relation to the nine core processes there are key areas of drama and theatre which are of particular interest to the Dramatherapist and to Dramatherapy.

- The process of entry into and playing of character
- The process of entry into a theatrical/dramatic world and state
- Theatrical/dramatic communication
- The relationship between the 'theatre frame' and 'life frame'. By this I refer to the differences, similarities or parallels between an event taking place in someone's life outside Dramatherapy, and an event taking place or being represented within the parameters of the Dramatherapy session
- The performance process. This refers to the means by which a performance is created. There are several routes for this. The most common process consists of; identification of play/content to be performed, casting and rehearsal, fixing of rehearsed work into a final form, performance showing with audience, repetition of performance, ending of performance.
- The audience and the process of witnessing in theatre

From this background I will describe a series of processes which are crucial to the effectiveness of Dramatherapy work. I have presented the above areas to indicate the theatrical origins of many of these processes. They illustrate how the healing potentials of drama and theatre are realised through Dramatherapy. The nine core processes are:

- Dramatic projection
- Therapeutic performance process

- Dramatherapeutic empathy and distancing
- Personification and impersonation
- Interactive audience and witnessing
- Embodiment: dramatising the body
- Playing
- Life–drama connection
- Transformation

Each area will be defined in turn, then a piece of practice will be analysed in terms of the processes. This is intended to give a specific illustration of how the theory of the processes can be used to understand how specific pieces of Dramatherapy practice are effective.

Dramatic projection

Wilshire, in *Role Playing and Identity* (1982), discusses the relationship between the stage space and audience in a fashion which helps to see the ways in which dramatic projection relates to much Dramatherapy practice. He says that one of the constant attractions and needs for theatre is that we see ourselves 'writ large'. Wilshire considers this to be fundamental to the way we see and comprehend ourselves: 'to come to see oneself is to effect change in oneself in the very act of seeing' (1982, 5).

This refers to the change in the way we understand or see ourselves which can accompany a shift in perspective. It also refers to another phenomenon which can occur in theatre. As an audience member views an actor, a number of processes occur which seem to both involve and disengage them concerning what is happening on the stage. In some instances the audience member develops a relationship with one or more of the characters, or with the narrative action as experienced through the characters. Two of these processes could be described as being identification and projection.

We may, as audience members, identify with the characteristics of one of the personae on the stage either through motivation, experience or attitude. Accompanying this may be a projection. We project our own motivations, feelings and experience into the mould the actor provides for us. As a result of the content and action we witness, we may shift our relationship with the projected feelings during or after the engagement with the performance. This may, in turn, affect the way we understand and feel about the parts of ourselves which have been engaged with the projection.

A part of our relationship with the performers and the performance may be a playing out of these projected feelings. A dynamic can be played out between our projected desires and the potency of the stage events to both involve and to interact with these projected feelings through the possibilities they invite and frustrate. This act of seeing/witnessing and projecting is, according to Wilshire, a fundamental part of the dramatic process. Projection in Dramatherapy differs from theatre in its context and purpose.

As discussed above, we 'stand in with' the character and at the same time 'maintain a distance' as an audience member. This is true in a theatre setting and in a Dramatherapy session. An actor takes on a role, involves the self and projects the self into the role. They stop being themselves and yet remain themselves. Audiences in theatre project themselves into the dilemmas and emotional situations of characters. Similarly, in Dramatherapy individuals can take on a fictional character or role, they can play with small objects, create scenery or enact myths. At the same time as assuming a different identity, they project aspects of themselves into the dramatic material. A theatre in miniature is created within the group and within the self.

The classic Freudian position sees processes such as projection and identification as primarily defensive processes. For Dramatherapy, though, the importance lies in the way in which this phenomenon, of dramatic projection, creates a vital relationship between inner emotional states and external forms and presences.

Dramatic projection – summary

1 Dramatic projection within Dramatherapy is the process by which clients project aspects of themselves or their experience into theatrical or dramatic materials or into enactment, and thereby externalise inner conflicts. A relationship between the inner state of the client and the external dramatic form is established and developed through action. The dramatic expression enables change through the creation of perspective, along with the opportunity for exploration and insight through the enactment of the projected material.

2 Dramatic projection enables access to dramatic processes as a means to explore the issues which the client has brought to therapy.

3 The dramatic expression creates a new representation of the client's material.

4 The projection enables a dramatic dialogue to take place between the client's internally held situation or material and the external expression of that situation or material.

5 Both through the expression and the exploration a new relationship to the material can be achieved by the client.

6 From this, the reintegration of the material can occur, within the new relationship.

Therapeutic performance process

The therapeutic performance process consists of the ways in which performance is reached within the framework of Dramatherapy. There are factors which differ considerably in terms of the duration and intensity of these ways, but a basic process is at the heart of performance within Dramatherapy. Therapeutic performance is the process of need identifying, rehearsal, showing and disengagement within Dramatherapy. Clearly this definition parallels that of a theatrical performance, but it achieves different meanings and potentials when considered within a therapeutic framework.

Within Dramatherapy the *need identifying* is the way in which a need to express material arises within a client or group. *Rehearsal* may be an internalised rehearsing, or may involve work with elements of stage craft which aim to find the dramatic expression which most satisfies client needs. The *showing* is the process of enactment or expression when the client shares the dramatic form or enactment with others or, in individual work, the Dramatherapist (see p. 111). *Disengagement* is the means by which the client moves out of direct involvement with the dramatic material.

There are two main therapeutic effects within this performance structure. On the one hand the process allows the client to find expression for the material to be worked on, and the means for working with the material. The client can change their relationship to personal material by exploring the dramatisation during the rehearsal and showing. For example, this can occur through the client taking on different roles within an enactment, or by the client directing alternative ways of the action taking place. The emphasis here is upon the exploration of the content which the client has expressed.

For some clients the *process itself* may be therapeutic. no matter what the content, the movement from need identifying to rehearsal to showing may be the main therapeutic work. By engaging in the physicalisation or representation, a shift in the client's relationship to the material may occur. For example, merely by creating or taking part in an enacted myth or story which has connections to a problem they are encountering, a client may gain insight into their life experience (see Chapter 10).

The process of working with others in creating a dramatic expression may have therapeutic effects. The relationships formed with other group members and the Dramatherapist during the creation of enactments may begin to reflect the way the client experiences others or forms relationships outside the Dramatherapy group. This may enable difficult relationship patterns to be reworked within the comparative safety of the Dramatherapy space.

Within Dramatherapy, performance need not have the connotations and conditions of much theatrical performance in terms of a clearly defined situation involving audience and performer. The detail of the process may vary widely according to the approach taken. In some contexts the work may relate to highly formal, traditional forms of theatre: utilising an existing script, the memorising of text, scenery. In others, the work may be entirely improvisatory, or use play materials such as a sand tray and toys. The work may end in a performance shown to others in the group, or shown outside the group. It may involve a brief showing of improvisatory work as it is in progress.

For some situations the work remains unseen by others, and the showing here becomes the client's sense of a completed action. For example, in play orientated work the client may involve themselves in solitary play with objects. Similarly, in group improvisation the material may not reach a point of 'showing' and not be performance orientated, the Dramatherapist may be the sole witness for the showing.

Therapeutic performance process – summary

1 Therapeutic performance involves the process of identifying a need to express a particular problematic issue, followed by an arrival at an expression of that issue which uses drama in some way. Here performance holds the primary role of creating access to, and allowing expression of, material.

2 The structure of need identifying, rehearsal and showing is a vehicle for exploration and re-exploration of a problem.

3 Disengagement is the means by which the client moves out of direct dramatic involvement with the material.

4 The performance process may be therapeutic in itself no matter what the content or subject matter brought by clients.

5 The client may hold a number of roles within the performance process. They may take on a number of the characters present in a particular

scene, or they may become a director of a scene, or become an audience member for a while. The holding of these roles may be in itself therapeutic in that it can offer the opportunity for a change in the relationship to the material, or change in perspective concerning the expressed material.

6 The client's engagement with the medium of drama through the performance process may enable them to experience their own creativity. They may then feel able to bring this creativity to bear upon the situation or problem they are focusing on within the drama. This creativity may also enable change to occur as the client is able to deal with the problematic material from a different perspective. For example, in life outside the Dramatherapy they may feel stuck with a problem. However, they may feel able to creatively engage with finding a solution or experimenting with new alternatives in the drama.

Dramatherapeutic empathy and distancing

Often empathy and distancing are presented as oppositional forces, two opposing processes within theatre and within Dramatherapy. I would argue that it is more profitable to see both as part of any reaction we have to a dramatic phenomenon whether in a theatre or a therapy group. One may be foregrounded more strongly than the other, but it would be inaccurate to describe a response as being completely distanced or completely empathised. These processes have been linked to mediation and the ways in which an individual relates to others and events in life: 'Healthy functioning requires a balance of feeling and thought' (Landy, 1986, 98).

Dramatic empathy refers to the creation of a bond between actor and audience. It relies upon the audience being able to identify with and engage their emotions in the characters portrayed. It also refers to the empathy which an actor creates within themselves to the role they are working with, as they look for points of identification and draw upon emotional resonances within themselves. This way of working and describing theatre is most commonly connected to Stanislavski's work or the 'Method'.

Distancing refers to a way of approaching drama and theatre related to Brecht's *Verfremdungseffekt*. The actor 'does not allow himself to become completely transformed on the stage into the character he is playing' (Brecht, 1964, 137). Rather than developing empathy and strong identification, the actor or actress is asked to emphasise their critical response; what they think, judge or wish to say about the role they play. The approach stresses the sheer theatricality of a production. It does not wish to create an illusion of reality, but rather to emphasise that what is occurring is a dramatic representation and not actual, 'Making people aware of the world of the theatre . . . There is a theatrical reality going on at each moment. A chair on the stage is a theatre stage' (Handke, 1971, 57).

In Dramatherapy these two phenomena are crucial to the effectiveness of dramatic portrayal, emotional engagement and disengagement. They are also central to the processes of gaining access to material and to de-roling or creating perspective to that material. The terms also create a framework for considering the level of engagement which a client has in relation to their material within Dramatherapy.

There is an emphasis within Western theatre upon emotional intensity as being a measure of a 'good response'. Within Dramatherapy this is echoed, but it is important to remember that both engagement and disengagement are present in theatre and drama, and that within therapy a distanced piece of work may be as important for a client as a highly involved, emotionally expressive act.

The form of dramatic material and structure used can encourage a particular kind of response. Some exercises and approaches encourage the development of empathy, others clearly encourage distancing. So, for example, a warm up linking the properties of a chosen object to that of the person or quality it is to represent would increase the client's empathic involvement with that object. A de-roling exercise describing the actual functions of the object, the object as that object (i.e. to stress the fact that a piece of wood is a piece of wood rather than something that is hard, unyielding, unresponsive and like a member of the client's family . . .) is more likely to increase a distanced response.

Many exercises can be used to create access to either response but the approach and context can emphasise empathy or distance. Role reversal or doubling, for example, may have the immediate effect of distancing the client by taking them outside the role they are playing and have started to become involved in. In a role reversal, for example, the client moves out of the role they are playing to briefly exchange roles with another during an enactment. Two people playing mother and daughter might swap their roles for a short period of time. However, the ongoing effect of that distancing may result in a greater empathic involvement with the role when they return to the action, so the role reversal may have increased the emotional charge and accuracy of the enactment. Similarly doubling may unleash unspoken or unacknowledged feelings which deepen the empathic and emotional response to the enactment. Alternatively role reversal can act as a device to distance a client who is perceived to be overinvolved in the depiction of a situation. The Dramatherapist needs to consider the specific context – the client's needs at any particular point in an enactment and the relationship of an exercise or activity to the empathy/distancing phenomenon.

Dramatherapeutic empathy and distancing – summary

1 Empathy encourages emotional resonance, identification and high emotional involvement within any work. The development of an empathic response to a role, objects or dramatic situations or dramatic activities may be the therapeutic work in itself. For example, some clients may have problems in developing relationships or dealing with others due to a lack of understanding or capability to empathise with another. The development of an empathic response during dramatic work can help to encourage empathy towards others in life outside the Dramatherapy group. Empathy often plays an important part in warming up clients to engage with the material to be worked with. This is the case both for clients who are working on their own material, or for people who will act as doubles.

2 Distancing encourages an involvement which is more orientated towards thought, reflection and perspective. In Brecht's terminology the client functions more as a reader to the material presented. This is not to say that the client becomes disengaged, but that they are involved with material from a different perspective. In some situations the use of a distancing approach can help a client create perspective on themselves or an issue – the capability to develop such a response may be the therapeutic work in itself.

3 Both processes can refer to clients whether in an active engagement with the dramatic material or as witness/audience to the material. The functions of empathy and distancing within Dramatherapy are related but different for 'actor' and for 'audience' member.

4 Within any one reaction or engagement, the client is likely to experience aspects of both processes and this can be used to fuel development and movement within the Dramatherapy session. Often the tension between the two, or movement between the two, can create the dynamic of change which is essential to the work being undertaken. For example, moving under the skin of a role by playing the part and then looking at

the role during de-roling can engender insight and a changed perspective upon the role and the situation the role has encountered during the enactment.

5 The level of response, of empathy and distance, within an enactment or dramatic activity can be utilised as a tool in the assessment of a client's relationship with the material they present.

Personification and impersonation

Dramatic representation refers to the means chosen to express material within the Dramatherapy session. There are two particular aspects which are common within practice; one might be best described as 'personification', the other as 'impersonation'.

Personification is the act of representing something or some personal quality or aspect of a person using objects dramatically. The literary definition of personification is 'an inanimate object or abstract object is spoken of as though it were endowed with life or with human attributes or feelings' (Abrams, 1981, 65).

So, for example, in *The Two Gentlemen of Verona* the clown Launce could almost be beginning a family sculpt . . .

> I'll show you the manner of it. This shoe is my father; no, this left shoe is my father: no, no, this left shoe is my mother; nay that cannot be so neither:- yes, it is so; it is so; it hath the worser sole. This shoe, with the hole in it, is my mother, and this my father . . . this staff is my sister, for look you, she is as white as a lily and as small as a wand.
>
> (II, iii, 15ll.)

'Impersonation' refers to processes such as the impersonation of one person by another, creating a persona, or the Brechtian demonstration of a person. In Dramatherapy this would involve the improvising or role playing of an imaginary character or a person taken from the client's life experience. Landy has defined impersonation as the ability 'to fashion a personality' through taking on and playing out various personae or roles (1994, 30).

Within Dramatherapy the means of dramatising and enacting material which needs to be worked with is wider than role taking or the traditional representation of character in Western theatre. Role is only one small aspect of the range of representative forms which an enactment within Dramatherapy can use.

The client has a variety of expressive forms to choose from to represent the material they are bringing to therapy. Esslin divides dramatic forms into two areas: of expressive techniques based on the use of the body itself, and the materials which can be carried on the body (1987, 61). For the client in Dramatherapy this would mainly include the mimetic expressions produced by their own body, face and voice, the use of space and interaction with others, the use of make-up, mask, costume, or the use of objects and props.

Personification and impersonation – summary

1   A client represents a feeling, issue or person, themselves or aspect of themselves within a dramatic framework. They do this usually by impersonation – depicting something or playing a part themselves, or by personification – using objects (e.g. toys or puppets) to represent the material.

2 This entails the following process:

- The client has an emotional need to represent through drama an issue they bring to therapy. This may be a clearly identified subject (e.g. an oppressive boss) or a less defined emotion (anxiety) which results in an initial exploration through improvisation and the arrival at a personification or impersonation.

- The entry into an imaginative relationship with the representation: e.g. with a created character or with objects used in playing. The creation of a state of sufficient interest and distance for an imaginative relationship to take place is a crucial part of this stage of the process.

- The creation of a context for the impersonation or personification to be developed in and through (e.g. a scene is created, or other characters are introduced).

- The development of the representation through drama (e.g. through improvisation or the creation and enactment of scripts or stories using the personifications or impersonations).

- The exploration of the meaning of the personification or impersonation for the client, during and/or after the development. This exploration also occurs for those taking part as witnesses or other actors involved.

- The leaving of the active representation and the completion of the relationship within the particular activity.

3 Impersonation and personification provide a particular focus for the client's expression and exploration of problems and issues.

4 Impersonation and personification enable the client to experience what it is like to be another, or to be themselves playing another. This connects to the process of creating empathy and can help in developing the ways a client relates to others. It can also assist in the process of seeing a problematic situation from the point of view of another.

5 The involvement of fictional or imaginative material through the personifications or impersonations can create opportunities to transform and explore the issue in a new fashion. The fictional world created can give permissions and allow explorations which the client might censor or deny in their everyday life.

Interactive audience and witnessing

In this process 'audience' refers to a role, 'witnessing' to an action.

Witnessing is an important aspect of the act of being an audience to others or to oneself within Dramatherapy. Peter Brook, in his essays 'The World as Can Opener' and 'Entering Another World', gives a warning and a condemnation which is pertinent to the Dramatherapy group. He warns against experimental theatre work without audiences present, where 'Sincerity is to make a closed world where you use theatre forms, improvisations, etc. for exercises for yourself'. This is 'a terrifying situation ... highly destructive' (1988, 127). In many ways his description here could be seen to refer to Dramatherapy's expectations of the benefits to be gained by clients where Dramatherapy exercises are used 'for yourself'. He says that 'It really denies the whole existence of theatre' (1988, 127). One of the fundamental condemnations he makes of this situation is the absence of audience. Brook sees the audience as giving theatre its fundamental meaning (1988, 234). In the 'heat' of the encounter between audience and performer, the 'peak' experience is achieved. He describes the encounter as 'a meeting, a dynamic relationship' between the prepared (performers) and the not prepared (audience) (1988, 236).

In saying these things he echoes many theatre practitioners, such as Brecht and Boal, in the emphasis upon the audience/performer encounter as being a crucial core to theatre. It would be possible to fit Dramatherapy into Brook's description of the audienceless theatre scenario. Indeed, this is one of the most undeveloped areas of Dramatherapy thought and practice. Much consideration has gone into the dramatic work that occurs for those involved in the enactment, but much less has gone into the consideration of the notion of audience in Dramatherapy. Key theoretical texts, such as Schattner and Courtney's *Drama in Therapy* in both volume I and II (1981) or Robert Landy's *Drama Therapy* (1986), have no index entry under 'audience' whilst 'role', 'props', 'acting', 'catharsis', 'chorus', 'play', 'theatre games', 'costume', 'scenery' are all included. So, is the aspect of the theatre phenomenon which gives it its 'fundamental meaning' as absent as these indexes would suggest?

I would argue against Brook, proposing that the function of the audience, or witnessing, is present and crucial within Dramatherapy group work, but that it manifests itself differently, and has a different function than it does in theatre. I would not say that Dramatherapy, by remaining in a closed group situation, misses the 'heat' of the central encounter, which he assigns to be the essence of theatre. Rather I would argue that it is present in a number of ways, and provides an important function in the Dramatherapeutic effect and the work of therapeutic change within a group.

Earlier I defined the act of witnessing in Dramatherapy as being an audience to others or to oneself within a context of personal insight or development. In Dramatherapy both aspects of audience – witnessing others and the opportunity to witness oneself – are of equal importance. Within much theatre work there is a shift in these areas from the rehearsal phase to the performance phase. In the first phase the actors and director act as an audience to their own work, the future audience being present as an anticipation. In the performance stage there is a shift whereby the main response is that of the audience present at the performance. Within Dramatherapy work this shift does not occur in such a marked fashion, except in cases where a performed piece is part of the therapy. In ongoing Dramatherapy work it is unusual for there to be an audience called in to witness the work.

In Dramatherapy the audience phenomenon is present in a series of possible interactions between group members, and between group members and facilitator. Both aspects as outlined above – that of the rehearsal phase and of the performance phase – are paralleled within these interactions, but their form and effect shift.

I have summarised the process as follows:

For the client within Dramatherapy:

- the client can function as a witness or audience to others' work
- the client can become a witness to themselves: for example by the use of doubling or role reversal, or by use of objects to represent aspects of themselves.
- the client can develop the 'audience' aspect of themselves towards their experience, enhancing the capability to engage differently with themselves and life events.
- the experience of being witnessed within a Dramatherapy session can be experienced as being acknowledged or supported
- the projection of aspects of themselves or aspects of their experience on to others who are in an audience role (e.g. other group members or the Dramatherapist) can help the therapeutic process by enabling the client to express problematic material.

(Jones, 1993, 48)

Witnessing in Dramatherapy can take place briefly, as one person observes an improvisation of another or others; as the group witnesses the improvisation of a small group or pair; or in a more sustained way as during an individual's work, when group members and the therapist become audience to the role play or enactment which emerges.

The degree of consciousness of the role of audience can vary greatly. It does not have the formality of many theatres where the audience area is clearly demarcated, separated off with curtains, seated in rows, etc. It may change from moment to moment, the client in Dramatherapy is a participant observer to themselves and to others. At one moment the client working on material may be at the centre of an enactment, the next they may be in an audience role, or doubling. Similarly, someone as an audience member can find themselves shifting as they are suddenly asked to double or to play a role in someone else's enactment. The client is called upon to act and at the same time to witness; at the same time they are the audience and yet are not the audience to themselves.

The audience–performer relationship can be slight, with no areas being clearly demarcated or no clearly defined roles. Alternatively the role of audience member can be clearly delineated within Dramatherapy, the area in which the clients who are to engage in enactment being clearly marked, with roles clearly differentiated. This creates a different relationship between those who are engaged as actors in drama and those in an audience position. In the latter situation more distance is created between one state and the other, and the act of witnessing is made more visible. This can serve a number of purposes: the creation of safety, the enhancement of boundaries concerning being in and out of role or the enactment, to heighten focus and concentration, to heighten the theatricality of a piece of work. The shift from audience to actor can act as a pivot for change, enabling perspective and insight.

The audience's presence can be used in a number of ways – as support, as confronter, as guide, as companion, as a pool for individuals to take part in enactment. For example, as recipients of projection the audience can be seen as punitive, as judgemental, as all-understanding, as competitors.

The nature of the audience can be significant in the dynamic of the group – just as the fantasy of the individual client, concerning the type of audiencing they are subjected to, is of value to the work. The identity which a group or individual assumes when in audience role is interesting in terms of the dynamic: some groups may become punitive, divided, etc.

Interactive audience and witnessing – summary

1 Witnessing is the act of being an audience to others or to oneself within Dramatherapy. Both aspects are of equal importance.

2 The audience in Dramatherapy is interactive and has little of the formal demarcation of place and continuity of role of traditional Western European theatre. Within one session the client can experience both audience and performer roles and functions.

3 The audience–performer relationship in Dramatherapy consists of a series of possible interactions, e.g.

- being witnessed by other group members or by the facilitator

- witnessing others

- the client witnessing themselves (e.g. through video, role reversal or being represented by objects)

4 The audience can play an important part in the processes of dramatic projection, the dynamics of the group and in the creation of perspective and support.

Embodiment: dramatising the body

In theatre the body expresses an actor's imagination, and helps actors to discover and express their imaginary ideas. The audience is engaged by an actor's bodily expressions through movement, sound and interaction with others. For most forms of theatre and drama, in all cultures, the body is the main means of communication. The actor discovers and expresses roles, ideas and relationship through face, hands, movement, voice – the body. The audience will experience theatre primarily as these bodily expressions in the stage space.

In Dramatherapy the dramatising of the body is of similar importance. This concerns the way in which an individual relates to their body and develops through their body when involved in dramatic activities within Dramatherapy. Embodiment in Dramatherapy involves the way the self is realised by and through the body. The body is often described as the primary means by which communication occurs between self and other. This is through gesture, expression and voice (Elam, 1991). Attention is given to the ways in which the body communicates on an unconscious, as well as conscious, level.

Sociologists have considered how identity is connected to the ways in which the body is presented in social space. Some consider that the self presents selected personae in different situations and arrives at a sense of identity through bodily expression and behaviour in relationship to others.

Courtney (1981) has stressed the importance of the connection between the body, action, change and drama. Witkin has described the way we encounter ourselves and the world in terms of the 'intelligence of feeling', of two kinds of response or 'performance knowledge'. One kind of responding to the world is the immediate experience of an event, the other is the way a more general or abstract understanding is constructed from the experience. Courtney goes on to argue that in drama the body plays a particular role in the way we know ourselves and respond to the world. He says that, when an individual is involved in drama, knowledge is gained primarily by and through the body in action: 'Dramatic knowledge is gained not through detachment, but through an actual, practical and bodily involvement' (1988, 144).

By physically participating in a dramatic activity the body and mind are engaged together in discovery. Issues are encountered and realised through physical embodiment – they are made and encountered through the body. In Dramatherapy this physicalised knowing and being within a dramatic representation of a problem or issue makes a crucial difference to the verbal recounting or description of a client's material.

As Courtney says, the acted out embodiment of an issue involves a bodily experiencing of the material *in the present*. It means that through embodiment the client presents and encounters their issues in the 'here and now'. A deepened exploration can occur as Witkin's (1974) two modes of experiencing are combined within the Dramatherapy session.

On the one hand, the client, in physically portraying material in acting, explores something through immediate, bodily experience. In addition the client can reflect upon the material. Embodiment in Dramatherapy is the client's physical encountering of material through enactment, and combines the knowledge to be gained through sensory and emotional feeling with the knowledge to be taken from more abstract reflection.

Much theatre involves the hiding of an individual's identity, and this is true in a wide variety of cultures. Dramatherapy uses this notion of theatrical transformation to achieve personal change. As will be described in Chapter 7, the creation and entry into a dramatised or disguised self through enactment is used in Dramatherapy to achieve change. This process concerns the way in which freedom to explore personal material can be created within the changed, disguised use of the body. In taking on a dramatic identity an individual can move, speak, respond and feel differently. The physical changes can create a freedom from the usual identity a client holds and from their usual codes, rules, patterns of experiencing the self, relationships with others and situations. This freeing can open up the opportunity for new ways of being, behaving and relating. In turn this can begin to offer opportunities for the client to connect the experiences made whilst in disguise, or in dramatic identities, with those in their real life. The physical change in identity and experience in the dramatic world can result in changes in the client's usual identity and real life.

Embodiment – summary

1 The way the body relates to an individual's identity is an important element in Dramatherapy work.

2 On a general level embodiment concerns the way a client physically expresses and encounters material in the 'here and now' of a dramatic presentation. This participation results in a deepened encountering of the material the client brings to therapy. Hence the use of the body in Dramatherapy is crucial to the intensity and nature of a client's involvement.

3 There are specific ways in which this process relates to change in Dramatherapy.

- The first area involves clients in developing the potential of their own body. Here the body is focused upon in terms of dramatic skill. Dramatic work focuses upon aiding the client to inhabit or use their body more effectively. This might, for example, concern communicating with others more efficiently. This is related to the area described by Jennings concerning people who have 'difficulty in using their bodies in positive, effective and creative ways' (1975, 27).

• The second area has as its main focus the therapeutic potentials and benefits of the client taking on a different identity within the Dramatherapy. Within this area the self is transformed by taking on a different bodily identity. This transformation can result in insight, new perspective and release which can result in changes in the client's life outside the created identity, in the client's own life. For example, the client might grant themselves new permissions in terms of their relationship to their body.

• The third concerns work which explores the personal, social and political forces and influences that affect the body. Here Dramatherapy offers the opportunity to explore areas such as body image or emotional traumas related to the body.

Playing

Play in Dramatherapy refers to processes which involve both children and adults, and refers to the following:

• a general attitude or framework which the experience of Dramatherapy can encourage: playfulness
• the use of play as an expressive form within Dramatherapy
• the use of a developmental model of play within the process of therapeutic change in Dramatherapy
• the creation of a play space in the Dramatherapy session

Playfulness and the play space

The creation of a play space in Dramatherapy involves the creation of an area set apart from the everyday world, and has specific rules and ways of being. The client in Dramatherapy can be described as having a playful relationship with reality. This does not necessarily refer to a humorous response to real life. Playfulness in Dramatherapy concerns the way a client can enter a state which has a special relationship to time, space and everyday rules and boundaries. This state is often associated with the spontaneity and creativity frequently linked to playing.

Play content

Play activities are part of the expressive language and therapeutic process in Dramatherapy. The early stages of sessions often contain play in the form of games, and warm up activities are often developed from or inspired by games. The creation of a playful frame or space is often achieved through the use of play activities. For some groups, play language is an appropriate language to work with. Many see play as a part of dramatic language.

Developmental playing

Dramatherapy makes use of developmental ideas or models of playing. These models recognise that play develops in most cultures along continua of increasing complexity. Though the specifics of the continuum may vary, the notion of development is used in two ways. One is to help in the development of play/drama skills or the broadening of the client's expressive range. It can be helpful to understand developmental sequences as this can help to provide a framework to inform what an individual or group might be able to explore or develop into next in terms of play or drama work. The second acknowledges a connection between the developmental stages in play and particular stages of cognitive, emotional or interpersonal functioning.

Development in playing processes can often be accompanied by changes in cognitive, emotional and interpersonal developments. Hence the client, for example, can develop emotionally or cognitively through the crossing of developmental drama stages in Dramatherapy.

A developmental perspective can also involve interpreting a client's problem as concerning a blockage or problem at some stage in their life. Cattanach describes this as 'a stage in our journey where we got stopped and got stuck' (1994, 29). Dramatherapy's use of play can involve the re-creation of a state where such a block occurs, and the reworking of that stage in a more satisfactory way.

Playing – summary

1 A state of playfulness is created whereby the client enters into a special playing state. The Dramatherapy session is a space which has a playful relationship with reality. The relationship is characterised by a more creative, flexible attitude towards events, consequences and held ideas. This enables the client to adopt a playful, experimenting attitude towards themselves and their life experiences.

2 Play is seen as part of an expressive continuum – as a part of drama. As such it is a specific language (e.g. object play, toys, games) which can be a part of the way a client explores or expresses material in Dramatherapy.

Play content in Dramatherapy usually includes play with objects and symbolic toys, projective work with toys in the creation of small worlds, rough-and-tumble play, make-believe play involving taking on characters and games.

3 Playing also involves a developmental continuum. This continuum is often connected to cognitive, emotional or interpersonal development. For some clients in Dramatherapy, the therapy will consist of moving through a new developmental level. For example, for a client with severe learning difficulties, the therapeutic work might involve engaging in a shift from one level to another. This might be a change from playing in a solitary fashion to co-operative play. This change would entail a therapeutic shift in the way the client can interact with people and with their environment. They begin to be aware of others, and to use objects in interactions with others rather than staying involved in solitary activity.

4 For other clients, playing might be a way of returning to a developmental stage in childhood where a problem or block occurred. The playing process within the Dramatherapy session would aim to revisit that aspect of themselves and their life and to assist the client in renegotiating the developmental stage.

Life–drama connection

In some performances or enactments there is a clear split between the theatre world and real life – in traditional Western plays, for example. In others drama and life might be said to intermingle for some or all of the time: an example of this might be certain types of festival or carnival. In yet others drama and theatre are given the function of reflecting on society or life: political theatre, certain forms of ritual expression or puppet shows in some cultures have this function. Courtney (1983) has described actors as being in a liminal state – 'betwixt and between'. They move into a fictional world to perform, and yet they come from and return to 'ordinary' life.

In Dramatherapy there is an intimate connection between life and drama. This is intentional and is essential to the process of change in Dramatherapy. If the connection did not exist then the client might be able to create and maintain a separate Dramatherapy world. This could be counter-therapeutic. Any change, any new way of being, insights, new relationships or discoveries might be contained discreetly within the Dramatherapy space. The client would not be able to bring life experiences into the Dramatherapy, nor would they be able to take the experiences within the Dramatherapy into their life outside the session or group. A number of authors have likened the dramatic state in therapy to Winnicott's notion of a 'transitional space' (Winnicott, 1974) – a realm which occurs between subjective and objective worlds. Blatner and Blatner, in making this comparison, refer to a 'fluid dimension' in psychodrama, where reality becomes malleable and hence safer, enabling 'creative risk taking' (Blatner and Blatner, 1988a, 78).

The notion of a life–drama connection acknowledges the therapeutic potentials of bringing life into contact with drama within a framework of intentional personal change.

Life–drama connection – summary

1 At times within Dramatherapy the work involves a direct dramatic representation of reality: for example in a role play of a specific life event, or the improvisation of an experience.

2 At other times the actual dramatic work will have an apparently indirect relationship with specific life events. Examples of this might include the re-enactment of mythic material, or performance-art-based work which uses abstract or non-specific movement and singing.

3 Many activities make a number of different kinds of connection simultaneously. A realistic role play of an interaction between a client and her mother, exploring an unresolved problem might have a number of significances. To the client presenting the material, to the other actors and to the audience, the interaction, might symbolise a struggle between two aspects of the self, personified by the mother and daughter, for example.

4 At times the life–drama contact will be conscious and overt for the client. They might decide on an issue from their life and proceed to create a dramatic expression deliberately linked to it. However, the client might proceed into a piece of work without knowing what the contact with themselves or their life might be or become. They might, for example, spontaneously create a story which is enacted. Only during or after the enactment might the connections with themselves be made. A client might be working in someone else's drama. They might have been asked to play a role or to improvise with another client's material. During this involvement in another's work, issues might arise spontaneously which connect to their own life. For some clients, the experience of the drama, rather than a cognitive acknowledgement, is the connection between the enactment in the Dramatherapy and their life outside the

group. An activity might involve a change in the way they respond to a situation, or the way they feel about an issue. This change might not be made overt within the session or even be conscious.

5 The fact that the Dramatherapy space is connected to, but not part of, everyday life is important to some clients. Artaud has spoken of the need for 'true action' in theatre. By this he means that, in some theatre, the freedom can be taken to act 'without practical consequences' (Sontag, 1977, 177). Solomon has spoken of Dramatherapy in a similar way. It must be '. . . sufficiently removed from reality so that unconscious motivations can find gratification without the anxiety and hazard attendant upon actual gratification' (Solomon, 1950, 267).

6 In some work the life–drama connection will be constantly acknowledged. This would be important for clients whose relationship with reality might be confused or tenacious. For others, as in the Case Study 'The Prince In the Tower' (see pp. 224–229) it might be important to work in a way which has little direct acknowledgement of the life–drama connection.

Transformation

A number of authors and practitioners point to transformation as central to any theatre or drama event. Transformation can be seen within a great many aspects of dramatic and theatrical processes. It can refer to the transformation of human being to player/performer, or to audience member, of objects or props into representations of other things, for example. Schechner (1988, 110) identifies two kinds of theatrical transformation. One involves the displacement of antisocial/injurious behaviours by ritual gestures and displays. The other is the transformation of events into fictional representations acted out by invented characters. Evreinov goes so far as to place it at the centre of all theatre:

> Transformation . . . is the essence of all theatrical art, [it] is more primitive and more easily attainable than formation, which is the essence of aesthetic arts.
>
> (1927, 25)

Read Johnson, in discussing Dramatherapy, says that human consciousness is always transforming, 'as the stream of inner life shifts, ebbs and flows' (1991, 285). He parallels this with a dramaturgical model of the self. An individual should not be seen as 'a character in a play, but an improvisation . . . an active constructing of experience that is taking place all the time, a becoming, not a being' (1991, 286).

Within Dramatherapy dramatic processes facilitate this 'becoming', this development of the client through transformation. Transformation refers to the changes in state which the client experiences through the enactments in Dramatherapy. These changes in state are therapeutic.

Read Johnson describes this as a dynamic relationship which is created between the internal feelings and images of the client and the characters, activities and relationships within the Dramatherapy (1991, 291). He describes a transformative series of stages. Within the Dramatherapy, the client

- expresses the material,
- confronts and remembers unhelpful or unresolved issues
- works with them

Johnson analyses this in terms of

- owning the experiences
- actively engaging with them in dramatic form
- resolving and integrating the material

Dramatic representation and exploration in Dramatherapy can be described as a reorganising, a rearranging of material. Often this transformation can be experienced as destructive. Anderson says that growth is the 'disintegration of one way of experiencing' something (Anderson, 1977, x). Koestler echoes this, saying that creative development involves a temporary disintegration of the traditional forms of reasoning and perception: 'A de-differentiation of thought matrices, a dismantling of its axioms, a new innocence of the eye, followed by liberation from restraints . . . and a re-integration in a new synthesis' (Koestler 1977, 5).

Transformation in Dramatherapy – summary

1 Life events are transformed into enacted representations of those events.

2 People encountered in everyday life are transformed into roles or characters.

3 Objects are transformed into representations of something, or are transformed by being given significances which are additional to their concrete properties.

4 Everyday life experiences and ways of being are brought into contact with dramatic ways of perceiving and dealing with experiences. The life experience can be transformed by this different, dramatic reality.

5 The everyday, usual ways of experiencing the self and events are altered by the use of dramatic language. The self can be described through an enacted story or through a puppet. An event can be improvised rather than lived, for example. This means that the life event takes on the improvisatory qualities of enactment. It can be experimented with and altered through the playing and re-playing of the experience. The dramatic language can transform the experience as it opens up new possibilities of expression, feeling and association.

6 The process of being involved in making drama, the potential creative satisfaction of enactment, can be transformative. In part this is due to a transformation of identity – the artist in the client is foregrounded within Dramatherapy. The creation of dramatic products, the involvement in dramatic process, can bring together a combination of thinking, feeling and creativity. This combination has a transformative potential as the different aspects of a client's way of apprehending and responding to themselves and the world – thought, emotions, creativity – are brought together. Often these aspects can become separated, fragmented. In Dramatherapy the client is often called upon to bring these elements together.

7 The relationships which the client forms with the Dramatherapist or with other group members can be experienced as transformative. Past relationships, past events and past ways of responding can be brought into the present of the Dramatherapy group. Here they can be reworked within the drama and the relationships within the group.

Case study 5.1 The Fire Demon

This following describes the sixth session from an ongoing Dramatherapy group of twelve people attending a psychiatric day centre. The sessions lasted for two hours. The majority of participants were living in the community. The centre's work involved a psychodynamic approach, with an emphasis upon counselling and group work. In addition to Dramatherapy clients attended verbal group therapy and some attended art or music therapy.

In the previous week clients had used provided objects such as string, buttons, plasticine and wood. They sculpted the objects to show a situation and feeling in their life which they thought was difficult. These had then been discussed in the large group.

Each client had then taken the identified feeling and had used a selection of small objects to tell a fantasy story in which one or more characters experienced their initial feeling. The story had to be about someone or some thing. It needed to contain the feeling, a problem encountered and the problem overcome. They were told that the next few weeks would be spent in enacting and exploring these stories.

One person, whose initial feelings were 'sad' and 'defenceless', chose a lake, a boat with a hole in it, a cat, a wet ball of wool and a packet of cigarettes. Another who identified one feeling – pain – chose a car wheel, a drill, a bandage and a torch.

The sixth session marked the beginning of the enactment and exploration of these stories. One of the clients, Gina, said that she wanted to work with her story. Previously she had not participated in many activities. Her reaction to myself, as therapist, had been often hostile, saying on two occasions 'You can't help me.'

Gina cast the group. A series of chairs were set out, one for each character or element of the story to be played. One person she asked to play a bird, another two were villagers. She used a series of boxes and wooden poles to represent a forest and a large cardboard box to be a mouth. One person played the role of an anxious heart which was at the centre of the forest. The other group members sat in a designated audience area.

She sculpted the group, placing each person in a shape within an area which was indicated by her, at my request, as the enactment area. She decided that she wanted to play the fire demon in her story.

The fire demon was extinguished. All its fire had gone. It had lived inside a fire made of wood taken by the villagers from the nearby forest. The villagers had stopped feeding fire to the demon and it was slowly going out. It would soon have gone out altogether but at the moment it was a bit smoky. The demon's heart was at the centre of the forest but she was too frightened to go into the forest. She was frightened because if she became fiery she might set fire to the forest and her heart might be burnt up, too. No one would help the demon because they were frightened of her flames. The bird visited the clearing where the demon lay but was too frightened and flew away. With her last breath the demon called out to the bird who at first stopped at the top of a nearby tree. The demon asked the bird to help her to find the heart. The bird agreed and together they went into the forest. The bird flew overhead, helping to find the way to the heart. When the demon found the heart it stopped being so anxious and the demon smouldered rather than burst into flames. She could put the heart back inside her body because her body was no longer on fire. Gina's movements as the demon had been sluggish, hesitant. At this point she gave a brief performance of walking with her returned heart. She walked through the forest with confidence and pride.

At the close of the enactment, people sat on chairs still in role and talked about what the story had been like from the perspective of their character or element. They then left the chairs, leaving the parts they had played, physically shaking their bodies. Each player sat on a cushion near to the chair they had just left and said their own name to the audience. They then said anything they wanted to about what it was like to play the part they had just left. Care was taken to speak as themselves and not as the role they had played.

Gina said that she felt that the bird was something she needed. As the fire demon she felt that her heart was somehow separated from her – she couldn't say exactly how, but that it was part of her lack of feeling. She said that it felt good that the heart had wanted to come back, that it had stopped being anxious. She said at times she felt that her feelings were so fiery that no one wanted to come near her. Other clients shared their feelings – one man who had played the bird said that it had given him a positive feeling to be useful, to overcome fear. Another client said that as the heart she had felt depressed and the feeling was still with her, but not in a way that felt overwhelming – it had connected to her own story.

Audience and clients who had played in the story gathered together in a circle and time was left for people to speak about the session. This lasted for about twenty minutes. Some of the audience members shared the feelings that the enactment had evoked for them.

In future weeks Gina was to reflect further on the story and to create further work based on these themes. Other clients worked with the stories they created in a fashion that was similar to Gina's.

Gina became involved in the work through *dramatic projection*. The small objects and the different enacted parts of the story took on elements of her own personal material. This did not seem to be an entirely conscious process. Though she chose the basic feeling which was reflected in the story, the plot, the characters and the feelings within the tale all could be said to have arisen without direct intention to reflect elements of her own life or inner dilemmas.

The personal material was realised through the processes of *personification* and *impersonation*. Objects took on acted personalities (such as the heart or the forest) and were used to construct the story. Impersonation occurred in the enactment of the villagers and the fire demon. An *empathic* response was created between Gina and the fire demon and the other elements in the story, between the players and the parts taken on, and between the audience and the enactment. This took place as Gina doubled the characters and elements at the start of the playing, as the characters spoke in the chairs and as the playing developed. *Distancing* was used in the de-roling process.

Embodiment occurred as the players entered physically into role – it was especially interesting to note the way in which some of Gina's feelings were highlighted in her initial sluggish depiction of the demon and in the change when the heart returned. The *life–drama connection* was present in the way the story began with one of the client's feelings, the way the story, when told and enacted, took on feelings, dilemmas and issues relevant to Gina's life and in the way she was able to begin to make connections in de-roling and the completion of the session. An additional aspect might be considered to be the way in which the relationship Gina had with myself as therapist (previously characterised by her feeling that 'I' could not help her) might be present in the relationship with the bird. She said herself that this echoed the way in which she didn't like to accept help. My relationship with her, and the relationship between the bird and the demon, might be seen to be a life–drama connection in that it might reflect the way she had formed relationships in her life concerning 'help'. The story seemed to allow Gina, as the demon, to begin to rework this, to permit some assistance.

Transformation occurred in a number of ways. One occurred as the objects were transformed into elements of the story and as metaphors for aspects of the clients' lives. As clients transformed their usual identities into the story impersonations and personifications, another occurred. An additional level of transformation concerned the ways in which the transformations in the enactment reflected actual and potential transformations of clients' personal material. For example, the transformation of the relationship between the bird and the demon, or the demon and the heart, seemed to have importance for Gina, for the players involved and for the audience.

Witnessing occurred as Gina saw the way her own life was reflected in the objects and in the enactment. It was also present in the way the group were able to actively participate in the work through verbal feedback, through taking part in the enactment by playing parts and in the connections they were able to make and begin to acknowledge between the enactment and themselves. Gina was able to give herself freedoms to consider new ways of being and relating within the story and within her playing of the demon, as she had a '*playful*' relationship with personal themes and issues. This was due to the playful space and the permissive nature of the dramatic world created. The *therapeutic performance process* occurred as the need identification stage took place at the start of the session, and as clients identified feelings and constructed their story elements. Rehearsals took place as the stories were created and as the players moved into role within Gina's work. The performance stage was the enactment of the story. Closure involved the point at which the narrative ended and players returned to their chairs. De-roling involved reflecting back upon the material, leaving the chairs, physical shaking, clients saying their own names and discussing the experience. The completion involved the group sitting down in a circle, leaving the audience/stage division, and reflecting on the session together.

Summary

The nine core processes described in this chapter serve as a framework within which we can understand and examine Dramatherapy practice. Though by no means exhaustive they aim to provide a way of seeing how drama and theatre processes are at the heart of Dramatherapy.

As Landy has said, Dramatherapy, though an 'interdisciplinary art and science', is primarily an art (1986, 229). The nine processes are rooted within drama and theatre yet they show how the inherent healing potential of the art form is marshalled and developed within Dramatherapy.

Part IV

Chapter 6
Dramatic projection

'It is characteristic of theatrical fictions that they are, curiously, acknowledged both as real and not-real.'

Courtney, 'Aristotle's Legacy'

Introduction

Projection involves the placing of aspects of ourselves or our feelings into other people or things. Usually it is an unconscious process. Aspects of projection are present in our everyday life; Main describes it as a 'normal mental activity' (Main, 1975, 64). It is a part of the way we relate to and understand the world.

One manifestation of this is the way we imbue other people or things with our own feelings. As psychotherapist Alice Theilgard has pointed out, a child might unconsciously project their own sadness into the sight of trees in autumn as they describe the falling leaves as a 'tree's tears' (Cox, 1992, 164).

Projection is often the inspiration for creative activity. Edvard Munch, in recalling the experience that led to the creation of his painting *The Scream* in 1893, describes a moment on a walk by a fjord when a sunset felt to him as if it were 'a loud, unending scream piercing nature' (Dunlop, 1977). One way of understanding this experience is to say that Munch is projecting his own feelings of anxiety and despair into the sunset. The act of creating this painting is, in part, a way of reproducing the projection and exploring it.

Shakespeare's Antony, as he senses his own declining fortunes, also looks into the sky; seeing in clouds the constantly shifting and dissolving forms of dragons, bears, towering citadels or mountains. As he describes the cloud forms to his fellow soldier, Eros, he realises that he is projecting a part of his sense of personal confusion and dissolution into them,

> My good knave Eros, now thy captain is
> Even such a body: here is Antony,
> Yet cannot hold this visible shape.
> (*Antony and Cleopatra*, IV, xiv, 12–14)

He is projecting his inner feelings into external forms. As he unconsciously projects his feelings, he is able to make a connection and to
gain insight into his situation – he realises that he, too, is unable to hold
his shape. This process of unconscious projection followed by insight
has parallels with Dramatherapy's use of projection.

Dramatherapy encourages the projection of an inner emotional trauma
or problem into a dramatic representation. It builds upon and uses the
everyday and creative aspects of this process to therapeutic ends. For
Dramatherapy the importance lies in the way in which projection creates
a vital and special kind of relationship between inner emotional states
and external dramatic form or presences. The projected material is
explored during the Dramatherapy and is engaged with as part of the
therapeutic work.

This chapter will explore the way projection occurs in Dramatherapy
and will detail the therapeutic potential of this phenomenon.

As an introduction to dramatic projection in Dramatherapy I want to draw
a parallel between Shakespeare's clouds and a moment in an ongoing
Dramatherapy group. It occurred in the fifth weekly session in a London
special school for children with emotional and behavioural difficulties.
A boy of 13, Peter, stands under a spotlight. He is dressed in a cloak
and is covered by a mask in the form of a shiny, totally black helmet,
twice the height of his head. In appearance it is not unlike those worn
by medieval jousting knights. The previous week he had spent over thirty
minutes colouring the helmet's card in several layers of vigorously
applied black wax crayon. No part of his face is visible. There is only
a small slit for an eyehole. A flap is hinged over the hole, and this is
attached to a string which the boy can pull down to cover his eyes
completely. As he turns round slowly to the group, he says, voice muffled,
'No one can be seen unless they kneel down first in front of me'.

This black helmet is linked to Antony's seeing himself through cloud
forms, in that they are both examples of dramatic projection. Like Antony,
the boy is interpreting an aspect of himself, though through the form of
the created helmet rather than through clouds. However, whilst Antony's
words to Eros might be seen to be part of an everyday process, for the
boy in the special school the act is more complex.

Antony's projection into the clouds gives him a momentary insight as
he connects it to his own life situation. For Peter, though, the projection
into the helmet is part of a process rather like Munch's in painting *The
Scream*. In creating and using the helmet within a Dramatherapy group
Peter is being encouraged to explore and develop the projection. A theme

was given to the group: 'difficult feelings and relationships'. Masks and costumes were made with the aim of looking at personal issues for group members within this area. As a therapist I was trying to help him find a form to articulate and examine a problematic aspect of himself.

This connection between inner problems and dramatic expression lies at the heart of Dramatherapy's use of projection.

Dramatherapy utilises the projective possibilities of theatre and drama in a number of ways. However, psychological and theatrical notions of projection differ from the way the process is used in Dramatherapy. What is the difference? How does Dramatherapy use this process to facilitate change? After discussing psychological and theatrical perspectives on projection, I will return to Peter and his helmet to answer these questions and to define dramatic projection within Dramatherapy.

Projection: a psychological perspective

Yalom in *The Theory and Practice of Group Psychotherapy* (1985) describes projection as an unconscious process which consists of 'Projecting some of one's own (but disowned) attributes onto another, toward whom one subsequently feels an uncanny attraction/repulsion' (1985, 117). It is possible to identify a series of key stages which describe projection as understood within psychotherapy.

Firstly, the 'projector', or client, experiences unmanageable feelings. Secondly, there is an unconscious fantasy of putting this unmanageable feeling/state into another person in order to dispose of it or to make it manageable. Thirdly, there is an interactional pressure, with the unconscious aim of making another person have these feelings instead of the client.

The emphasis here is upon projection as a defence mechanism within therapy. It is seen as a way of denying feelings by putting them outside oneself. The aim of the psychotherapy might be to enable the client to achieve insight into this process and to re-engage with the disowned parts or feelings through discussion and analysis.

Dramatherapy's relationship to projection differs from this. Whilst the area Yalom describes forms a part of the way the process is utilised within Dramatherapy work, the description of projection needs to be broader. Landy points out that, from the classic Freudian position, concepts such as identification and projection are primarily defensive processes. He adds that for the Dramatherapist they can be utilised differently: in the creation of a 'balanced form of therapeutic dramatisation' (1986, 74).

Dramatherapy emphasises the ways in which projection can be linked to dramatic form to enable a client to create, discover and engage with external representations of inner conflicts. This is the 'therapeutic dramatisation' identified by Landy. In Dramatherapy, projection becomes expressive rather than being exclusively defensive. The owner/client still puts their difficult feelings outside themselves – but they are placed into dramatic forms. The client can then engage with these forms during the Dramatherapy sessions.

This means two things. Firstly, that projection becomes a way of enabling drama to take on the potency and quality of the client's inner feelings. As we shall see, it also means that this can be followed by the projection being explored through dramatic forms such as role, masks, puppets or play with objects.

There is a key difference, then, between psychotherapy and Dramatherapy in this area. Psychotherapy focuses upon projection as a defence mechanism. Dramatherapy emphasises its role in helping the client to project their problems out into dramatic material. This creates a means to both express and explore the client's difficulties.

Projection: a theatrical perspective

Wilshire, in *Role Playing and Identity* (1982), discusses the relationship between the stage space and audience in a fashion which can relate to much Dramatherapy practice. He moves from the commonplace, that one aspect of our attraction to and need for theatre is that we see ourselves 'writ large', to say that drama and theatre are fundamental to the way we see and comprehend ourselves; 'to come to see oneself is to effect change in oneself in the very act of seeing' (1982, 5).

Why do we 'see ourselves' in theatre? What has this to do with 'change'? I would argue that projection is an important part of seeing oneself in theatrical performances. As Holland has said, 'We find in the external reality of a play what is hidden in ourselves' (Holland, 1964, 347).

I would also suggest that both actor and audience participate in projection when they are involved in theatre.

An actor projects: the legacy of Lear

An actor may identify with the characteristics of a role they are playing either through motivation, experience or attitude. Accompanying this may be a projection. This means that aspects of the actor's feelings or personality which are denied, repressed or unwanted can be brought out by the role they are playing. In this way actors are projecting aspects of themselves into the role. The actor Brian Cox, in playing King Lear for the Royal Shakespeare Company, describes how he was 'personally affected' (Cox, 1992, 57) by this process.

His own fears became projected into Lear's situation and experiences. Cox sees himself as connected to Lear's situation 'as I am, too, a relatively old man'. In acting out the role he begins to project his own fears of rejection by loved ones in old age into Lear's situation. The playing of the role starts to cause him discomfort. His personal desire for acceptance seems to come through in his strong response to Lear's 'being endlessly rejected, rejected, rejected and that rejection gets to you' (Cox, 1992, 57). He still seems involved in this projection: 'I've still got a lot of Lear hanging around me which I haven't got rid of; a sense of physical old age, a sense of my body, all kinds of things which I find a real burden; the legacy of Lear' (Cox, 1992, 57).

This example shows how an actor can project his own fears into a role. The role can amplify projected, unexpressed feelings about the self. Cox, though, is left with the projection unresolved, hence the sense that Lear still 'hangs around' him; the feeling of physical old age, rejection and of needing to be rid of something. The term 'legacy' denotes something which is bequeathed to someone after their death. The role of Lear is dead to Cox in that he is no longer playing it, but the projection is left with him. Clearly, mere acknowledgement of this projection is not enough to end Cox's distress.

This lack of resolution, of a 'burden' still carried, demonstrates how in theatre there is no real opportunity to work with the projection – to explore it in terms of the actor's personal material. Figure 6.1 summarises this process: Cox's own fears are projected into his exploration and performance of Lear, but he remains 'stuck', with the projection unresolved.

Cox's experience also illustrates a fear often expressed in hospitals when a client is involved in Dramatherapy. The fantasy of professionals and clients alike is often that the client's projection into a role will merely be an amplification, that it will aggravate or encourage a problem rather then help to alleviate it. Brookes describes this situation in her production of Marat/Sade in a Massachusetts psychiatric hospital:

> One nurse asked, 'What kind of part does Jack have?' He had a leading role and I described what his character was like. 'Oh no!' she protested. 'That's how he is around here!'
>
> (Brookes, 1975, 433)

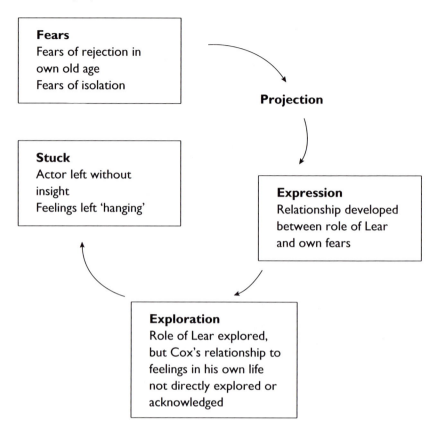

Figure 6.1 Brian Cox and King Lear

I would argue that this is more a problem for theatre rather than for Dramatherapy. Theatre form enables the expression of projection, but does not allow for the experience to be worked with or resolved.

The projecting audience

There are fundamental differences between the way in which an audience member and an actor experiences projection. An actor projects directly into the role they are playing: the audience member is witnessing the roles and projects at a distance. The process is, however, a parallel one. As audience members we can pour our own motivations, feelings and experience into the mould the actor provides for us.

An audience member can project their own feelings or situation into a character or scenario occurring on the stage. As an audience member

I may desire the characters or the narrative to develop in a certain way; to follow a certain course of actions to satisfy my projected feeling. Hence the activity on the stage, once my projections are involved, may develop a dynamic relationship with the parts of myself I am projecting.

This act of projecting is a fundamental part of the way actors and audience become involved in theatre. The role invites both to project aspects of themselves which may be denied expression in everyday reality. The difference with Dramatherapy is in the context, purpose and potentials of this process.

The chief difference between theatre and Dramatherapy here is that the Dramatherapy experience allows for the exploration and resolution of projections whereas the theatre only invites an expression of the projected feelings.

Dramatic projection in Dramatherapy

This section will attempt to define 'dramatic projection' in Dramatherapy. This will be followed by a description of the ways in which projection is used within a variety of Dramatherapy techniques.

Case study 6.1 Peter and the Helmet

Peter attended a special school for children with emotional and behavioural difficulties. One of the behavioural problems he was presenting with was a way of relating to others which was chiefly characterised by violence and withdrawal: he refused most contact with adults and peers. His relationships with his peers mainly involved aggression and violence, both verbal and physical. Verbal interactions would be mainly kept to commands or orders. He had a history of truanting from schools and of absenting himself from rooms. His interactions with others were characterised by silence and avoidance of eye contact. Any attempt to discuss or explore these areas would be met by Peter's flat denial of the behaviour. He had, however, participated in a series of drama classes offered by one of the teachers at the school. His teacher and educational psychologist agreed to his participation in a Dramatherapy group. The main aim of the work was to explore relationships through the creation of costumes and performance art.

By the fifth session the group had made masks and costumes, and had engaged with a number of activities which explored the theme of 'difficult feelings and relationships' as mentioned earlier (see p. 131).

The mask material and the cloth used to make costumes acted as a way for Peter to create forms reflecting the theme. He was able to make his own design or interpretation, developing from the activities we had introduced to the group which had initially explored the theme. The mask and costume aimed to reflect his inner emotional preoccupations rather than any brief given to him by staff or other group members.

Peter was able to project the aspects of himself he verbally denied into the forms. He made a cloak which was decorated by the repeated screen-printed image of a clenched fist. The helmet described earlier was also designed by him to go with the cloak. After costumes had been created, the group were encouraged to improvise a series of interactions using abstract movement as well as stories which explored aspects of their costume's qualities. Characters were created based on the costumes and masks. Short improvisations developed from this.

The character he developed was an increasingly exaggerated persona based on some of the attributes mentioned earlier: aggression, silence, the rigid controlling of interactions. An example of this was that the eye flap would be shut down suddenly to end conversations, another was that the cloak had magical controlling powers. As described above, he would not express his problems by talking about himself with the staff. This work gave him the opportunity to express the aspects of himself which were problematic, which seemed to restrict his ability to relate to people. The improvisations helped him to project these parts of himself into the helmet and cloak. Each improvisation was completed by a clear time when the pupils left the characters they had been playing. This was followed by a space to talk about the characters and what it had been like to play them.

Two main outcomes were achieved by Peter. One was that the sessions enabled him to de-role and to discuss the character of the dark helmet. He was later able to talk about the relationship of the dark helmet character to himself in his everyday life. Hence, the previously censored aspect of his life and behaviour had been made accessible to reflection.

The improvisations led to the creation of different, alternative ways of behaving with the helmet. The improvised stories witnessed a change in the role of the helmet, becoming less extreme. Following the discussions about the dark helmet, Peter began to give the character alternative ways of behaving. It became more involved in the action, it began to act together with other characters – planning plots, co-operating in ventures. Again we were able to discuss these different ways of relating with Peter in terms of the relationship between the helmet and his life outside the session.

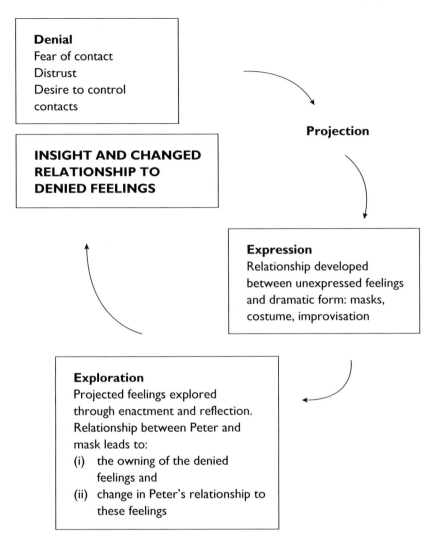

Denial
Fear of contact
Distrust
Desire to control
contacts

**INSIGHT AND CHANGED
RELATIONSHIP TO
DENIED FEELINGS**

Projection

Expression
Relationship developed
between unexpressed feelings
and dramatic form: masks,
costume, improvisation

Exploration
Projected feelings explored
through enactment and reflection.
Relationship between Peter and
mask leads to:
(i)   the owning of the denied
      feelings and
(ii) change in Peter's relationship to
      these feelings

Figure 6.2 Peter and dramatic projection

The second main outcome, then, was that Peter was given the space to work beyond his stuck modes of relating. The projection of inner fears and fantasies into outer dramatic material gave an opportunity to gain access to locked, fixed behaviours. It also provided the means to create a distance to look at the material and an avenue to experiment in order to alter and change the problematic area. This new access also led to discussion within Peter's work with the school's educational psychologist.

A significant part of Peter's difficulty seemed to be a verbal denial of any problem in his life. Whilst he manifested complete distrust and fear of others and excluded contact with them unless on his terms, he rigorously denied this. This created a 'stuck' situation. In the Dramatherapy group Peter was able to project aspects of himself into the dramatic form. He was able to both explore and develop this projection by taking roles, creating masks and costume, and improvising. Through de-roling and separating from the projection he was able to talk about aspects of himself. Through experience and exploration he was able to change his awareness and understanding of that part of himself.

Figure 6.2 illustrates Peter's experience. It can be compared with Figure 6.1 relating to Brian Cox's work with Lear. Cox is 'stuck' at the end of the process: the experience ends with no exploration of his own feelings. Peter's situation enables him to explore his life: he can gain insight into his experience.

It is possible to formulate a basic description for the way the process of projection is utilised in Dramatherapy. Peter's work illustrates many aspects of this. Box 6.1 is a summary of the basic stages in the process of dramatic projection in Dramatherapy.

Box 6.1 **Dramatic projection in Dramatherapy**

- Dramatic projection within Dramatherapy is the process by which clients project aspects of themselves or their experience into theatrical or dramatic materials or into enactment, and thereby externalise inner conflicts. A relationship between the inner state of the client and the external dramatic form is established and developed through action.

- Dramatic projection enables access to dramatic processes as a means to explore the client's material.

- The dramatic expression creates a new representation of the client's material.

- The projection enables a dramatic dialogue to take place between the client's internally held situation or material and the external expression of that situation or material.

- The dramatic expression enables change through the creation of perspective, along with the opportunity for exploration and insight through the enactment of the projected material. Both through the expression and the exploration a new relationship to the material can be achieved by the client.

- From this, the reintegration of the client's projected material can occur, within the new relationship.

Dramatherapy, projective techniques

Dramatic projection in Dramatherapy can occur in a number of ways. There are aspects which are primarily of use with regard to testing, diagnosis and assessment. Others are relevant to techniques and approaches within ongoing work. All areas, however, can be divided into the creation of projective dramatic vehicles, the use of these vehicles and the ways in which meaning is taken from the experience. The dramatic vehicles include play work with objects, sculpting, improvisation in movement and character, puppetry, script and mask. Many of these areas are core activities within Dramatherapy and are considered elsewhere in this book. For the purposes of this chapter I intend to concentrate on the ways in which the various activities can be considered within the process of dramatic projection.

Testing

Chapter 12 contains a wide variety of assessment and evaluation activities and areas of practice which are related to dramatic projection. Here I will only touch on the basis of much of this work – projective testing.

The 'projective' test makes use of aspects of the phenomenon of projection. In this, individuals are given a stimulus which is seen as comparatively neutral, or, as Singer describes them in *The Child's World of Make Believe* (1973) 'relatively ambiguous stimuli', such as ink blots or sets of models or dolls. The client is then asked to make up a narrative or to give interpretive material in whatever way they choose. The notion here is that the client is presented with materials designated as neutral, vague or ambiguous – giving what Millar describes as 'a minimum of objective information' in which it is 'assumed that an individual's production will necessarily reflect his/her own emotional preoccupations' (Millar, 1973, 148).

Dramatherapy's use of projective testing consists of the creation of dramatic forms which operate as these 'relatively ambiguous stimuli'; the enabling of the clients to utilise these stimuli as projective tests; and the engagement with conclusions or meanings from the results.

Small worlds

The creation of miniature dramatic worlds or play worlds has a long history within therapy and analysis. Klein, in her psychoanalytic work with children, used spontaneous play and projective play. Millar (1973, 226) says that spontaneous play was used by her as a direct substitute for the verbal free association used by Freud in his treatment of adults. Klein assumed that what the child does in free play symbolises the wishes, fears, pleasures, conflicts and preoccupations of which they are not aware. The therapist is given roles by the child which reflect other people/ feelings towards them. These are linked to the problems the child is encountering. The therapist's function is to make the child aware of this by interpreting the play for them.

The process consists of the stages outlined in Box 6.2.

Box 6.2 Dramatic projection and small worlds

- Client experiences problem, or is encountering unconscious material which is problematic.

- This is projected into play material or into the relationship with the therapist during play.

- Therapist makes interpretations of the client's play or the relationship which is emerging between client and therapist.

- Client becomes aware and conscious of the material and is able to effect change.

Klein used toys in her work. These mainly consisted of representations of family figures for projective play. Techniques and approaches included:

- play to communicate with the patient
- play as a talking point/play for the social situation it can create
- restricting the child to few toys
- encouraging the child to re-enact certain scenes known/suspected to be traumatic

Lowenfeld's World Picture Technique is a particularly precise way of working with this concept. It utilises similar notions relating to therapy and play within a structured format. The projective material here consists of miniature replicas of people, animals, fences, means of transport, houses and 'unstructured materials' such as Plasticine, paper and string. Water and sand trays are made available, and the child is told to play as they would like. The child is then asked to explain the world built to the therapist and to say what will happen next.

Lowenfeld (1970) refers to her tools as a multidimensional language, requiring no special skills. The work aims to facilitate 'expression of concepts, and of inner experiences which are outside the framework of even "fantastic" drawing and modelling'.

The method of introduction has two parts, 'The bridge' and 'Picture thinking'. The basic notion is that child and adult live on opposite sides of a river, they are separated by a gap in understanding. Both child and therapist are to build a bridge across the river together. The child's attention is directed towards the sand tray, the therapist demonstrates that sand can be moved and that water, or the blue base of the tray to represent water, can be used. Next, the child is shown the cabinet of toys, and is asked to make 'a picture' in the sand, using any or none of the objects provided. The child can use any other objects in the room. The therapist adds that this need not be a 'real' picture and that if it occurs to the child to use objects in an odd way, then they should do so.

Following this 'making', the therapist must find out the exact meanings the child gives to the materials, and the work is recorded through photography or drawing.

The World Technique can be divided into the phases outlined in Box 6.3.

Box 6.3 **Dramatic projection and World Technique**

- Introduction: client's use leading to familiarity, repetition and exploration through activity, a relationship is established with the materials.

- The client becomes deeply engaged in the projection of a revived expression of infantile processes.

- The client works out unconscious processes. The materials are used to express and explore the problem and are used in changing the client's relationship to the problem.

- The fantasy experience tapers, the materials becoming less and less absorbing for the client.

I would argue that the Dramatherapist can use the approaches described above. The area can be included within the remit of Dramatherapy in the same way that dramatic play can (see Chapter 8). The Dramatherapist, however, has the additional possibility to develop this work with small play worlds into additional dramatic expressions.

This area of work within Dramatherapy creates a theatre space in miniature. Within the therapeutic space the client and therapist work with dramatic representations using objects as the main medium. The technique has a more complex relation to projection than the earlier comparison with free association made by Millar (see p. 140). Bowyer rightly contradicts Millar's description of Klein's play work being analogous with free association, saying that this is an understatement. The area of work, including Lowenfeld's World Technique, creates 'a world in which the child lives through its stresses again sometimes over and over in a long drawn out process of working through' (1970, 109).

The use of small representational work creates a parallel but different relationship between the fictive, created world and the client than do 'larger' enactments in which the client uses their own body in a physical representation, or conceptualises on a 'life-size' scale. The following summarises the main four differences between small world work and 'larger' enactment in Dramatherapy:

• The client's relationship to the events or issues can be affected by the fact that the play world is a miniature representation of a much larger reality. The play world materials are small and can be easily moved around by the client. The client can feel more powerful, more able to physically change the materials than the life events or issues they represent. This in turn, through analogy, makes the client more able to feel empowered to make change in terms of the real events or issues.

• The objects chosen affect the client's awareness of the issue represented. For example, if objects already existing as a specific form (small dolls, farm animals) are deliberately chosen to represent an important other, or if they were chosen 'at random' and the significance is realised during the action/play, then the object's form will add an additional factor of awareness, another level of possible meaning to the work. Aspects such as its texture (e.g. soft, hard, furry), identity (e.g. cow, bulldozer, baby) or memory associations (e.g. a fond childhood memory attached to a particular kind of object, a dislike of sand or water linked to a particular experience) will affect the client's relationship to the issue.

This will result in a potentially different awareness of the original material being represented. Hence a truck representing a father has wheels, a gear, a horn, cargo, etc., which the father in real life does not possess. The fact that the truck as a dramatic object can be moved, can sound its horn, can break down and have a wheel changed, can reveal aspects of the client's feelings towards the father. The different shape, physical properties, context (in a sand tray), and position of the object in relation to other play objects may all give information. If a client chooses a furry elephant to represent a father, then different aspects of their relationship will be highlighted than if a hard, cold object such as a stone had been chosen.

• The cultural associations of clients concerning playing with objects will frame the experience. A common association is that object play is the domain of children, therefore associations for the client may be linked to this area – with their own childhood, or children with whom they have some current or previous connection.

• The relationship between therapist and client shifts as the object world becomes a key part of the language of the work. Objects may represent the client's perception of aspects of the relationship between therapist and client.

In Dramatherapy it is also possible to work with this notion of the small world as part of the dramatic continuum. Peter Slade (1981) makes a division between projected play and personal play:

> Projected play . . . with apparatus and sand trays . . . [and] personal play, where the child must take on a role and test out the responsibility for moving and communicating as in real life.
>
> (1981, 194)

I do not like to make such a clear division between projected work and other dramatic areas. I prefer the notion of continuum described later (Chapter 8), as this permits the movement into a different part of the expressive range without demarcating one area as being 'projected' and another as not being part of projective experience. 'Role . . . moving and communicating as in real life' (Slade, 1981, 194) can be as much a part of projected work as any other aspect of the dramatic medium. If this is accepted then it sets up the possibility of a further dramatic relationship with the client's small world of objects. The work with objects can be developed into role play, improvisation and movement activities. This can be used to amplify, extend, initiate and develop the small world work.

Puppetry

Puppetry in Dramatherapy can be considered as an extension of this kind of object work. Within Dramatherapy the puppet can become a vehicle for projection in much the same way that an object can. The issues discussed above concerning the possible projective processes can be considered as appropriate for puppetry. The physical and imaginative properties of the puppet invite a way of involvement which lies between the object and the use of improvisation. As described in the Chapter 8, (see p. 193), the puppet may be seen as a progression from the symbolic use of objects in play. So in projective use, the puppet can be seen as a progression from object usage, rather than a completely different area of practice.

Having said this, there are important differences. The body of the client may be engaged physically. For example, with a glove puppet, the hand of the client is involved. With others, such as rod puppets, the relationship is through manipulation of the puppet through rods. The shadow puppet is again manipulated by rods, and can be seen in reverse against the screen, but cannot be seen 'face on' by the manipulator. This kind of engagement affects the projective work. For hand puppets, the physical act of having the hand inside the puppet will engage the operator in an intimate relationship which enhances empathy between operator and puppet. For rod puppets the physical presence of rods attached to the limbs means that the fact of the manipulation is constantly visible and the manipulator has a clear statement of their power to shift limbs whilst maintaining distance. This will create a mixture of feelings regarding empathy and distance.

Larger than life puppets, whose size is greater than the size of the puppet operator, can change this projective relationship. They offer potential projections in areas such as clients' feelings of being overpowered or issues regarding parental authority.

A puppet can move in a way which most objects in play cannot. There are specific cultural associations of the ways in which puppets 'act'. This means that the client will usually have a set of expectations which differ from the way they would relate to object play. These usually include areas such as the urge to bring the puppet to 'life' through drama, the production of voice, the attribution of human or animal characteristics. The engagement with puppets is potentially strong in terms of dramatic empathy, and this is likely to be stronger than most object play work. The puppet, then, within projective work, can be seen as a form which invites strong empathy, which inherently invites less distance than object play, which involves dramatic possibilities and which carries with it a clear process of physical relationship (e.g. hand, rod, shadow). The quality of clients' projection into the puppet may, therefore, differ from projection into objects.

Masks

Ensor, the Belgian painter, acknowledged as the inventor/precursor of Expressionism, has described the mask as an empty shell for a soft creature to hide in. There are parallels between this process and the use of masks in Dramatherapy. In terms of its relation to dramatic projection there are three main points to consider. The first is that, as in object work, the form of the mask affects the nature of the material projected by the client into the form. Hence a blank mask will enable the client to project one kind of experience, whereas a mask of a clown might bring out a different kind, and a client's own decorated mask might bring out yet another.

The second concerns the paradox which Brook speaks of, that the 'mask is the expression of somebody unmasked' (Brook, 1988, 219). The creation of a second skin, as it were, means that the client can present a part of themselves through the mask. The presence of the mask creates a sense that this is not really themselves, but rather the mask that is speaking or moving. This enables the client to project into the mask feelings or ways of behaving specifically to do with the part of them which is highlighted by the personality of the mask. The mask creates a freedom to express material which would be repressed within the client's usual presentation of their identity. Hence the mask can enable a client to project aspects of themselves usually denied or hidden: the mask unmasks.

The third relates to the way the mask encourages a projection of a focused aspect of the client's personality or experience. The selective quality of the mask – its fixed form – means that the one frame is presented, rather than the continuous moving and shifting of the natural face. The effect of this is that one aspect or facet of the client is high-lighted to the exclusion of others. This means that the client is invited to present a concentrated, heightened part of themselves.

The mask, then, encourages a concentration upon a particular aspect of the self, along with an emphasis on the expression of parts of the self usually denied expression.

Script and story

In Dramatherapy clients can use an already existing text or can create their own script to work from. These are worked with so that the client can find their own associations, meaning or interpretation. This might develop into improvisation or work on the text which further explores the association. The emphasis becomes less on the intention of the author or therapist and much more upon the themes or meanings which the client feels to be significant. Images, interactions, characters, reactions to the text can all be part of this. As detailed in Chapter 10, the text or story can take on personal meaning for a client. As Gersie has said, 'the potential for positive, projective identification between a story-character and oneself does inspire new ways of being' (Gersie, 1991, 242).

Theatrical play production includes the notion of interpretation of a text. As Esslin points out in *An Anatomy of Drama* (1978, 88), audiences are drawn to plays in part to see the particular interpretation an actor or director brings to a given text. So, in Dramatherapy, interest in projective work with a text relies on a process akin to the interpretive work undertaken by director or actor. The interest lies in the ways in which the client can use the text as material to project their inner preoccupations into, in order to use it as a means of self-exploration.

Summary

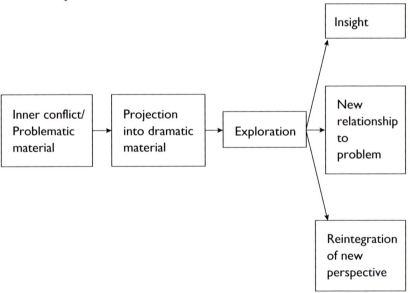

Figure 6.3 Dramatic projection in Dramatherapy

All the above areas – the creation of small worlds, mask work, improvisation, story and script – have a basic process in common.

Figure 6.3 shows the four key stages which are at the core of the way Dramatherapy relates to the process of projection. Despite the individual differences outlined above, at its simplest, dramatic projection can be described as a process which lies at the heart of all Dramatherapy. It enables the client to project inner conflicts into dramatic material and this allows the problematic area to be connected to the healing possibilities of drama. This chapter has illustrated some of the ways in which dramatic projection relates to the exploration of problematic material.

It is this process which enables the client to see and feel themselves in the drama that is created in the Dramatherapy group. Without this seeing and feeling there would be no potential for involvement or for change.

Chapter 7
The Dramatic Body

> The history of the theatre is the history of the transfiguration of the human form.
>
> Schlemmer in Gropius, *The Theatre of the Bauhaus*

Introduction

The early twentieth-century Bauhaus movement in Germany is primarily known for its work in art and architecture. However, its attempt to revolutionise culture extended to theatre in a way which provides a useful starting point from which to consider the body within drama and therapy. Oskar Schlemmer began work in the Bauhaus community as head of the scripting workshop, but he gradually transformed it into the Bauhaus 'Stage Shop', as the leader of the movement, Walter Gropius, describes it. The remains of the output of the Shop are with us in the form of writings, photographs and diagrams. The recorded images contain many of the costumes and productions of the Bauhaus, but all return to Gropius' central theatrical aim: to experience stage space through the body.

The photographs show strange creatures, part metal, part flesh, humans with limbs connected to spirals, captured by multiple exposure camera work. Gropius and Schlemmer produced a series of diagrams which attempt to illustrate the 'transformation of the body as it exists in theatrical space' (Gropius, 1979, 5). Schlemmer's acting forms depict figures from which emanate lines of power. Geometric waves emerge from the actor's chest and stomach (see Plates 7.1 and 7.2). The statue and the audience arena become a receptacle to be filled by 'the actor whose body and movements make him the player' (Gropius, 1979, 20). As the quotation at the start of this chapter states, theatre is seen by Schlemmer and Gropius as the transfiguration of the human form.

According to the Bauhaus approach the body changes when it enters dramatic space. The human figure and its expressions automatically change on stage so that 'each gesture or motion is translated in meaningful terms into a unique sphere of activity' (Gropius, 1979, 92). Even someone from the audience, if removed from their 'sphere' and placed

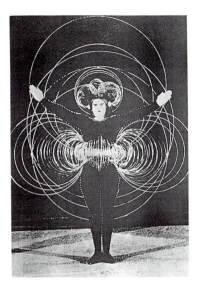

Plate 7.1 Schlemmer's body transformations in theatrical space (from Gropius, 1979), © 1961, Wesleyan University

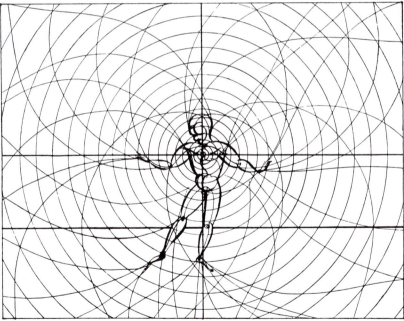

Plate 7.2 Schlemmer's body transformations in theatrical space (from Gropius, 1979), © 1961, Wesleyan University

on the stage, would be clothed in a 'magic nimbus'. The same change can happen if someone simply moves back a step in front of two or more curious spectators to act something out for them.

The building of the 'Total Theatre', which was to be the culmination of the Bauhaus ideas, was abandoned after 'Black Friday' which brought Hitler and the Nazis to power. The vision of the Total Theatre was not realised, and the ideas have never been brought to fruition. However, the Bauhaus experiments usefully introduced an approach to the body in dramatic and theatrical space which helps in the discussion of the Dramatic Body in Dramatherapy. The Bauhaus concern with the changes which occur in the body, and the way in which forces meet and emanate from the body, when someone is engaged in theatre, bring me to the key questions of this chapter: What changes occur in someone when they enter into enactment within Dramatherapy? What role does the body have within theatre, drama and Dramatherapy? What is the relationship between an individual's identity and their performing body?

The term 'Dramatic Body' refers to the body when it is involved in a theatrical or dramatic act. The Dramatic Body is a place where imagination and reality meet.

Actors' bodies express their imagination, their bodies help them to discover and express their imaginary ideas. The audience's imagination is engaged by an actor's bodily expressions through movement, sound and interaction with others. For most forms of theatre and drama, in all cultures, the body is the main means of communication. As the artist might work with brushes, paint and canvas, so the body is the chief means of theatrical expression. The actor discovers and expresses roles, ideas and relationship through face, hands, movement – the body. The audience will experience theatre primarily as these bodily expressions in the stage space.

In Dramatherapy the body of a client is of similar importance. As will be explored later, in a Dramatherapy session an individual might find their body wearing a mask, its shape disguised by cloth, represented by a painted Body Map image, covered in paint, or entering a different bodily identity through taking on the character or role of another. A disguised client, after an improvisation, summed up many of the issues concerning the body in Dramatherapy when she observed, 'It felt like me, but it wasn't me.' She felt herself to be a part of the disguise, but also recognised some kind of difference. Courtney (1983) argues that the body is important in exploration and discovery within drama.

This chapter will explore theoretical and practical issues concerning the body, identity and enactment. The Dramatic Body will be defined and its relationship to Dramatherapy practice described. In this way the chapter intends to detail the reasons why the body can be a primary focus of therapeutic change in Dramatherapy.

Background to the Dramatic Body

The body and identity: an overview

The body and its relationship to the 'self' and to society has been the focus of discussion and debate in a number of disciplines – from theology to medical science, psychoanalysis to anthropology.

Four main aspects of this debate are especially important in the consideration of the Dramatic Body in Dramatherapy:

• the relationship between the body and an individual's identity
• society's regulation of the body
• bodily expression and communication
• the role of the body in the construction of a social persona

Psychoanalysis (James, 1932; Deutsch 1947, 1952; Lowen, 1958) and object relations theory (Krenger, 1989) have suggested a relationship which connects body, emotion and identity. Rossberg-Gempton and Poole (1991) summarise the psychoanalytic approach as follows: the mind and body is seen as a functional unit. Unconscious material can be physicalised through bodily expressions that are orchestrated by the ego. They add, however, that, though bodily movements were considered to be important, 'therapeutic improvement could not be realised until the client could verbalise feelings associated with those movements and the accompanying bodily sensations' (1992, 40).

This position is echoed by some dance movement therapists. Siegal (1984) states that 'because a person lives with, in and through the body, their total being is affected by life's bodily experience'.

The self is often seen to be realised by and through the body. This is usually presented as a relationship which involves duality or tension. The Christian tradition, for example, is permeated by the individual's battle between Body and Soul (Marcuse, 1969). Freudian consideration of the body in works such as *Totem and Taboo* (1950) emphasises the tension within individuals between gratification and social regulation. Nietzsche (1967) and Walter Benjamin (1955) both point to a division in bodily expression within societies – between the Apollonian and the Dionysian. Apollonian expression emphasises the rational, discursive and analytic. Dionysian expression is characterised by rapture, sexual ecstasy and the frenzy of the body in dance. They discuss the tendency of societies to emphasise one of these modes of bodily expression at the expense of the other.

Turner (1982) reflects upon the history of this duality concluding that in Western philosophy and theory the body/self relationship is one in which the body appears simultaneously as constraint and potential (Turner, 1982, 4). The potential refers to the body as a means to express, discover and develop the self. Constraint can be understood as the ways in which the body is regulated and restrained by self and society. This constraint is often allied to a perceived set of limitations or regulations put upon the individual (Scheflen, 1972). Feminist social theory (Mitchell and Rose, 1982) and the writings of Foucault (1976), for example, point to the ways in which society constrains and uses the expressions of the body. Sexual activity, public and private expression, family, social and economic behaviour are all analysed in terms which ally suppression of the individual with suppression of bodily actions and expressions.

Within Western culture, then, the relationship between an individual's identity and their body can be characterised by a tradition of duality. In all the material described above there is a tension indicated between identity, body and society.

The body is often described as the primary means by which communication occurs between self and other. This is through gesture, expression and voice (Elam, 1991). Attention is given to the ways in which the body communicates on an unconscious as well as conscious level (Lorenz, 1966; Argyle, 1972). Douglas, in works such as *Purity and Danger* (1966), has indicated how the body communicates in a metaphoric way. The body is also seen as a surface which is used to mark identity in terms of social status, age, gender and religion through marking and clothing (Polhemus and Benthall, 1975). This approach focuses upon the body as both the key to communication and as a primary aspect of an individual arriving at a sense of identity. The body communicates the individual's identity to others. It is also seen as a means by which the individual arrives at a sense of their own identity and as an expressive medium through which society and the individual connect.

Sociologists have considered how identity is connected to the ways in which the body is presented in social space. In particular, Goffman has analysed the role of the body in the construction of a social persona (Goffman, 1972). In his work the self presents selected personae in different situations and arrives at a sense of identity through bodily expression and behaviour to others.

The Dramatic Body: key themes

Passions in space: bodily communication in drama

In theatre, character portrayal is made in part by the actor's physical expression. The signs which an audience or other actors react to is given through the body (Elam, 1991; Frost and Yarrow, 1990). As we have seen, sociologists, psychoanalysts and anthropologists treat the body as an agent of communication: 'Body movement can be regarded as a communication of the mores, customs and role relationships found in a particular culture' (Lomax, Bartenieff and Paulay, 1968). Within theatre form this process is seen to be heightened. In much drama and theatre theory the body of the actor is seen as the centre of a powerful impulse extending outwards as a heightened focus of communication (Artaud, 1958; Brook, 1968; Grotowski, 1968). Lecoq describes this process beautifully in the intensity of his performed mime:

> What we give to the public comes from within. There's a link, a reverberation between inner and outer space. If I make a physical action – pulling or pushing – it's analogous to internal emotion, love or hate . . . I indicate passions in space.
>
> (Lecoq in Frost and Yarrow, 1990, 101)

The body is given heightened permissions and qualities of communication – a simple pulling or pushing brings out inner feelings in an intensive way. I also want to note the primacy Lecoq gives to the body in the act of theatrical communication. The importance of the body as communicator in theatre can be seen in the Polish semiologist Kowzan's work. He lists thirteen sign systems involved in stage presentation (1968), of which eight concern the body: facial expression, gesture, movement of actors in dramatic space, make-up, hair, costume and two aspects of vocal presence.

As in the Bauhaus images, the body is seen as the primary means of theatrical communication: in addition, the entry into dramatic space is perceived to involve a strengthening or changing of the body's communications.

The lying truth

A constant theme within drama's relationship to the body is that of truth, deception and the paradox that truth may come from and through deception. A strong part of theatrical and dramatic form involves the hiding of an individual's identity. This is true in a wide variety of cultures from the Padstow Horse, the mudmen of Asaro, Africa (Schechner, 1988, 127), Ryszard Cieslak in *The Constant Prince* (Grotowski, 1968, 29–31), or Robert de Niro having to increase his body weight by 28lb to play Jake La Motta in *Raging Bull*. All take the physical form of an individual and transform them within the drama into a different shape or manifestation. Eyes, expression, bodily movement, posture, weight, skin scarring, cloth, make-up and mud – all are used to acknowledge physically, and to create, a dramatic identity which belies the natural state and form of the person who is acting.

Theatrical training in many cultures involves the teaching of the body to dissemble its usual movements when in dramatic mode. Examples of this include the Elizabethan dance theatre with its 800 mudras or syntactic units (64 limb movements, 9 head, 11 kinds of glance) and Indian classical theatre (Yoshihiko, 1971). I would argue that Western naturalistic acting can also be seen to be within this framework of the lying body; that the body is also disguised. The actor is taught, and expected to perform on stage, within certain systems of bodily alteration. The most obvious are costume and make-up. In addition, though, the actor is taught to dissemble through body posture, movement, facial expressions and characteristics.

The paradox here is that much theatre and drama aims to reveal truths to its audience – about life and the society it is part of (e.g. Sophocles, Shakespeare, Ibsen, Brecht, Boal). The actor often works within a framework of revealing greater truths: yet they do so by – literally – lying with their body. It is as if theatre disguises individuals in order to reveal truths. The disguised state allows the actor to have the freedom to reveal truths.

Another aspect of this paradoxical process can be seen in Grotowski's work in physical theatre (Grotowski, 1968) and in some of the Odin Theatre's current work in Scandinavia (Barba and Savarese, 1991). In Grotowski, the idea is that the body of the actor becomes a medium through which 'inner' material can emerge. The basic notion here is that the true self is hidden or disguised by the everyday uses of the body. The actors, as they are in a heightened state, can transform themselves in order for inner truths to become visible. The everyday identity of the actor is disguised in a role or dramatic presentation – in this specially disguised state the body is a vehicle for revelation and emergent truth.

As we shall see, for Dramatherapy this paradox is also present. The client, in creating bodily disguise for their everyday identity, is able to engage in personal revelation which would not usually be possible.

Constructing the Dramatic Body

Certain traditions contain a rigorous training for the body. Kathakali, for example, has numerous exercises for the eyes and face. Boys begin training for six years between the ages of 8 and 16, and their bodies are 'literally massaged and danced into shapes suited to Kathakali' (Schechner, 1988, 270). The training is seen as an important way of enabling an individual to enter into a dramatised self. Boal, in his *Poetics of the Oppressed: Experiments with the People's Theatre in Brazil* (1974) gives a rather different perspective on the relationship between self, Dramatic Body and training. He, too, speaks of the necessity of training the body, and it, too, is done within a context of control. However, he seeks to enable the spectator to become the actor, seeing it as a journey from the passive reception of a product to the state of becoming the producer of that product: 'To control the means of production, man must, first of all, control his own body, know his body, in order to be capable of making it more expressive' (Boal, 1974, 125).

Boal sees the body in drama as the key to meaning, understanding and power. The first three of Boal's four stages of transforming the spectator to actor concern training the body. He calls these 'Knowing the body', 'Making the body expressive' and 'The theatre as language' (1974, 127). By this work he aims to enable participants to become aware of their own bodies. This involves finding the possibilities for positive expression and the 'deformities' (1974, 128) which society and the individual's work imposes on the use they make of their bodies.

So, here, two aspects of the trained body in theatre and drama are highlighted. The first concerns the way training is often connected to the creation of a special theatre language and theatre identity for an individual – a separate Dramatic Body. The second is that training can alter the expressive possibilities of someone's body for performance purposes. In turn, this can lead to a greater awareness of the body for an individual.

The Dramatic Body in Dramatherapy practice

In its work with the body Dramatherapy uses a variety of approaches and techniques. These can be divided into three main areas. Each area is not totally separate from the others, but should be seen as an aid to help describe different aspects of practice in relation to the Dramatic Body.

The first area involves clients in developing the potential of their own body. The second has as its main focus the therapeutic potentials and benefits of the client taking on a different bodily identity within the

Dramatherapy. The third concerns work which explores the personal, social and political forces and influences that affect the body.

Developing the potential body

In the first area the emphasis is often upon the client inhabiting, or using, their own body more effectively. This might be the main therapeutic aim. In other situations, however, this 'inhabitation' might be preparatory work. For example, until a client can inhabit their own body they will find it difficult or impossible to develop their body's capability to represent another identity through the key processes of personification or impersonation.

Whether as preparation or as the main focus with the therapy this work usually concerns the areas listed in Box 7.1.

Box 7.1 **Main areas of concern – the potential body**

- the developmental level of the client's relationship with their body
- the range and quality of communication a client can achieve using their body within dramatic activity
- the range and quality of the client's physical relationships with others within dramatic activity

---

Presenting problems here include clients who are experiencing difficulties owning or relating to their body. This might happen, for example, after a stroke or as a result of trauma. Clients might be experiencing difficulties around the physical use of their body in terms of motor skills. Issues might concern the use of their body in everyday relationships with others. This might include, for example, people who have been in long-term hospital care who are moving into the community, and whose social skills have not had the opportunity to develop due to institutionalisation.

In general this area of Dramatherapy is appropriate for people who experience difficulties because they have not developed their body's range of relationships and possibilities. A developmental issue may be present as a problem. (For further details on developmental levels concerning the body in Dramatherapy, see Chapter 8.)

With some clients this area might remain the chief focus of the work. For example, a problem might be located in the way a client uses their body in communication. The Dramatherapy work might be to aim to enhance the individual's ability to communicate with their body.

Case study 7.1 The Potential Body

In a psychiatric hospital within a programme of rehabilitation a Dramatherapy group was operating for six individuals. The aim was to complement the group members' move into community care. The role of the Dramatherapy group was to enable people to communicate more effectively, and they had identified goals for each individual. Many of these concerned the rudiments of establishing relationships with others. Most individuals expressed anxiety about this, and many had few experiences of relating to people outside ward settings. It was inappropriate to engage directly in playing out situations in role. Assessment work had established that people were not able to communicate with their own bodies effectively, and mimetic skills were minimal.

The initial focus was upon the relationship clients had with their own bodies. Individuals seemed to express their lack of skills and their anxiety by the avoidance of eye contact and mumbling speech. Games and activities were used to encourage people to begin to relate differently to their body. One game involved swapping seats with someone by making eye contact with them. Others involved moving through different imagined substances, stretching and physical exercises which encouraged a range of bodily expressions. This progressed to activities designed to lengthen and maintain eye contact, and which developed effective posture in miming. The group developed a vocabulary of mimed emotional body positions – 'closed', 'open', 'confident', 'reticent'. Clients attempted the enactment of simple conversations. They stayed themselves, rather than taking roles, but played different emotions such as 'bored' or 'interested' in the interactions.

The group talked about the different reasons why someone might want to communicate, and what someone might try to communicate. These scenarios ranged from the need to ask for a ticket on a bus, to the need to communicate in establishing potential friendship and conversation. Discussion followed the improvisations. Individuals talked over how the enactment had felt and how effective they considered they and others had been in using their bodies. Areas such as eye contact, voice, and posture in communicating were looked at. The system outlined below was used to help structure feedback and monitor progress.

The Dramatic Body: meaning and communication analysis (Jones' adaptation of Kowzan's and Pavis' sign systems)

In this area of work five of the theatre areas described by Kowzan (Kowzan, 1968) are useful, in that they focus upon the body and communication in dramatic activity. The following system (Boxes 7.2–7.5) is an adaptation of Kowzan's classification of sign systems in the theatre and elements of the Pavis questionnaire for performance analysis (Pavis, 1985). It aims to aid group members and Dramatherapist to assess and monitor progress in the ability to create meaning and to communicate effectively with the Dramatic Body within Dramatherapy. Each criterion is assessed in terms of low, sound and high efficacy. The meaning of the terms 'high', 'sound' and 'low' are discussed with the group.

In the case of the group described above we used a combination of self, peer and therapist assessment and feedback. They decided with myself that 'high' (H) would mean that the area was highly effectively handled, 'sound' (S) meant that there were some key areas which could be improved, and that 'low' (L) indicated that the area wasn't effectively handled and would need to be looked at in some detail. A form was given out to each person after the group and therapist had agreed upon an improvisation concerning communication between two people. The results were both used as feedback and as a way of helping each client to form new goals in terms of communication.

Box 7.2 **The Dramatic Body**		Tick one box	
Facial Expression:	L	S	H
– emotional range	☐	☐	☐
– production of intended expression	☐	☐	☐
– effective reception (by others) of expression	☐	☐	☐
– effective reading of others' facial expression	☐	☐	☐
– appropriate response to another's expression	☐	☐	☐

Facial Expression (Box 7.2). The specifics of each area are selected in collaboration with clients. Each area is given a number of specific focuses. So, for example, emotional range can be allocated a series of emotions which clients feel to be important – happiness, sadness, anger, interest, encouragement. Discussion around the rest of the group reading the emotion and the intention of the client producing the expression can then develop into work which explores responding to others' expressions or feelings.

Box 7.3 **The Dramatic Body**	Tick one box		
Gesture:	L	S	H
– range of gestures or postures to express intended emotions	☐	☐	☐
– effective reception (by others) of these postures and gestures	☐	☐	☐
– effective reading of another's gesture	☐	☐	☐
– appropriate response to another's gesture or posture	☐	☐	☐

Gesture (Box 7.3). Here the group might choose to look at postures and gestures that are encouraging or welcoming, at the difference between a closed posture/gesture and an open one. Other areas might concern communicating anger, engaging someone's interest or attention, or the assertive use of gesture and posture.

Box 7.4 **The Dramatic Body**	Tick one box		
Movement in dramatic space:	L	S	H
– range of movements	☐	☐	☐
– social use of space between people	☐	☐	☐
– use of space as intended	☐	☐	☐
– recognition of others' movements	☐	☐	☐
– recognition of others' use of space	☐	☐	☐

Movement (Box 7.4). In this the group looks at walking, approaching someone to engage with them, avoiding contact with someone. In terms of social space, exploration might concern areas such as distance and proximity when engaging in conversation, or movement in space with strangers as compared to with friends.

Box 7.5 **The Dramatic Body**	Tick one box		
Voice (words and tone):	L	S	H
– range of vocal expression	□	□	□
– communicative effectiveness	□	□	□
– accurate reading of others' vocal communication	□	□	□
– appropriate vocal responses	□	□	□

Voice (Box 7.5). The group explores different feelings and contexts in terms of the way the voice is used. Areas such as public and private, shouting and whispering, the relationship of speaker to the receiver (e.g. friend, stranger) can be explored. The effectiveness in terms of whether the voice could be heard, whether it was too loud for the situation, is established. This can develop into the group trying to read people's feelings through their voice and to consider the way to handle spoken responses.

Summary: the potential body
In this way of working, then, the Dramatic Body is being used to effect change in the way someone relates to their body in everyday life. The Dramatherapy space and dramatic activity allows the individual to discover potentials and ways of using their body. The drama activities can also have a training aspect, as the improvisation helps new skills in voice or in gesture to develop. Through dramatic projection clients become personally involved in the impersonations or personifications they create. The client can develop a new relationship to their body and to the way they relate to other people through their body. The client's Dramatic Body is given different permissions than their everyday body. The client's relationship to their own body is transformed by the enactment in Dramatherapy. Through the life–drama connection the work in the Dramatherapy group can affect the client's life. The client can begin to assimilate aspects of the new relationship they are making with their body in Dramatherapy into their everyday life.

Body transformation

Body transformation in Dramatherapy refers to an aspect of the adoption through a dramatic act of a change or alteration in identity. This adoption is shown to others and experienced by the client through their body, through embodiment. The client may take on a different character through impersonation, or may alter their usual identity in some way. This may involve the use of the body to represent a thing or quality – the client's body might depict water moving, or personify 'temptation', for example.

Prerequisites for body transformation

To achieve transformation into another persona in Dramatherapy, it is necessary to have a certain level of skill and capability. It is necessary for the client to be able to inhabit their own body sufficiently to be able to take on another identity. This means that they must be able to recognise body parts as their own and to identify their body as a whole as themselves. The client also needs to be able to move in and out of playing someone or something else without confusion or distress. In addition the individual must be developmentally able to take on a character, different identity or different characteristics (see Chapter 8). Before attempting any work which involves transforming the body, it is important to establish the above capabilities.

Preparation

One aspect of this work involves looking at and developing the client's mimetic body skills. These are summarised in Box 7.6.

Box 7.6 **Mimetic skills checklist**   Tick appropriate boxes

Can the client:	A	B	C
• mime imaginary objects?	☐	☐	☐
• mime physical activities? (e.g. climbing, eating)	☐	☐	☐
• mime sensations? (e.g. feeling cold, hot)	☐	☐	☐
• mime emotions? (e.g. feeling sad, happy)	☐	☐	☐
• mime more abstract qualities or phenomena? (e.g. darkness falling or electricity)	☐	☐	☐

A = Yes   B = Some evidence   C = No

These skills need to be developed in solitary activity as well as in improvisation with others, with attention being paid to the client's capability in communicating the mime and understanding others' mimetic communications.

In addition, it is necessary to establish the client's relationship with movement in portraying a different identity. This includes their capability in creating a movement vocabulary and repertoire in relation to depicting the way others move: walking, sitting, expressing feeling. The use of movement which is not naturalistic needs to be established: fine and gross motor capabilities, abstract movements, movements from particular cultural styles.

The client's vocal range will also need to be considered in terms of the way they use their voice. Can they explore different ways of producing sound, projecting the voice, reproducing speech patterns, rhythms or words of others/reported speech?

It is important to establish whether the client can combine these skills into the coherent portrayal of another identity and whether they can improvise with others whilst portraying a different identity.

The body transformed
The transformation of the body into being able to take on other qualities, or those of other personae, can be used in Dramatherapy in a number of ways.

By taking on other personae through impersonation or personification, permissions concerning the client's relationship with their body can occur. The distance achieved by taking on a different identity can enable them to experiment with alternative ways of using their body. The experience of being in character can also allow the client to discover things or allow access to repressed issues.

Case study 7.2 The Body Transformed – Climbing a Mountain

In a special school for adolescents with emotional and behavioural difficulties we were exploring the way people related to each other. The general physical language of the group towards each other was of aggression and violence. This reflected the way they dealt with relationships outside the group. Through adopting different personae in an improvisation about climbing a mountain, themes such as responsibility, care, lack of care were dealt with. Individuals took it in turns to play different physical roles such as 'leader', 'irresponsible clown', 'trouble-maker', 'dependable'.

By alternating roles each member was able to play different physical characteristics. This enabled individuals to widen their repertoire of body language in relationships. Physical aggression was contained in certain role characteristics whilst others permitted individuals to express different ways of relating to each other. The roles gave permission for this type of bodily behaviour to be experienced in the group.

Case study 7.3 The Body Transformed – Falling Backwards

During an improvisation a client chose the character of someone who was severely debilitated, who constantly fell backwards, and whose body had to be continually 'rescued' by the group in that it had to be carried, bandaged, cared for. She said that she had not deliberately chosen the bodily characteristics, but that they 'came from nowhere'. During the improvisation, and in reflection afterwards, she became distressed as the improvisation had enabled her to contact two important aspects of herself which, she felt, were present in her life but unacknowledged by her. The first was that the character had taken on many bodily aspects of her mother. The second was that she realised how familiar the feeling of having her mother present within her own body was. This was accompanied by the realisation that, like her mother, she herself used her body to manipulate and control people in her life.

In speaking about the character afterwards she said that she wished to own her own body more thoroughly. This insight proved a starting point for further work where we explored her body through character improvisations. The example shows how the taking on of a physically different identity in a transformation can help the client to gain insight into the relationship between their own body and identity.

Summary: the body transformed

The importance of the shift which can occur when the client enters into their Dramatic Body was noted earlier (see p. 155) as being important in Dramatherapy. In this work the shift is the main focus of the therapeutic work.

It is important that the moving into and out of dramatic space and the dramatic body is marked. Through dramatic projection the client has invested the impersonation with a high degree of emotional charge.

De-roling from characters or creations is important in order for the client to re-inhabit their own body and to consider the relationship between the 'two bodies'. From this point integration of elements of the Dramatic Body into the client's usual body (the life–drama connection) can occur.

The work might be completed in the re-learning of the way the body can be used. Alternatively, this might be the springboard to look more deeply at how this situation has arisen and to look at the client's experience of their body in a more exploratory way.

Bodily memory and the two bodies

Within Dramatherapy the client can explore the relationship with their body in terms of the problematic memories and experiences with which their physical self connects. On occasion a particular exercise can evoke a particular strong or difficult feeling or response. This might be to do with an experience which occurs in the present for the client or it may be one which is rooted in the past or a combination of contemporary and historic issues. Social and political forces at work in the client's experience of their body might also be important to consider.

This might be worked with in a number of ways – the basic task in this area of work is to find the appropriate dramatic vehicle which enables the client to explore their experience of their body.

The work of the group might concern people's relationships with their bodies in terms of body image. The focus would be upon the exploration of the forces which have shaped the problem. The aim would be to enable the client to achieve a different relationship with their bodily selves through the dramatic work.

This kind of work is often undertaken with people who have body related problems such as eating disorders, or those who are experiencing physical symptoms which might be linked to emotional trauma or difficulties.

Case study 7.4 Body Map

A client had drawn a life-size representation of their body. Within this they had drawn a map, consisting of painted textures or images to represent aspects of their body. For example, the stomach was painted as a forest, the hands as bright red. She then dramatically explored the map, personifying different aspects by touching the part and speaking as if she were the red hands, the forest. This developed into the different parts communicating with each other. The work explored elements of her relationship with her body image.

The created image acted as a script and as a way of physicalising abstract, often unconscious, feelings and aspects of her experience of her body. The change enabled by the creation of this dramatic body map enabled the client to explore her relationship to this dramatic image and enactment. It created a perspective, the changed experience of painting and enacting the body enabled a new set of perceptions to occur. Much of the work of the Dramatherapy here was upon reintegrating the enacted body with the client's actual body and self.

This example illustrates how important it is in Dramatherapy to consider the point made earlier (see p. 156) – that the client must feel able to identify and inhabit their body. If this were not the case then work such as this could result in the individual feeling dislocated or dissociated from their body. It also highlights the importance of reintegrating the enactment with the individual at the end of the session. If this does not happen then the client is not offered the opportunity to return to their own body and self and to relate to the dramatic creation.

Summary

The body is the main tool of communication and expression in drama and in Dramatherapy. It is the chief means through which individuals express themselves – and make contact with others.

The use of the Dramatic Body in Dramatherapy is typified by a series of changes:

- The physical body of an individual essentially stays the same when in and out of dramatic mode. However, when an individual enters into a dramatic act or space, a change in the way the *individual experiences* their body and the relationship between their *body and identity* can occur.

- The change involves a *shift in behaviour* and *relationship* to body, self and others, due to the kinds of rules and boundaries within a drama space. These rules usually differ from those in reality outside the drama.

- The client is perceived to be in a *heightened* or *special state*. This involves an alteration of perception, a change of focus and responses, the sharpening of senses.

- The sense of identity of an individual can be *altered* by physically changing appearance and body language in dramatic activity.

- The *way others perceive and relate* to the individual's body and identity can alter. This is the case whether people are engaged directly with the individual in the drama, or indirectly, as audience members.

- This change involves *transformation* due to a different language of gesture and expression being used. This language is due to training and theatrical traditions and can involve impersonation and personification within Dramatherapy.

- As an individual's body becomes involved in dramatic acts it can lead to an *increased awareness of the body's range and potential.*

- By involving their body in drama an individual can become more *self-aware* in terms of being able to look at their own body, their relationship with it, and the social or personal forces affecting it.

For the Dramatherapist it is important to acknowledge not only what the body can do in terms of performance possibilities, but what occurs to the individual's identity in relation to their body whilst engaged in enactment within Dramatherapy.

The Dramatic Body as defined above seeks to describe the relationship between an individual and their body within drama. Three main ways of working have been described in this chapter: one involves developing the 'potential body' of the client through enactment in Dramatherapy, a second involves transforming the body through dramatic forms, the third concerns the way in which Dramatherapy can evoke and work with memories linked to the body.

Chapter 8
Play and playing

What the child likes most is the theatre, that is to say, the transformation of actuality as given from without, into something that he himself creates.

Evreinov, *The Theatre in Life*

Introduction

Play is a close relative to drama and is a source for both content and process within Dramatherapy.

Evreinov speaks of this close relationship between play and drama in his discussion of the Soviet Malachie-Mirovich's work on the educational value of toys: 'All children have the ability to create a new reality out of the facts of life' (1927, 36). The child plays naturally, without instruction, creating their 'own theatre', proving that 'nature herself has planted in the human being a sort of "will to theatre"' (1927, 36).

It is interesting to note how many key figures within the development of Dramatherapy began their initial thinking and work in the areas of play and dramatic playing with children. From Moreno's work with children in Viennese parks in 1908 to Slade's work with Child Drama and initial use of the term 'Dramatherapy', the inspiration for the use of drama as therapy has been found in play. Play has a great deal of relevance to the therapeutic use of drama. Blatner has spoken of the 'common basis of drama, psychodrama and the play of children' (Blatner and Blatner, 1988a, 51).

For the Dramatherapist and for the client in Dramatherapy play is a part of the expressive range which can be drawn on in creating meaning, exploring difficulties and achieving therapeutic change. Crucial to this relationship is the way in which the client finds meaning in play processes.

Play has been seen to have a healing quality. In Dramatherapy individuals and groups can reflect upon and deal with encountered problems by playing.

Case study 8.1 The Falling Man

One of the best studies of this phenomenon was made by Brown, Curry and Tittnich (1971). They described how a group of school-children witnessed an accident – a man, working on lights, fell twenty feet and was killed. The incident occurred only a few feet away from where a dozen children were playing. Their teachers recorded the play of the children, aged between three and six, for a number of months after the incident, and studied the play and the children's feelings.

They found that for months afterwards the children's play reflected the incident. Children played falling and jumping, referring to falling on their head, asking questions such as 'Where's the body? We have to go to hospital and take the body', giving instructions such as 'Fall like that man' (1971, 29). In their play they used details of the accident such as bleeding eyes, nose and mouth, wearing hard hats and hospitals. A variety of dangerous situations concerning falling and death were created – for example, a cat was shot dead and fell out of a tree; a group of boys played out an incident repeatedly for many months in which one of them fell and died, was taken to hospital and examined with stethoscopes.

The staff described the play as being a way for the children to accom-modate the experience, to deal with the stress and shock, to adjust to and accept the death they had witnessed and the fears it caused in them. The play is a natural way of exploring and resolving the experience. Simply to talk about the experience would not have allowed the depth of participation and the working through of feelings and fantasies in enactment.

Dramatherapy utilises this natural process of play as a means of dealing with trauma or life problems. However play relates to Dramatherapy in three particular ways.

- The first concerns the way in which *playfulness* and the general process of playing can be the vehicle of therapeutic change within Dramatherapy.
- The second relates specifically to the notion of *developmental play* and drama. Here both are seen as parts of a continuum of different devel-opmental stages. The continuum relates both to assessment and to the way change occurs for clients in Dramatherapy.

• The third focuses upon *content*. Play involves particular areas of content and has a particular way of articulating that content. For example, in many cultures play usually involves certain subjects, certain recognised forms of expression, along with rules regarding that expression. Play also has a special relationship with reality. In Dramatherapy this content, form and relationship with reality become particular ways for the client to express and explore experiences.

What is play?

A twentieth-century perspective

Huizinga defines play as a free activity standing consciously outside 'ordinary' life, as being 'not serious' but at the same time absorbing the player intensely and utterly. In his often quoted phrase, play 'is an activity connected with no material interest and no profit can be gained by it. It proceeds within its own proper boundaries of time and space according to fixed rules and in an orderly manner' (Huizinga, 1955, 13). Since his seminal work, *Homo Ludens* (1955), debate and research have pointed to evidence which suggests contrary interpretations of playing. Indeed Dramatherapy has an ambiguous relationship with Huizinga's way of framing and defining play. Whilst, as this chapter will show, the qualities which Huizinga describes as 'absorption', the notion of discrete boundaries of time and place, and the standing outside of ordinary life are all highly relevant to Dramatherapy's connections with play, the notion of no profit, no material interest and the implication of a distance and irrelevance to ordinary life must be called into doubt if play is utilised within a Dramatherapy framework.

In the twentieth century our understanding of play has shifted. A number of different fields have re-examined play – from biology, psychology and psychotherapy to anthropology, from economists and large marketing companies to educationalists. This has resulted in new approaches to describing and defining play. These changes have provided insight into the way play relates to psychological and emotional development, to learning and to creativity. This reframing of aspects of play is relevant to the way it has come to be used in Dramatherapy.

Psychoanalytic theory's impact upon play has been considerable. Its emphasis is upon play as a way of mastering and dealing with traumatic experiences and in its influence upon individuals' psychological maturation and development. This approach has been developed by Klein (1961), Winnicott (1953, 1974), Axline (1964) and Erikson (1963).

For example, as described in Chapter 6, Klein used spontaneous play as a substitute for verbal free association. She included miniature toys in projective play within the psychoanalysis of children. Erikson's work concerned the way in which psychosexual conflicts of children are reflected in their play with toys (1963, 80). Neubauer encapsulates the central concerns of this way of approaching play in his definition. Play is an expression of wishes and fantasies; 'it is an enactment of these wishes in search of fulfilment; and it is an awareness of its own unreality' (Neubauer, 1987, 8).

Especially important to Dramatherapy are Winnicott's notions of transitional objects and phenomena and the consideration of potential space in relation to play (Winnicott 1953, 1966). The area of play and objects are seen to be the origin of creativity by him:

> The baby begins to live creatively and to use actual objects to be creative into. If the baby is not given this chance then there is no area in which the baby may have play or may have cultural experience.
>
> (1966, 371)

Play began to be analysed as a factor in intellectual development. It was seen to reflect and contribute to the maturation of a child's thought processes. Piaget (1962), a key advocate of this view, outlines a series of cognitive stages linked to types of play and a child's age. These are summarised in Box 8.1.

Box 8.1 **Piaget – play as a series of cognitive stages**

sensorimotor (practice play) – 0–2 years
preoperational (symbolic play) – 2–7 years
concrete operational (games with rules) – 7–11 years.

He stresses play's role in children's assimilation of information and the accommodation of their experiences of the world.

Other areas of the analysis of play have included analysis of its role in social development by Parten (1932), Erikson (1965) and Howes (1980), and as practice for adult life (Groos, 1901).

Play has also been re-examined within the field of education. In the United States John Dewey emphasised 'learning by doing' and Winifred Ward in 1930 published her influential *Creative Dramatics*. This way of seeing play was linked to the child-centred learning theories of Rousseau, Froebel and Pestalozzi. They redescribed play as a way of encountering and learning about experience rather than as a recreational or marginal activity.

In England practitioners such as Slade, Way, Heathcote and Bolton linked play and drama, emphasising the importance of the educational value of dramatic play and of process rather than of creating a product such as a performance. The role of playing in developing reading, writing and language development has been demonstrated (Garvey, 1974; Pellegrini, 1980) For educationalists play is a way of learning about, testing and making sense of the world, exploring the self and its relationship to the environment.

Within many of these new approaches play is often defined as a series of different stages which develop in psychological and creative complexity. A number of different models exist and an important area for Dramatherapy within these developmental descriptions is the relationship between drama and play. Play is seen both as an area in its own right and as an early form of drama – at one end of a continuum of complexity (Courtney, 1981; Smilansky, 1968). In this way play develops many of the functions and capabilities which are present in drama. It is often divided up into a developmental sequence of sensorimotor play, symbolic play, dramatic play and drama.

Box 8.2 encapsulates the concerns of the key aspects of this new framework.

Box 8.2 **Dramatherapy – important play areas**

• play as a way of learning about and exploring reality
• play as a special state with particular relationships to time, space and everyday rules and boundaries
• play having a symbolic relationship in relation to an individual's life experiences
• play as a means of dealing with difficult or traumatic experiences
• play's relationship to an individual's cognitive, social and emotional development
• play's connection to drama as part of a developmental continuum

Meaning and play

Case study 8.2 Girls' Play in Silwa

A study of Egyptian children in Silwa describes how girls often engage in play representations of adult women's activities and ceremonies. The play involves making straw figures, bedecked in bits of cloth as men and women and children, and with the help of stones, building a house. All the details of an event or ritual 'are played out in a make-believe way, thus marriage, circumcision, cooking and social meetings are all imitated' (Ammar, 1954, 119).

This process can be described as the child playing out events they have witnessed in order to master and learn how to come to terms with them. The child's experience is seen as an essential part of assimilating and accommodating reality – what things *mean* to the child.

Shaw describes a key connection between play, the development of intelligence and the creation of meaning. The kind of experience described above is grounded in a form of 'symbolic transformation' of 'experiential data (overt enactment of the "as if")' (Shaw, 1981, 72) which she says is essential to the development of human intelligence and is a fundamental way by which the child makes and finds meanings in the world they encounter.

A similar position is taken by Bolton. Early play is typified by an individual finding meaning in the world about them in solitary or parallel play. Bolton describes the development of more complex forms of play into drama as focusing around a shift concerning the *communication* of discovery and the mutual finding of meaning. In dramatic play the child does not only involve themselves in a solitary discovery but in a mutual one which involves the sharing of meaning discovered through an enactment. Bolton stresses the importance of interaction and acknowledgement of meaning in dramatic play, indicating a self-consciousness and desire to articulate. There must be 'some significance related to the concrete action that all participants can share' (Bolton, 1981, 185).

Blatner and Blatner also emphasise the meaning-finding process in play and drama. From a psychodramatic viewpoint they equate the notion of play activity as an arena to sort, solve and resolve, with the space later taken by drama. The dramatic mode is seen as an adult equivalent of child's play. Play is marked by the child's struggle with understanding and emotionally apprehending the world, a clarification of problems and testing of new approaches. Blatner and Blatner describe make-believe play as an arena in which children test out their experiences and abilities. They go on to say that 'in adulthood this becomes the activity of drama' (1988a, 50). The aspect of play whereby a child reproduces experiences of reality symbolically, mentioned by Shaw and Bolton, is developed by Blatner and Blatner in terms of its potentials for healing and therapy: 'Drama is a more mature extension of the natural phenomenon of play, and this capacity for symbolic manipulation of experience is . . . important . . . in psychosocial healing' (1988a, 75).

Winnicott describes play as an area of 'potential space', essential for the infant to establish relationships between the inner world and outer experience: 'play is, in fact, neither a matter of inner psychic reality nor a matter of external reality' (Winnicott, 1966, 368). This space is one in which a negotiation between personal identity and surrounding world takes place in terms of meaning and relationship.

This creation of a special state which has a symbolic framing relationship with reality is part of the way the client finds meaning in Dramatherapy. The areas of communication, the manipulation, mastery and coming to terms with reality and the notion of testing and assimilating which typifies the state of playing are all relevant to the way play manifests itself in therapy. The following example illustrates these aspects of play in a therapy context.

Case study 8.3 The Bear and the Fox

Loewald, in 'Therapeutic Play in Space and Time' (1987), describes how a client, Paul, in his fifth therapy session, takes a bear hand puppet and gives her a fox puppet. The bear bites and kills the fox. The bear puppet continues to kill for a number of weeks: 'At each session he was the invincible and evil minded bear . . . the persons I was assigned to were always hunted and killed' (1987, 182). Eventually the bear allows some of the other puppets to survive 'just so there would *be* a next time' (1987, 183). Loewald understands this to indicate Paul's working through the 'mutual anger' (1987, 186) of his relationship with his mother. The bear is seen as part-Paul, part-mother – the play expressing at the same time both anger and fear of anger. Paul develops a routine at home with a stuffed animal called 'Foxy'. Paul warns that the animal can still be be 'nice and nasty' but his mother is asked by him to feed it, talk to it and tuck both himself and Foxy into bed. This is described by his mother as a significant change, the 'most intimacy Paul has allowed . . . for a long time' (1987, 186).

In part this case could be understood to demonstrate Paul playing out of his fears of his own and his mother's anger. The bear's destructiveness might be interpreted as anxiety over fears of being overwhelmed by anger, of annihilation. The fox and the bear puppets are used in the therapy to express and master the fear. Paul discovers and allows the possibility of survival – some of the puppets live, there will be a 'next time'. This is followed by a *rapprochement* as Loewald calls it: Paul transfers the fox puppet used in the therapy to a stuffed 'Foxy' in his real life. The link between the discovery that relationships other than one involving anger can be had with the bear might be said to be connected with the way Paul uses the stuffed animal to negotiate a shift in his relationship with his mother.

Here is an example, then, of the creation of the special state of play in therapy. Paul creates a symbolic framing relationship with aspects of his life which are problematic. He uses the playing within the sessions to parallel and manipulate elements of his life and to come to terms with his and his mother's anger. In a sense the playing enables him to master his feelings and to test out a new way of dealing with his feelings and his mother. Eventually he is able to test this in reality.

'The Bear and the Fox' supports Blatner's suggestions that play helps children to find meaning, to understand and emotionally apprehend what is happening to them.

The creation of meaning in play is crucial to all three areas of Dramatherapy identified at the start of this chapter: to playfulness and the general process of playing, the developmental framework and play content. The main aspects of meaning-finding through play illustrated by Paul's work with the bear and the fox puppets and relevant to these three areas are:

- the symbolic transformation of experience
- finding meaning in the world
- sorting, solving and resolving
- mastering and learning
- negotiating a relationship between inner and outer reality

Cultural factors in play

Cultural and socio-economic factors relating to play are important for the Dramatherapist to consider. A degree of research has been undertaken into the different cultural forms, processes and societal significances given to play, similarly into the different ways children and adults relate to play given their social and economic position (Sutton-Smith, 1972, 8).

The conclusions drawn from the research vary widely. Some researchers have explored cultural and socio-economic differences according to notions of 'deficit'. This considers the ways in which specific processes such as dramatic play or play with objects are inhibited within certain cultures or within socio-economic status. For example, children in some cultures are considered as an 'economic asset' and participate in work which depletes playing. Adult attitudes in actively preventing children from playing are considered in some studies such as Levine and Levine's exploration of Gusii childhood in Kenya (Levine and Levine, 1963, 9). In other cultures play is described as being essentially absent (Ebbek, 1973).

The methodological approach of some of these studies has, however, been questioned. Fein, Stork and McLoyd have criticised the stance taken by researchers as inadequate: 'If lower-class pre-schoolers and children from non-Western societies have not been observed to engage in rich fantasy play, it is only because we have not used the right methods or techniques to discern their play' (Johnson, Christie, Yawkey, 1987, 145). They advocate a research orientated towards considering difference rather than deficit and cite more recent studies such as 'An Examination of Afro-American Speech Play in Integrated Schools' or, in 1986, The Anthropological Association for the Study of Play's, 'Play in the Desert and Play in the Town in Bedouin Arab Children'.

For the Dramatherapist it is crucial to contextualise play within cultural difference. The use of dolls, objects, space, relationship differs between cultures. Feitelson (1977) has discussed the different roles of toys and objects in some Middle Eastern and African societies and in North African and European immigrants in Jerusalem. A child originating in a home or culture where objects do not have a primary role in playing will need to be worked with in a different way to one who does not come from such a background.

Play and Dramatherapy

Play in Dramatherapy refers to processes which involve both children and adults. Playing has a part in all Dramatherapy work in that it is usual to involve clients in forms of playing as part of the Dramatherapy. This occurs on a *practical* level in that many warm ups involve forms of playing – such as games. The Dramatherapy work might use play activities and processes as a mode of therapeutic intervention. It also occurs on a *conceptual* level: Dramatherapy can be said to involve clients in a playful relationship with themselves, other group members and reality.

However, it can be argued that play in Dramatherapy is clearly not the play which a child engages with in the spontaneous circumstances of natural play within their usual environment. In Dramatherapy aspects of our understanding of the way play functions are separated and emphasised. The notion that a natural play state is totally re-created within Dramatherapy is an incorrect assumption. Play within Dramatherapy occurs within specific boundaries and frameworks which differ from those in which the child will usually play. The condition aimed for is related to, but different from, a child's usual play. This chapter aims to identify this difference, to describe how Dramatherapy connects with and uses play and play processes, and to examine technique in this area of practice.

Overview: key concepts

The area of play has come to have considerable influence within Dramatherapy, both in terms of the understanding of the general processes at work and in the development of specific methods linked to playing. The following discusses key conceptual areas in the relationship between play and Dramatherapy: playing and playfulness, play content and the 'play shift' and developmental issues.

Playing and playfulness

In Dramatherapy the creation of access to 'playfulness' is often central to the therapeutic work. Access to playing can form a way of engaging in spontaneity, it can form a route to becoming creative. This process can be seen as therapeutic in itself. This access can form the main aim of the therapy, in that the creation of spontaneity can be therapeutic. Playfulness in Dramatherapy can enable the client to engage with self, others and life in a spontaneous way. This allows the group or individual to engage creatively and playfully with problematic material where before they have been only able to be stuck and uncreative in response to problems.

Play content and the 'play shift'

For children and adult clients play is important as an area of content and in discovering meaning within Dramatherapy work. Play is characterised by specific activities and by particular kinds of relationships between individuals and the way they deal with the world around them. These activities and relationships form one key area of the way play features in Dramatherapy.

In 'Play Behaviour in Higher Primates: A Review' (1969) Loizos tries to define the function of play within primate play. She says that it is a 'behaviour' which borrows or adopts patterns that appear in other contexts. In their usual place these patterns appear to have immediate and obvious ends or goals. She states that,

> When these patterns appear in play they seem to be divorced from their original motivation and are qualitatively distinct from the same patterns appearing in their originally motivated contexts.
>
> (Loizos, 1969, 228–229)

Here, then, emphasis is placed upon a shift in meaning – a *'play shift'*. Whilst many of the forms or structures of real life are retained in playing, the intention is different. Piaget (1962) has said that in play the individual's interest is transferred from the goal to the activity itself – to enjoyment of the pleasure of play itself.

David Read Johnson has allied the play space with the Dramatherapy group. Both are 'an interpersonal field in an imaginary realm, consciously set off from the real world by the participants' (Read Johnson in Schattner and Courtney, 1981, 21). Schechner echoes this, paralleling the workshop experience with play. He says that the workshop is a way of playing around with reality, a means of examining behaviour by 're-ordering, exaggerating, fragmenting, recombining, and adumbrating it'. The workshop is a protected time and space where 'intergroup relationships may thrive without being threatened by intergroup aggression' (1988, 103–104).

In Dramatherapy this paralleling of reality within a playing state is important. The notion of a 'play shift' is the fulcrum of Dramatherapy's use of play. In play, as described by Loizos and Piaget, elements of real life are retained but they are subjected to different motivations – enjoyment, exploration, assimilation. The play shift involves reality being taken into the play space and treated in a way that encourages experimentation and digestion.

In Dramatherapy the mode of play is used to enable a further development of this 'play shift'. This process is directed towards intentional change.

Developmental approach

As described above, the twentieth century has seen a great deal of study into the developmental processes which are marked by play and which are aided by play processes. These concern the cognitive and psychological development of an individual. The psychological, cognitive and emotional developments which are enabled by play (or which accompany playing) form the third area of importance of play's relation to Dramatherapy.

Play is seen as the precursor to the development of drama. As figures 8.1–5 and Tables 8.1 and 8.2 indicate, a clear connection can be made between activities described as 'play' and 'drama'. They form a continuum of increasing complexity and richness of meaning. The Dramatherapist works with a dramatic continuum. The detail and processes involved in this continuum are important for the Dramatherapist to understand and utilise in their work. This chapter will describe the notion of dramatic development and its main uses in Dramatherapy.

Dramatherapy practice and play

The general process of play as a vehicle in Dramatherapy

At the start of any work in Dramatherapy it is important to discover the play language of the group. This involves seeing whether a group plays or not. If it does, how does the playing occur? If it does not, how does the absence of play manifest itself? From a diagnostic perspective, the issues which are presenting as problems may be manifested through play language.

This is followed by the consideration of whether play processes can be utilised as part of the therapeutic work to be undertaken.

The next aspect involves the position of play within the therapeutic work. This usually involves either the introduction of play processes and languages or the group's spontaneous use of play and playing.

This approach can be codified as a series of stages, which are summarised in Box 8.3.

Box 8.3 **Dramatherapy guide – discovering play language**

- Learning the language of play within a group. What is happening here and now?

- What is not happening or has not happened in terms of play? Are there elements of play content or process not occurring or seemingly unavailable to this group?

- In what ways can the play language be of therapeutic use to this group? (a) Are there ways in which playing can be therapeutically effective for the group?

(b) Can the developmental aspects of play/elements of play missing in the group be involved in the therapeutic work?
(c) Can the client use play as a way of communicating and exploring the problems they are encountering?

• How can the Dramatherapist create the conditions for effective play processes to be created within the Dramatherapy setting?

• How can the assessments concerning play connect with the aims of the Dramatherapy group and developing a potential play space and play activities within the Dramatherapy group.

• How can connections between the actual play within the Dramatherapy session with the client's life outside the play.

The above outlines the ways in which the general process of play features within Dramatherapy's efficacy. As described, there are specific areas of play and play process which are pertinent to Dramatherapy.

Play content in Dramatherapy

Landy gives play as one of the key areas of the 'media of the dramatic arts' (1986, 52) which inform the practice of Dramatherapy. He includes child play, especially dramatic play and the ability to play as an adult (1986, 56). Activities which are used within Dramatherapy include:

• sensorimotor/body play
• imitation activities
• play with objects
• play with symbolic toys
• projective work with toys in the creation of small worlds
• rough and tumble play
• make-believe play involving taking on characters
• games

Dramatherapy tends to echo Peter Slade's approach in seeing play as a beginning and as a part of dramatic activity (Slade, 1954). In some work the activity is mainly focused in play activities, in others there can be a mixture of play and more developed dramatic activities such as role play.

The use of play space in Dramatherapy

Creation of play worlds

In Dramatherapy one of the important aspects of play is the notion that entry into play means an entry into a specific 'special' state and space. Most authors dealing with play concern themselves with this phenomenon, though stressing different aspects.

Feitelson and Landau (1976) have commented upon cultural differences regarding play space, writing about Kurdish immigrants in Israel. Authors such as Cohen (1969) and Ammar (1954) have also considered cross-cultural issues in the use and creation of spaces to play in. Sutton-Smith (1979) notes that cultural attitudes to play space differ, and that this affects the way space is used in play. Some cultures discourage play and adults are observed to actively disrupt the play space; in others, social patterns concerning work mean that children are involved in work from an early age (Levine and Levine, 1963). Sutton-Smith (1979) has argued that in such cultures physical space and time to play is minimised, 'The adults know what must be done to survive and they cannot afford the wasted time of child play' (Sutton-Smith, 1979, 6). However, this view is challenged by Schwartzman (1978, 192) who, in referring to a variety of cross-cultural studies of play, says that in virtually all cases where children contribute to the economy they devise ways to combine playing and work.

Play work in Dramatherapy echoes Griffing's four areas of preparation for activity. Griffing (1983) considers that in preparing for play an adult needs to provide four things: (i) time, (ii) safe space, (iii) appropriate materials, and (iv) preparatory experiences. Singer (1973) has said that physical space and privacy are prerequisites for imaginative play skills to develop. Some theorists say that children must have an 'as if' stance towards reality modelled or encouraged (Singer, 1973; Smilansky, 1968).

In a therapy situation the qualities of play can be produced, but though there are similarities there are also differences which are crucial to understanding the shift. Within Dramatherapy play processes are part of a deliberate therapeutic programme for working with the client. In addition an adult therapist will constantly be present within the play area.

The Dramatherapy session will produce the conditions necessary for play to occur. Much of the content will be identical in form and structure. However, they will occur and be contained within a therapeutic framework.

Stage one of the shift is the reproduction in play form of activities from or related to reality, which are played in a special time and place.

The activities do not have the same context – they are out of their usual framework.

Stage two in Dramatherapy involves the re-orientating of this activity within a framework which hopes to both keep the qualities of play and enable it to have new goals. These goals are to offer personal therapeutic change for the client.

When play occurs in therapy there are both similarities and differences with play outside of the therapeutic context. The similarities are that the session will produce the conditions necessary for play to occur mentioned by Griffing (1983), and that much of the content will be identical in form or structure. However, the form, structures and content of play are given a particular purpose. The use of play within Drama-therapy marks a formal shift, where play processes are part of a deliberate therapeutic programme for working with the client. An additional difference is that the Dramatherapist will constantly be present within the play area.

The following two case studies illustrate these aspects of the creation of the play world within therapy.

Case study 8.4 Jane

Cattanach describes how a client, Jane, who had been physically abused, creates a play space within the therapy. At first the time and space is tested by the client until security and boundaries are estab-lished. Initially she scrabbles with the toys, tests the space for safety. Cattanach reflects on the child's early experiences as 'Would I come again, when was a week later, why couldn't she control me and make me stay? Could she really trust me to come again with the toys? Of course not all adults tell lies' (Cattanach, 1992, 94).

It is easy to see here a number of the aspects of the 'play space' described above in action. Griffing's (1983) areas of time, space and materials are being set up and tested. The therapist's providing and holding of these areas, along with the client's scrabbling with the toy materials, might be seen to be part of the preparatory experiences. Jane's first session is 'chaotic'; at the close of the session she cries and screams (Cattanach, 1992, 94). This response continues. Cattanach reflects upon this: 'She was angry and refused to stop playing. Again I was firm and we kept the rules' (95). The therapist here is modelling the use of the special place by preserving its integrity. The preservation of the play space is described by Bixler as setting limits in which the client should not destroy property other than the play equipment, to attack the therapist, to stay beyond the time limit, to remove toys or equipment, or to throw them out of the room (Bixler, 1949, 1–11). Cattanach's work echoes these limit settings. After this initial creation and testing of the space Jane goes on to use family dolls to re-play experiences such as being repeatedly pushed into scalding water, achieving, according to Cattanach, a 'discharge anger and distress about her abuse' (1992, 95).

Case study 8.5 Paper and Objects

The Dramatherapy group took place in a community centre and had advertised for members. There were eight adults in the group, which had been meeting for seven weeks out of a total of twenty. Participants were invited to take a number of objects and play with them, noticing themes as they emerged and following wherever they wanted to. People could play on their own or with others.

Anna took several objects from the box and some tissue paper. She moved the objects around for a few minutes, trying out different ways of moving the objects, different combinations. She rejected some, putting them in a small pile. Eventually she covered one object with the tissue paper and placed the rest around them. The other objects were placed around the sheet of tissue paper so that their bases rested on its edges. Anna blew on the paper, but it couldn't move as it was held fast by the other objects. With a partner as witness she animated the objects. Firstly she gave voice to all the small objects around the tissue paper. They were all demanding, 'Give me my dinner', 'Make love to me', 'Help me I've fallen over'. She then fell silent, touched the covered object and said in a quiet voice, 'Help me. Help me', and tore the paper saying, 'She can breathe now.'

In this example Anna is playing with objects and paper. These activities are typical of object play in that materials are taken and their physical and representational qualities are explored. However, the playing activity takes place within a therapeutic framework. The goals of the play activity concern personal change. The therapist, in line with Griffing's (1983) four areas, has provided clear time, a safe space, materials and preparatory experiences. Anna connects the play work to personal material. She uses the playing to reflect a difficulty and to try out in the play world within the Dramatherapy a solution she could not yet try in her life outside the group. The Dramatherapy space created an opportunity for object play to occur. It also enabled Anna to play in a way which reflected her life and to use the play shift – the reproduction of her life in a way which makes 'playing around' with reality possible. Within this playing around the trying out of a needed change is allowed.

In both Jane's and Anna's work the playing that is facilitated occurs within a therapeutic framework. The processes which the clients are engaged in enables play to become a way for Jane to voice her abuse and for Anna to express her distress. Anna said that in playing she had no direct intention – she didn't know what would emerge. The paper and the objects soon became vocal – 'as if by themselves', as she said. The tearing of the paper as a response to the voices came, she said, 'suddenly, from nowhere'. Anna, on reflection, said that it felt 'wonderful' to do this. That something needed to be let out, she was holding too much. The tearing, though, made her feel sad – as if something had also 'been broken'.

Play occurs within a special created, facilitative context within Dramatherapy. In both examples the activities aim to explore problematic issues through playing within a therapeutic framework. Client and therapist together create play in order to express, explore and work towards a resolution of problems.

A developmental approach and the play–drama continuum

As described earlier there are many varying models of play development. Many include the notion of a continuum. Within Dramatherapy the consideration of play within a continuum is of use as an assessment tool, as a means of finding an appropriate developmental level of play to work with clients, and as a means of understanding therapeutic change.

As also noted earlier, play can be seen as a part of a continuum of development leading to drama. The continuum can be considered in terms of creative development, psychological development and skills development.

The play–drama continuum

Specific developmental stages have different implications for Dramatherapy practice, and are associated with different methods.

It is important to discover an appropriate developmental level for a group concerning their use of play and drama. Until the Dramatherapist has established the level at which the group appear to work, or might be able to work, or choose to work, then communication will be marred. The therapist needs to understand which areas of play and drama the group can best use to find meaning in. Schwartzman has pointed out that developmental notions concerning play are often culture-specific, and compares a number of different studies of play in different settings in her book, *Transformations* (1978). Authors such as Fortes present specific developmental studies of play. He considers the developmental stages of Talinese children's playing (1938). Irwin has pointed out that it is useful for the therapist to be aware of developmental levels to determine how an individual uses drama and play. Many clients and children, as she says, in the course of treatment, 'experience regression and/or fixation in both the form and content of their play' (1983, 105). The therapist's awareness of the developmental continuum from play to drama 'can help the therapist be sensitive to shifts in functioning and to deal with them . . . via appropriate media and materials' (Irwin, 1983, 150).

The following section gives a general overview of this process.

Summary of the play–drama continuum

Firstly, an individual discovers their body and is involved in a relationship with an important other such as a parent. At this level play involves the discovery of body parts and the body, along with contact with the important other. Later play develops to include forming relationships with concrete objects and the physical qualities which they possess – rolling, holding, dropping. This is followed by the development of symbolic play with objects, either as representative toys or as symbols with personal meaning. At first this is in solitary play or play with an important adult. This solitary play is usually followed by parallel play where a child plays with toys in a way which is similar to other children who are near, but individuals do not play together. The next phase involves playing together. This involves object play or brief sociodramatic play – activities which engage with playing other identities for a short while. The next phase involves the shift from dramatic play to drama. This concerns more sustained activities which involve taking on an identity in relationship with others. This is accompanied by more consciousness of showing activities to others and communicating the meaning of what is happening.

The above is intended as a general summary and is not intended to be seen as the only avenue of development for all individuals.

The following pages summarise key aspects of this developmental process as it relates to Dramatherapy. They are of two sorts, reflecting the main uses in Dramatherapy. The first, Figures 8.1–8.5, summarise the main aspects of the development along the play–drama continuum, and the second focuses upon two specific areas: character and object usage. The stages are summarised in Box 8.4.

Box 8.4 Key aspects of the play–drama continuum

- Sensorimotor play
- Imitative play
- Pretend play
- Dramatic play
- Drama

Figures 8.1–8.5 indicate important aspects of each stage. For example, the stage of 'Imitative play' is summarised by five areas (or stages) of capability, which usually follow on from each other.

For the Dramatherapist each stage should not be seen to be only appropriately worked with by the listed activities or areas, but, rather, seen as opening up additional areas of expression and meaning for the client. As the case studies show, the developmental stages summary is appropriate to groups irrespective of age. For people with learning difficulties the developmental levels are important as sequential steps, similarly for other groups for whom developmental progression is an issue within the Dramatherapy work.

Figures 8.1–8.5 are used both in aiding the understanding of the development of drama but also in ascertaining which activities can be undertaken by a group able to work at a certain developmental level. They do not aim to summarise development for all groups but provide general guidelines.

A summary of key developmental stages in terms of play, dramatic play and drama follows. Each area is given a title which indicates the main quality of the developmental stage, and key characteristics are indicated.

Sensorimotor play

Context

Jernberg typifies the sensorimotor stage as being concerned with 'movements through space and [the] handling of objects in the outside world' (Jernberg, 1983, 128). The following case study illustrates how this

Sound and movement
explores own body and
own body parts

Contact with and   **Locomotion**
physical exploration   rolling, crawling,
of **OBJECTS**   standing, walking

Physical relationship
with another

Figure 8.1 Sensorimotor play: motor play and use of physical properties of objects

sensorimotor stage can be present and important in the range of dramatic expression of adults within Dramatherapy work.

Case study 8.6 Ellen

'At one point Ellen brings her hands over her eyes as in a game of peek-a-boo. It is a playful gesture that makes us both laugh. I begin to relax, and forget some of my own fear as I feel . . . contact and exchange taking place between Ellen and myself. I cannot say for certain, but I believe she is experiencing similar feelings'.

(Schattner and Courtney, 1981, 72)

Here the expression primarily concerns 'Sound and movement' and 'Physical relationship with another', as noted in Figure 8.1. The sensorimotor play helps to establish relationship between the two clients, and to indicate that playful relationships and expression are possible in the Dramatherapy group.

Certain types of solitary play are also contained within this expressive range. This can happen in individual client work in Dramatherapy, or when an individual is engaged in individual play within a group. The following case study is from work with a group of adults with severe learning disabilities. Assessment had established that they could not engage in symbolic usage of objects, nor could take on identity. However, they were interested in objects and concrete properties of the things around them. They did not relate to others at all within the setting, and the group had been set up with an aim of helping to create more contact between the individuals.

Case study 8.7 Objects

Clients in a Dramatherapy group were working with objects, pushing and pulling them, rolling them over one another. For the first weeks the clients mainly kept the objects to themselves. I began to initiate relationship through objects – offering them, playing in parallel to clients with the objects. Eventually clients began to offer objects back to me, and began to play with objects I was using. Later in the work clients began to play with each other using the objects. All the activities concerned the concrete qualities of the objects – rolling, pushing, banging.

This is an example of sensorimotor based work in Dramatherapy where the use of objects remains concrete, non-symbolic. In working with client groups who are not able to relate to objects symbolically the work with objects' concrete properties can: (a) develop the client's ability to relate to their environment, (b) develop their repertoire of responses to the concrete qualities of the object, e.g. to move from pushing to rolling, throwing, catching, (c) develop their relationship to and with others as expressed through the use of the object.

Imitative play

Immediate imitation
of a gesture

Immediate imitation
of a sound

Immediate imitation
of a facial
expression

Immediate imitation of
movement of objects

Figure 8.2 Imitation: the brief repetition of phenomenon

Context

In this area of Dramatherapy work the emphasis is upon the therapeutic possibilities of the developmental range of dramatic imitation. This includes facial and bodily imitation, and the imitation of object usage.

Case study 8.8 Facial/bodily Imitation

In working with a group of people with severe learning difficulties, the work started with imitation of gesture, facial expression and movement. This established a relationship between group members and marked the early stages of contact and of playing. The work built up into playing with facial expressions – stretching the mouth, yawning in unison, opening the eyes wide. From this we worked with the development of an expressive range using the face and the body. Group members began to parallel each other's facial and physical expressions. The imitation of physical gestures and facial expressions was a way of developing a relation between group members and establishing language and a structure of interpersonal contact.

Case study 8.9 Imitation of Gesture

With an autistic young man a series of fifteen sessions were devoted to the establishing of relation through a language based on imitation and parallel movement. In all his contacts the young man would push people away if they came into close proximity. The Dramatherapy sessions were given the brief to try to help establish a form of communication which would help him to sustain proximity and contact. Developmentally the client could not engage in symbolic use of objects, nor could he take on characters. He did not use verbal language but could produce some sign language representing concepts such as 'biscuit' and 'toilet'. He could reproduce gesture. My work with him involved establishing contact through my paralleling or imitating some of his gestures; eventually he began to imitate gestures initiated by myself. Through this medium we were able to establish contact and to develop conversation.

Pretend play

Use of combinations of objects
to represent other objects
(e.g. pebbles to represent cakes)

Acting single pretend events
*(e.g. imitating drinking or
digging, not in a sequence)*

Functional use of
symbolic toys
(e.g. using toy phone)

Brief wearing of other's
clothes to signify imitation
of another person
*(e.g. father's hat to
indicate father)*

Use of body to evoke/
mime objects when not
actually present
*(e.g. hand to mime
an apple)*

Figure 8.3 Pretend play: the representational use of objects and beginnings of make-believe play

Context
Irwin describes the responses of a 5-year-old, Theresa, to the death of her mother.

Case study 8.10   Theresa

'She made a line of animals in the sandbox, led by the baby giraffe. The "mommy giraffe" had gotten killed by the "bad monsters" and the baby giraffe was leading "all her friends" into the forest to find the mommy and unearth her, to bring her back to life' (Irwin, 1983, 27).

Irwin interprets this as the child dealing with her pain, a denial in fantasy, and her own wish to bring the mother back. The child is revealing inner conflicts – between reality of her mother's death and the desire to deny that reality. Here pretend play involves combining objects, using them to depict simple events and the imaginative use of the giraffes. The expression of the child's feelings around the mother's death through the play materials gives both a means to express the feelings and a language to begin to work through them.

Dramatic play

Continuous portrayal of others – people, animals *(e.g. sustaining a series of activities as a fox)*	Complex play with objects *(recognising, acknowledging and interacting with others' use of objects)*
Mastery of gross and fine motor skills in evoking and using objects	Ability to use the body to pretend to be in a different, imagined reality
Acting out make-believe situations (a short sequence of events) playing self or other for less than five minutes	Ability to use objects as part of situations– props in make-believe play
Simple games involving play identities *(e.g. farmer and his wife)*	Appropriate response and co-operation with others during play

Figure 8.4 Dramatic play: sustained fantasy and enacted portrayal of others

Context

Case study 8.11 Amy

A child, Amy, used a doll's house to play out problematic issues concerning her mother. She would lock herself in the house, as the 'Mummy', saying that she couldn't possibly come out to the other children. Another time she locked all the children in the house to 'keep them safe from the slimy monster'. In another activity she insisted that another child should play mother and lead the children for a walk, single file, returning them safe to the house for tea.

Amy had been placed in care, her mother having frequently left her alone and locked in the house, and finally abandoning her totally. The Dramatherapy sessions provided her with an opportunity to play through these feelings with the other children. Issues about caring and uncaring were prevalent in the group. The children were able to hold characters for a brief period of time, to participate in an imagined reality and to work together in a scenario. The situations and identities were only held for a short period of time before they switched to a different situation. However, this amount of expression allowed the children to briefly play characters and to experience a different perspective. It also enabled them to pretend to be in situations which they experienced as anxiety provoking, and enabled us to play out and discuss their troubles. Through playing the mother Amy was able to explain her upset to us and to play through the traumatic events in her life.

Drama

Acting out make-believe situations
(A sequence of events) playing self
or other for more than five minutes

Can keep in role and deal with interations with others	Can develop a sequence of imaginary events with others connected to roles being played
Consciousness and use of audience performer space and relationship	Can devise themes and prepare plot for enactment
Ability to use script	Division of roles in making drama *(e.g. director/actor roles*

Consciousness of communication
to others of dramatic product

Figure 8.5 Drama: sustained enactment with consciousness of audience

At this level clients are able to sustain the kinds of enactment described in the chapter on role (See Chapter 9). Here complex engagements with dramatic representation of the self can be sustained.

Tables 8.1 and 8.2 give a different presentation of parallel material. They focus upon two key aspects of development in Dramatherapy – of character and of object usage. This is useful in both considering the level of dramatic language an individual can use, but also in considering where developmental progress can go, as the case study on p. 194 illustrates. The tables detail the order of significant developmental stages in two key areas of Dramatherapy – character or role playing and forming relationships with objects.

Table 8.1 Character portrayal

1	Body depicts different personae during solitary play: brief contact
2	Body depicts different personae during co-operative play – brief contact
3	Sustained bodily portrayal – holding of one persona – simple use of costume
4	Sustained recognition, engagement and co-operation with other character portrayals, physical imaginative coherence of character portrayals
5	Extension of bodily range and imaginative exploration of physical portrayal of character – complex use of costume
6	Articulated awareness of relationship/difference between self and character

Capability to discuss, reflect and alter portrayals

In this approach the therapeutic work is seen to include or focus upon a shift in developmental level which is therapeutic for the client. This can occur in a number of ways.

A client may have been locked into a particular developmental level of play. This level is connected to an absence in the relationship between the client and their identity, or the client in their relationship with objects or with other people. For example a client may not be able to relate to objects symbolically, or may not be able to engage in co-operative play.

The Dramatherapist needs to identify the level at which the client usually functions and to consider what is involved in the client's functioning at this particular level. The work becomes the creation of conditions or situations which can help the client to develop further or differently in terms of developmental levels – to enable the client's growth through entering into new levels of play. This means the creation of new kinds of relationships between self and object, or self and others.

The main focus, then, is on enabling the client to function at a different developmental level to the ones they are currently functioning at. In some cases this means the movement to a more highly developed state of functioning. For others it means the working through of a level of developmental play which was absented or malfunctioning. In addition this new way of relating or functioning can be paralleled in new ways of

Table 8.2 Object usage

I	Physical contact with offered object – hands, mouth, visual contact; holding/letting go
2	Exploration of physical properties of object – interest in presence/absence, movement
3	Solitary moving of objects in relation to each other, focus on physical properties – manipulating, stacking, gathering
4	Giving meaning to single objects – using single object as if it were another object: e.g. block of wood as car; using symbolic toys e.g. coffee pot and cup to simulate pouring and drinking coffee
5	Combining objects into scenes – e.g. doll drinking; solitary make-believe play using objects in this way
6	Parallel play – using similar objects in play to others nearby, but no interpersonal contact in playing
7	Social play including using objects in association with others in a common activity
8	Using objects in play where they function as props to assist role and narrative – e.g. bags, wigs, clothes
9	Objects as dramatic personae – e.g. puppets Objects as props in drama – realistic and symbolic Objects as costume and disguise – e.g. mask

learning to relate to self, object or others outside of the realm of play itself. The play process becomes linked to emotional, cognitive, social and emotional development.

Case study 8.12 Developmental Play

Sandberg describes a client, aged 13. He was anxious about drama, and his expressive range was unable to sustain concentrated dramatic enactment. For two months she works with short games, non-verbal transformation, short mimes, 'young tree, old tree, various animals' (Sandberg in Schattner and Courtney, 1981, 41). She describes the first long interaction in the second month, lasting virtually a whole session 'he took on the role of a kangaroo . . . He developed an unembellished plot of two kangaroos fighting for their lives against white hunters' (1981, 41).

Here Sandberg uses the understanding of developmental progression in her Dramatherapy work. The client initially works as a pretend play level – the use of the body to evoke/mime objects when not actually present, acting single, pretend events. This is the level at which he can find meaning. The client, as he gains confidence and skill, develops on to dramatic play – sustaining portrayal of the kangaroo and involving a simple sequence of events.

The client or group often parallel the stages of this developmental notion, needing to work through various stages before reaching a state where they can begin to use dramatic form fully – this may be learning or re-learning skills or a way of approaching being with others, or it may be linked with regression occurring within the group (e.g. refusal to work with any objects as symbolic, rejecting from the group).

Summary

Drama and play are part of a developmental continuum. As a part of this continuum play is included in the expressive language which the client uses to create meaning and explore material in Dramatherapy.

For clients in Dramatherapy, playing is a way of discovering or creating access to their own spontaneity. For some clients this process forms the main therapeutic benefit within Dramatherapy.

Dramatherapy creates a playful relationship with reality. The Dramatherapy space enables clients to play with elements of their life – to rework issues, to try out new configurations or possibilities. This can be described as a 'play shift'. This playful exploration can produce changes which can be integrated into the client's life outside the Dramatherapy.

The understanding of a developmental continuum from play to drama can assist in assessment and evaluation work. It can also help to find an appropriate expressive level for clients to work with in Dramatherapy.

Cognitive, emotional and social development can be worked with using a developmental understanding of the play–drama continuum. Changes in the dramatic developmental level that a client is able to use in Dramatherapy, for example, can be accompanied by cognitive or social changes for clients.

Chapter 9
Role

Rain-stopping magic is made by pouring water on red hot stones
... the rain is not just represented, but is felt to be really present
in each drop of water.

Cassirer, Language and Myth

Introduction

An enacted role is a dramatic persona assumed by an individual within
theatre. The term 'role' has also become used as a way of describing
and analysing identity in life, not in theatre alone. Moreno (1960), for
example, identifies three main types of roles – somatic, social and
psychodramatic – which cover all of the possible aspects of an individual's identity. Somatic roles include activities such as sleeping and
eating, social roles include family, economic and occupational spheres,
whilst psychodramatic roles are those of fantasy and internal life. Landy
has described the role as a container of the thoughts and feelings we
have about ourselves and each other, as a basic 'unit' of personality. An
individual's self consists of a number of roles or units. Any role has
specific qualities providing uniqueness and coherence to each of these
units (1994, 7).

The work of Mead (1934) and Goffman (1959) has become influential
in Dramatherapy's approach to role. Mead's notion of the self is that it
is developed through social interaction; an individual's identity is seen
as constructed through the roles they perform in various contexts.
Goffman's work describes individuals, groups and society using theatre
as a metaphor to help understand how self, role and other relate. These
writers, along with others such as Sarbin (1986), Sarbin and Allen (1968)
and Hampson (1988), have helped Dramatherapists to discuss the nature
of the self and identity, the relationship between role and personality,
between theatre and life (Read Johnson, 1988; Landy, 1994; Meldrum,
1994).

Within fields such as psychodrama and social psychology the role in
therapy is usually allied with dramatised role functions. Within
Dramatherapy, role is not confined to dramatic ways of working with

role functions. It is used in its wider sense, describing a fictional identity or persona which someone can assume, and is also a concept used to understand the different aspects of a client's identity in their life as a whole. Both therapist and client can take on fictional roles during a Dramatherapy session.

Role has been a part of theatre throughout its existence, though the functions and ways of creating roles have changed radically from culture to culture and from age to age. As was mentioned in Chapters 1 and 3, the adoption of role is connected to healing in a number of cultures. A significant development which has occurred mainly in Europe and the United States has been the use of dramatised role work within psychiatry and the field of mental health.

Contexts for role in Dramatherapy

The enacted self

Any work with role in Dramatherapy makes the assumption that the self can assume different, fictional identities. The development of this notion in Dramatherapy is that the fictional self can be enacted. A dynamic tension is set up between the enacted fictional self and the client's usual identity, and this dynamic, active relationship is seen as the basis of therapeutic change in role work within Dramatherapy.

The creation of enacted roles occurs in three ways within Dramatherapy:

1 The client assumes a fictional identity which is not their own (e.g. another person, an animal or object, an abstract quality).

Case study 9.1 Ballet Dress

In a Dramatherapy group a young woman, Popi, had selected an important object which she was attached to. From her childhood she selected a ballet dress which her parents bought her. It was too small and she never wore it, but kept it. Even after leaving her parental home she still had it with her. She said she didn't know why that was. In the group Popi took on the role of the dress. She firstly indicated its shape by mime, and then mimed placing the dress in the centre of the group. Popi then stepped into the space where the dress had been put and, as she did so, took on the role of the dress. Speaking in the first person she began by describing her texture, where she was in Popi's flat and what Popi felt about her. The group helped her to improvise and to explore the role by asking her questions. The direction of the role work began to turn towards the dress's feelings about being too small, being never worn, and eventually towards the parents who bought the undersized dress for Popi. The reason it was never taken back to the shop emerged and the needs of the parents to keep their daughter smaller than she really was began to be voiced.

2 The client plays the role of themselves in the past, present or future (e.g. the client plays themselves at 10, at the present time, or confronting their employer next week).

Case study 9.2 Secret

Nosmul has written a short script at the start of a session. A theme in the group has been secrets, keeping them, divulging them. He reads the script with another group member. The final section of it is as follows:

MOTHER: I want that key. Give it to me now.
NOSMUL: I don't have the key.
MOTHER: I think you do!
NOSMUL: No! It's my box!
MOTHER: Let mummy have it now.
NOSMUL: It's my box.
MOTHER: Don't be silly. Children shouldn't have secrets from their mummies.

This is a scene from Nosmul's childhood, when he was 8 years old. Nosmul then took on the role of himself at 8. A group member played his mother. They ran the script through and then improvised from the point at which the script ends. The first time Nosmul gave the key and then came out of role, saying he wanted to try again. On the second time, as the script ended and the improvisation was about to begin, he stopped the role work and said, 'It's no good'.

3 The client deliberately isolates a specific aspect of themselves or their identity. The highlighted aspect or characteristic forms the basis of a created role (e.g. a role function such as 'Daughter' or 'Leader', or a characteristic such as 'The part of me that wants to sabotage my life' or 'The part of me that wants to leave hospital').

Case study 9.3 Red Mask

At the end of a Dramatherapy group for staff members in an inter-
mediate treatment setting a senior social worker sat by a chair on which
lay a mask. The social worker had made the mask and developed it
into a role: the aim of the group was to explore the dynamics of the
unit in terms of staff relationships and staff/client relationships.
The group had all made masks depicting specific group dynamic roles.
The social worker's mask was bright red and its allocated role title
was 'Aggressor'. The group had improvised being on an island
together. Jim talked to the mask about how it represented his fear,
the part of himself that was both frightened of the violence he works
with but that also wanted to be violent. During the improvisation
on the island the role he had taken and expressed whilst wearing the
red mask became the most powerful within the group. He joined with
the 'Saboteur' in such a way as to ensure that any of the tasks which
the group tried to achieve were blocked. So building a hut, looking
for water, finding things that had drifted ashore from the wrecked ship
they had arrived in – all remained unachieved.

Why should the dramatising of the self or aspects of the self be therapeutic?
Schechner (1988) sums up our role taking capability in a way which
indicates a part of the answer: 'Unique among animals humans carry and
express multiple and ambivalent identities simultaneously'. Part of the
therapeutic possibilities of enacting the self concerns the quality that
Schechner indicates: we are *conscious* of having *potential identities*, and
we relate to these in an 'ambivalent' way – we *reflect upon* these identities
and *express ourselves* through them.

Dramatherapy's approach to role in both theory and practice has been
strongly influenced by thinking in theatre, psychology, psychodrama,
dramaturgy and anthropology. In creating a context for the discussion
of Dramatherapy practice and role, the next section will illustrate these
influences.

Ecstasy and rationality

Wilshire (1982) discusses role by analysing its function in theatre. He
considers the involvement of audience and actor in creating enacted
roles as reflecting a basic human trait. When acting or watching theatre
he describes those involved as being in a trance-like 'primal mimetic

absorption in types of being and doing' (Wilshire, 1982, 23). Within the area of role this issue of 'primal absorption' is a focus of much debate.

The discussion of this area concerns:

- the level of our emotional involvement when we play or witness roles in theatre.
- the relationship between the usual, everyday self and the enacted self; the degree to which the usual self becomes lost or submerged in the enacted role.
- the nature and qualities of the way the usual self reflects upon the enacted self.

Often this issue is debated in terms of 'ecstasy' and 'rationality' (see Chapter 11, and Jennings, 1987; Scheff, 1979). Ecstasy refers to a sense of being 'taken over' by a role or dramatic experience – of being 'lost' within it. Schechner refers to both Balinese trance and Stanislavski's approach as being linked by this ecstatic approach to enactment: 'performing by becoming or being possessed by another' (1988, 177). Coult, of the UK's alternative performance company, Welfare State, describes this way of working as 'the inducing of trance-like states in which reflection, reason and awareness are suppressed or abandoned,' (Coult and Kershaw, 1983, 27). Rationality refers to the analytic, rational, thought-orientated aspects of role taking and playing. In this way of seeing role taking, emphasis is placed upon the degree to which the role taker stays aware, reflective and analytical of the role playing during and after enactment.

These two notions of ecstasy and rationality are often used as oppositional criteria in the analysis of the processes involved in playing a role. To what extent is the role taker immersed in the role? What levels of contact do they have with their everyday, usual identity? To what extent do audience members become emotionally involved or rationally engaged?

Theatre theorists and practitioners discuss role within this dialectic. Within certain types of theatre, absorption is so total that the actor claims to have lost a sense of any identity outside of the role. A drama student in Mast's study of acting described this process: 'You're no longer yourself ... You are the medium of the character you're playing ... you're no longer yourself so you shouldn't be looking at yourself' (Mast, 1986, 158).

Brechtian-influenced theatre aims for a more rational approach and experience for actors and audience. The actor constantly thinks, and tries to stay outside the role, reacting to the role. In the creation of an enacted role the actor must remain intellectually aware, and a minimum of the experience of ecstatic merging with the role must occur. This relationship is seen to lead to political, social and personal change.

Johnson and Johnson (1987) define the taking on of a role in 'role play' within a strictly rational process. The role taker stays fully aware of the reason for the activity, and is open to cognitive learning processes. The work is skills orientated, role playing is a tool for 'bringing a specific skill and its consequences into focus, and this is vital for experiential learning'. It is 'intended to give . . . experience in practising skills and in discussing and identifying effective and ineffective behaviour' (1987, 24).

Boal, in *Games for Actors and Non-Actors* (1992), aims for a more balanced relationship between immersion and disengagement: 'The rationalisation of emotion does not take place solely after the emotion has disappeared . . . it also takes place in the emotion. There is a simultaneity of feeling and thinking' (1992, 47).

Within role work the two states are seen by some to co-exist. This is reflected in Garvey (1977) and others' observational work on children taking roles in play. Garvey describes two kinds of communication. One sort is communication within the played role – the role, as it were, talking. The other is communication outside the role. Exchanges occur about the play activity – comments on what to do next, how to deal with problems in the play. This is referred to as 'metacommunication'. Though these observations concern play and not theatre, the existence of this metacommunication could be seen to indicate that a natural co-existence can exist between immersion and disengagement in playing a role.

It becomes clear that the relationship between 'ecstasy' and 'rationality', the levels of absorption in the enacted self, vary enormously. Factors affecting this are in part cultural, in part concern the intention of the entry into role, and in part concern technique. For Brecht, for example, the onus on rational process connects to the intended outcome of cognitive, political change. For Johnson and Johnson (1987) the emphasis is upon a rational learning process. Intention, technique and 'levels' of ecstasy and distance are connected in relation to created roles.

In Dramatherapy a balance is sought. Immersion and rationality together affect an outcome where feeling and thought are united. During a session, however, the balance of ecstasy and rationality in terms of role work might vary enormously. Some techniques used by Dramatherapists emphasise a distance from a role, others encourage a high level of immersion. For Dramatherapy it is important to note the centrality of the 'ecstasy'/ 'rationality' issue. Of equal interest to Dramatherapy is the connection outlined above – between intention, levels of involvement and technique. The relationship of these areas to Dramatherapy will be returned to later in this chapter.

Breach, disturbance, change

The capability to assume a different persona is often linked to disturbance or breach. Identity has been defined as being reliant upon an interconnected system of roles (Argyle, 1969). The coherence of the individual social role and its connection with other roles is crucial to the functioning of societies and to the individual's well-being (Brissett and Edgeley, 1975). From this point of view the health of any society and the effective functioning of an individual in terms of their sense of identity are interdependent. Argyle, a major proponent of this view, asserts that social organisations consist of a number of individuals interacting in a regular manner. The description of this regular pattern is made possible 'by means of the concept of role which [is] . . . defined . . . as the modal behaviour of occupants in a position . . .' (Argyle, 1969, 277).

When involved in drama or in enactment, an identity is shifted. This can cause disturbance. By 'shifted', I mean that the individual does not respond or act in the way they usually do. They do not consider themselves to have the attributes and qualities normally ascribed to them. To a small or large degree, they have shifted their identity. A small degree of shift might involve someone acting as themselves, emphasising or taking on different characteristics. This could take the form of acting as yourself but playing a specific part of your personality – a 'Mother', or a 'Blamer', for example. A larger shift might involve playing the role of a rhinoceros, complete with costume.

Theatre is often associated with this sense of disturbance in relationship to role taking. The European medieval Feast of Fools is one example of this, when social roles were entirely reversed within the Festival Drama (Southern, 1962).

The enacted self is linked to breach and disturbance by a number of authors. Within this approach to examining role the shifting in identity in taking on a role is seen as a way of responding to crisis. A special set of circumstances exist in reality and the recourse to an enacted identity is a response to this. The shift is seen as redressive and this pattern is often present, for example, in Shakespearean disguise. Becker describes the performance of Wayang, a traditional form of shadow puppetry, as a way of society dealing with political or spiritual crisis: 'a way of subduing or at least calming down dangerous power' (1979, 34). Turner describes a process of 'social drama' in certain cultures, which is used when 'the peaceful tenor of a regular norm-governed social life is interrupted by the breach of a rule controlling one of its salient relationships' (1974, 37). Here a drama is used to deal with and manage the disturbance.

The contemporary experimental theatre company, Welfare State, see their work within this pattern of a response to disturbance. In its residencies and performances the company describe themselves as 'working in a real world' (Coult and Kershaw, 1983, 12) in which dramatic myths and rituals are absent – these are forms 'rooted in society's real needs' (1983, 12). Welfare State seek to bring together theatre, carnival and festival to the everyday world of 'social living'. The contact with the world of theatre creates access to the disturbance of 'the transforming power of the imagination that makes change possible' (1983, 13).

In terms of Dramatherapy this connection of the enacted self to disturbance and to change is important. It is usually due to some disturbance in their lives that individuals attend Dramatherapy. The way that taking on role functions in Dramatherapy can be seen within the chain of connections made above is as follows:

Disturbance/crisis – role entry and exploration – alternatives sought – change

There are two additional elements which are especially important within this way of looking at role and Dramatherapy. The first involves noting that entry into role can often be experienced as socially and individually disturbing. It marks an experience outside the usual framework by which an individual is known to others and by which individuals know themselves. The second is that entry into an enacted self, a dramatic role, is, within certain disciplines, seen as connected to creating a space which is separate from usual reality to redress problems or difficulties.

The temporary change of identity gives permissions and alters the experience of self and others in a way which is seen to help bring about difference and change.

Self, learning and exploration

As discussed in Chapter 8 the taking on of roles can be seen as a capability which marks the development of certain social and psychological processes. These include the ability to develop relationships with another, the ability to identify with others and their emotional perspective. It can mark the development of social skills, cognitive perspective taking and moral reasoning:

The act of consciously transforming their own identities into a variety of make-believe identities may hasten the decentration process, thereby promoting perspective taking and a number of other cognitive skills.

(Johnson, Christie, Yawkey, 1987, 102)

Wilshire (1982) has echoed Evreinov's (1927) ideas concerning the essential nature of drama in human development. He places role taking and imitation in a context of learning: 'bodies biologically human learn to become human persons by learning to do what persons around them are already doing. The learning body mimetically incorporates the model' (1982, 116).

Blatner and Blatner place role taking and playing in the context of learning to creatively explore reality and to deal with problems encountered in the world. They see this, in terms of Winnicott's ideas concerning the individual's creation of 'transitional space', as an important developmental stage. Role playing takes place within a realm between what they call 'subjective' and 'objective' worlds, 'the relatively fluid dimension where people can utilise the potentialities of their imaginations. It is more explicitly expressed in drama, which allows it to be more consciously manipulated . . . safer . . .', and enabling 'creative risk taking' (Blatner and Blatner, 1988b, 78).

Role approaches, structures and techniques: a review

The previous section showed how assumptions concerning rationality and ecstasy, change and disturbance, learning, exploration and identity related to different ways of looking at the experience of taking on roles.

This section considers the relationship between assumption, structure and technique. It states the basic assumptions concerning role within a particular field and considers how the structures and techniques of the practical use of role in drama and in therapy relate to these assumptions. It also aims to help to differentiate Dramatherapy's assumptions and method from other areas using role.

Dramatherapy will be contextualised within other major fields which use role practically. Three areas which are closely related to Dramatherapy's use of role will be considered: theatre, psychodrama and the use of role in social skills training.

Theatre

In theatre the creation of roles focuses upon performance. A basic structure underlying most theatre productions in relation to role taking can be summarised as in Figure 9.1.

Selection ⟶ Audition ⟶ Roles ⟶ Rehearsal ⟶ Fixing ⟶ Performance
of text   allocated   of roles   of   of roles to
                                             roles   audience

Figure 9.1 Theatre role

Of course theatre is extremely varied in its different approaches and forms. Some practitioners do not fix performances; rehearsal processes vary enormously. An actor might create their own role through improvisation, a director might want the actor to play a specific interpretation, they might use personal experiences from life to create the role, or might work in a way which focuses upon more objective technical delivery of a role. Figure 9.1 seeks to summarise a process common to a number of approaches.

The general focus of the theatre process is normally upon a performed interpretation of a role. The actor, usually in conjunction with a company and a director, works to link their personal creativity with an agreed aesthetic. The aesthetic concerns the intention of the performance and the style of the performance (Classical or Kabuki, Noh or Agitprop). It also includes the style adopted in relation to the way the theatre performance communicates to the audience – realist, symbolist, interactive or naturalistic.

Psychodrama

Psychodrama sees the client's presenting problem in terms of role. The enacted role, in classic psychodrama, is the main means of treatment and resolution of this problem. Its methodology and philosophy (Moreno, 1983: Moreno and Moreno, 1959) understands psychological problems and illness in terms of role. The way psychodrama sees the relationship between self and reality has role at its centre. Whether focusing upon group or individual process, a classical psychodrama aims to identify a protagonist and frame the presenting difficulty within role in a 'role analysis'. The main elements identified by Moreno as essential to psychodrama – protagonist, director, auxiliary, audience and stage – serve to explore and redress the client's issues and difficulties through the creation and interaction of enacted roles. Blatner identifies role taking as the 'key skill' (Blatner, 1973, 108) for the client. In his analysis of the ways psychodrama operates, he selects a series of scenarios to illustrate the breadth of practice. These relate to clients' problems or issues in relation to reality testing, subconscious desires, trauma, psychosis and behaviour. In each situation the client's taking on a role or roles is the main means of therapeutic intervention. Role in psychodrama can be seen to be at the centre of client diagnosis, a client's expression of a problem and the treatment or therapeutic work undertaken in relation to that problem. The basic structure concerning role in psychodrama can be summarised as in Figure 9.2.

Protagonist and ———→ Problem framed in ———→ Expressed and explored
problematic issue   terms of role   in role playing
identified

———→ Catharsis – ———→ De-roling/ ———→ Sharing – talking
             emotional   leaving the   about role
             release in role   enacted role   experiences

Figure 9.2 Psychodrama role

Social sciences

In the social sciences emphasis has been put upon role work as a tool in learning and re-learning:

> In role playing, trainees practice the part they are going to play in a classroom situation, and are given some kind of feedback on their performance.
>
> (Argyle, 1969, 402)

Role is worked with in a 'role play' and is usually highly focused upon a set subject. The main concern is often with the effective psychological or social functioning of an individual, group or organisation. In part, role

Problem ——→	Problem ——→	Learning ——→	Role ——→	Role
perceived	framed	task	Play and	problem
	in terms	through	learning	resolved in
	of role	role play	takes	individual's
	and	formulated	place	life
	learning			
	need			
	identified			

Figure 9.3 Role and role play in social science

as a concept is seen as a framework to use in appraising an individual's functioning. The practical application is through role play used as a means to redress any perceived problems relating to psychological or social functioning.

For example, an individual might face problems in dealing with other people in social situations. Role play would be used to try to establish the most effective techniques to deal with these problems. The playing of roles would be used to try to establish and practise a new way of behaving and dealing with others in social situations. The expectation is that the new way of relating, created within role playing, would be transferred to the individual's everyday life.

The emphasis in approach is not upon the psychotherapeutic exploration of psychodrama, nor on the creative, aesthetic emphasis within theatre. The individual is seen in terms of a series of interrelating roles. Each person has a number of roles which they play. This gives an individual a sense of who they are. The roles others play are a means of understanding who they are. People relate to each other through the roles they play. Roles are seen as a function, essential to a sense of personal identity and equilibrium. The practical use of enacted roles through role play becomes a way of redressing an individual's social or psychological problems and these problems are seen as issues concerning the way the roles function. Examples of this include Maier's (1953) work on leadership, and Morton's (1965) work in a psychiatric hospital.

Dramatherapy

In contrast to theatre's relationship to role, Dramatherapy does not usually have performance or creative expression as a primary focus. Even when a performance occurs within Dramatherapy it is not the main goal. The focus of Dramatherapy would lie in the therapeutic benefits to be gained by the creative process of role taking and the performance. A performance in Dramatherapy is a means to a therapeutic end. Exercises and techniques may seem the same on the surface, however, when seen in terms of context, intention and effect, the experience of theatre is different from that of Dramatherapy.

For example, an actress may be preparing a role in a theatre production. In doing so she may consider her personal response to the role, the ways in which her feelings and her life experience connect to the role. In preparing for performance, in rehearsal, she may use aspects of her life consciously or unconsciously within the playing (see 'Gertrude and Hamlet' on pp. 5–6). In Dramatherapy a client might also prepare a role for performance, drawing upon aspects of their life experience.

The key difference is that the action of taking on a role and connecting it to personal process in Dramatherapy directly aims to engender therapeutic change for the client. This alters the experience, function and goal of the exercise. The actress will go on to perform her role, her delivery may be enhanced by the exploration and it may incidentally have an effect upon her life outside the theatre. The primary goal of role creation for her, though, is to bring about the effective, creative communication of her role to an audience.

There are parallels between the uses made of role by theatre, psychodrama, the social sciences and Dramatherapy in that the basic pattern of the role play in the social sciences, Dramatherapy and psychodrama show

---

Client issue or ⟶ Connection to ⟶ Approach ⟶ If role is an
problem   Dramatherapy   selected   appropriate
                   media and   as appropriate medium, a
                   processes   to client needs method is
                                                   chosen

e.g. ⟶ role play ⟶ De-roling ⟶ Assimilation

⟶ mask and role

⟶ script ⟶ performance

Figure 9.4 Dramatherapy and role

the undeniable influence of Moreno. The boundaries and relationship between psychodrama and Dramatherapy is still developing.

For psychodrama and for the social sciences' use of role, an individual or group problem is identified primarily in terms of role, and techniques and structures which focus upon role are used to redress the problem. This is not the case with Dramatherapy. A problem may present itself in role terms, but the Dramatherapist would consider the spectrum of dramatic processes and expressive languages to find a way to express and work with the problem or issue.

A Dramatherapist might see mask, improvisation, script writing, the use of existing scripts, performance of a play, costume making or scenery building as a means to enable the client to explore or resolve a problem. Role might form a part of the way the Dramatherapist works. For example, the presenting issue might be explored firstly through play orientated activity and then move into role play. This, in turn, might lead to the creation of a piece of work based in performance art.

In addition the Dramatherapist might enter into role within the therapeutic work. This might be in order to take part in a role play – to assist in the exploration of the material which the client is bringing. The entry into role by the therapist might also concern the exploration of transference issues which the client is experiencing. Landy has given a detailed account of a therapist in role in his 'One on One' essay, where he plays the role of an elephant in relation to the client taking on the part of a mouse (Landy, 1989).

So role in Dramatherapy is part of the expressive canon which the client and therapist can utilise. It might be used as the main way of working or in combination with other methodologies. In addition, Dramatherapy does not necessarily frame the presenting problem in role terms. An example of this might be the way that issues are considered within a developmental framework, as described in Chapter 12.

The process of the work would not need to have the structure of the classic psychodrama or the role play. These structures might be used. However, the client's need is considered in the light of a variety of dramatic processes. For example, the client might only need to *create* a role for the therapeutic work to be completed. No role playing with others or catharsis is needed. A role might be developed over a number of weeks through a variety of media until the client has worked with the issue or problem sufficiently. The traditional role play is a part of the process which Dramatherapy draws on, but it is not the only or main role process which is used. All theatrical, dramatic and therapeutic possibilities of the role are utilised according to the needs of the client or group.

Dramatherapy practice and role

Within Dramatherapy there are different approaches which emphasise particular aspects of role taking and playing. For example, Landy stresses the importance of distancing (1986) and the notion of a role inventory or taxonomy as a framework for Dramatherapy (1994). Jennings stresses the importance of developing the client's role repertoire (1987), whilst Grainger considers the more absorbed, ecstatic, ritualistic aspects of engagement with role (1990). Read Johnson considers the nature of role in terms of the therapeutic potentials of transformation (1988). Emunah and Read Johnson (1983), Jennings (1992) and Mitchell (1992) consider role within a performance and paratheatrical context within Dramatherapy. Meldrum has discussed Dramatherapy's approach to the relationship between self and role (1994).

Landy (1994) sees role as the primary component of healing in Dramatherapy and has developed an approach rooted in this area. The form of the work takes an approach which initially involves the naming of a role, taken from a taxonomy of roles created by Landy. Each individual has a system of roles. The work involves 'reaching in' to the system and extracting a role, 'a single aspect of personality' (1994, 46). This develops into the playing, working through and exploring of the role followed by reflection and the eventual integration of any change into the client's life. The presence of the taxonomy of roles aims to underpin role work, providing a systematic presentation of the role choices it is possible to make.

There is a basic pattern to all role taking in Dramatherapy, which Figure 9.5 summarises.

Enrolement ⟶ Dramatic activity ⟶ Disengagement ⟶ Assimilation
extends/explores   from role

Figure 9.5 Pattern of role taking in Dramatherapy

Enrolement

Enrolement is the process through which a client enters role. This may happen spontaneously: a client may simple begin to play a role. In a similar fashion the Dramatherapist may invite the client or clients to 'show' or to act rather than to describe something verbally. If this happens it is usually within a group who have experience and skills in drama or Dramatherapy. In some situations an individual might begin to act out a situation in this way but have insufficient impetus to sustain the role.

Box 9.1 Enrolement factors

- the concentration span of the clients
- the developmental level of the clients' use of drama
- the level of engagement and emotional investment
- the quality of creative involvement and skill
- the cultural background of clients in relation to theatre/drama traditions of role taking and playing
- the history of the group, previous experience of role work

This lack of impetus would usually be due to some or one of the following: a lack of interest, a lack of emotional engagement, too much emotional engagement, confusion or disorientation concerning the direction of the enactment, lack of concentration or skill, a psychological issue present as a resistance to entering into or remaining with a role.

Enrolement seeks to help clients move into role and to sustain the impetus of the role they are playing.

Before engaging in enrolement the group or individual's relationship to role work would be assessed (see Chapter 12). This would concern areas such as the developmental level of the client's ability to use drama and roles or the way in which they find meaning in dramatic expression in Dramatherapy. For example, an enrolement for an individual or for groups who are well versed in role playing who can sustain roles and create sophisticated dramatic interactions with each other would be run differently than for a group who are easily confused, have short attention spans with little role playing experience.

In some Dramatherapy activities it is not necessary to enter into interaction with other roles. However, in order to engage in substantial role activity, certain skills and specific capabilities are necessary. Box 9.2 helps to focus upon these skills and capabilities. It can be used in pre-role taking work to help establish whether individuals or groups might be ready to move into role work.

Enrolement activities need not have a clear goal in terms of aiming to create an 'end product' of a specific role. An enrolement can be

---

Box 9.2 **Pre-role checklist**   Tick appropriate boxes

A client can be considered ready to undertake
role work if they display a high proportion of
the capacities listed below: **A   B   C**
• can pretend an action   ☐   ☐   ☐
• can imagine what someone else might say   ☐   ☐   ☐
• can imagine what someone else might feel   ☐   ☐   ☐
• can imagine how someone else might respond
  to something   ☐   ☐   ☐
• can respond to others' imaginative ideas   ☐   ☐   ☐
• can communicate effectively with others   ☐   ☐   ☐
• can use objects as substitutes for other
  objects with an imaginative intention   ☐   ☐   ☐

A = Yes   B = Some evidence   C = No

---

completely exploratory, the roles developing out of the work. The enrolement case study comes from a group of six people meeting in a centre for substance abusers, and takes place early in the life of the group. Members had shown much interest and creativity in script and movement work.

Case study 9.4 Script and Enrolement

Group members had been developing work with script. The focus was on an imaginary conversation or interaction based around a word which represented a theme. This word could reflect something that the client had been working with, or which represented an area of difficulty. Rita had chosen 'No' and had developed this script:

A: Not here. Go over there.
B: Here?
A: No. That's not right. Go there.
B: Here?
A: No, no. That's not right at all. What is it with you?

Each group member had their own script. Rita had worked with her script, running exploratory improvisations, seeing what characters or roles came up as she played 'A' or 'B'. The script was worked with non-verbally, just using a series of body positions developing from the words. This was then taken further: from each body position the client could either speak a phrase from their script or could develop the script further. The series of body positions was then treated as an extension of the dialogue between the two roles, 'A' and 'B'. Rita's role came out with a series of negatives: 'I don't know' (her body crouched, arms tight around herself), 'Help me' (looking upwards), 'Leave me alone' (arms stretched out, pushing). Rita discussed what the script and positions reminded her of.

The material in the script was used in an exploratory fashion. It helped Rita to begin to identify the area of concern, encouraging her to begin to focus on an issue and to locate a feeling and a situation. Rita had previously talked about her difficulty in saying no to drugs, and how she had returned to the centre twice before this attempt to 'change my life'. From this point the role work went on to explore a series of issues concerning her desire to say 'no' and her inability to say it. No role was fixed beforehand; rather, roles emerged from the improvisations.

Cultural differences are an important factor to consider within role work. With some forms and traditions the emotional absorption and engagement of the player in the role is high; for others the emphasis is upon a more distanced relationship between player and role. The cultural background of a client may mean that their assumptions or approach to role may reflect a particular relationship to engagement and distance. Within much Dramatherapy a balanced state of engagement is aimed for, where 'the emotional and rational parts of the self are in balance' and the client is 'capable of feeling without fear of being overwhelmed by the emotion, and thinking, without fear of losing the ability to respond passionately' (Landy, 1986, 8).

An additional factor in enrolement lies in de-roling and the assimilating phase. Many structures for enroling are used again or used in reverse for de-roling.

The role of the Dramatherapist is to try to ascertain the emotional and creative/artistic needs of the group at the start of any role based work. If necessary they need to help to provide a structure to enter into role.

Role activity

At the end of enrolement the individual is engaged and involved in the role. The 'role activity' is any structure which enables the individual or group to explore and to develop the role. It will engage with the material which is presented by the client or clients and which the role activity aims to address. The role activity may have a single focus, a particular role or series of roles interacting together. It may move from a scripted role to improvisation to mask.

Within Dramatherapy, role activity can usually include the following:

- role sculpts
- role play
- improvisation
- work based on existing scripts
- enactment of scripts created by clients
- performance of a play
- role activity using media (masks, puppets)
- dramatic play

Processes such as doubling, the soliloquy and role reversal can be used within this expressive range.

The role of the Dramatherapist is to work with the individual or group to find an appropriate dramatic vehicle and process to meet the therapeutic needs of the client or clients. The following case study illustrates how Dramatherapy can combine a number of dramatic processes concerning role within its therapeutic work. The ensuing processes seek to meet the needs of the client within the forms of exploration and expression. Here role work in the form of role playing, story-telling, the creation of a symbolic, fantasy character and costume are combined. It takes place in an ongoing group of nine people in a psychiatric day centre. They had been meeting for ten months when the session took place.

Case study 9.5 Ana's Shadow, Role Activity

Ana presented a problem to the group. She had been invited to stay with her son and daughter-in-law. She could not bear to be in the same room as the daughter-in-law and had previously used her illness as a way out. Now that she was recovering, added pressure was being put on her, and she asked the group for support in saying 'No'. One of the group asked her what the problem was with the daughter-in-law. Ana said that 'There's something about her, I don't know what it is. I can't put my finger on it.' She said that she felt uncomfortable when with her: she felt 'in her shadow'.

I asked Ana if she wished to look at this further and she assented. We discussed the way we might explore the situation. I offered her a range of dramatic ways of working – including mask, story-telling or to look directly at what was happening by enacting a specific situation.

As mentioned above, the group had been meeting for some time and the clients were familiar with choosing their own route to working. I suggested that the image of the shadow might be one she could include in the work. After discussion with myself Ana decided to use sculpting and begin a realistic role play. She wanted the shadow to be a character present in the scene with herself, the daughter-in-law and the son. I asked her how the scene should be presented. She said she wanted three group members to play herself, the daughter-in-law and the son. The shadow would be played by herself, wearing a veil. This she formed out of some red cloth from the prop box.

Four chairs were placed to one side of the area where the enactment would take place, and an audience area was indicated by Ana. Prior to taking on roles, clients would sit in the four chairs, and these would also be used in the de-roling process, The group were familiar with this device. The enrolement consisted of sculpting and doubling. Ana used the group to sculpt a scenario: three clients were chosen by Ana to play herself, her daughter-in-law and son, and Ana sculpted them and put herself in the sculpt as the shadow. The scene took place in her own living room, the situation was a visit. Ana doubled herself, the son and daughter-in-law – she put her hand on each of the actor's shoulders in turn and said what she thought they were thinking and feeling. This was a way of starting to engage Ana and to brief and warm up the three other actors to their roles. She placed herself as the 'shadow' slightly behind the daughter-in-law.

When the playing started Ana was very disengaged at first and started to talk about other things, half in and half out of this role. It seemed as if she was losing her engagement with the material. Ana turned and looked at the group and myself, saying 'No. That's not right.' She added that this was exactly what happened: she couldn't actually confront the daughter-in-law. We re-played the scene and the same thing happened again. After being asked if she wanted to change anything she said that maybe it would help to talk as the shadow at first, alone. She said that she wanted to tell the story of the shadow herself and the others in the scene.

We paused the action as I discussed the way this would be done. Ana decided that she would hold the role of the shadow and that three people from the group would help to portray the story to the daughter-in-law, her son and herself.

The story told of how the shadow had lived inside other people's suitcases for all its life. It had been born into a suitcase and had slipped 'from one case to another' – never being owned. People would take it out and put it on with their other clothes without noticing it was there – but when they did they felt sad, confined, for no reason. They threw it away and left it until it managed to slip into someone else's case.

As Ana faced the family in role as the shadow, telling the story, she started to cry. At first she came out of role, but wanted to continue. From information that Ana had disclosed in the group some weeks earlier I knew that she had separated from her husband two years ago. He was now living with a woman with whom he had been having an affair during his marriage with Ana. I wondered at this point whether a part of this role of the shadow was to do with Ana's feelings concerning this loss, in addition to the loss she was experiencing in relation to her son. At the same time, the theme of being 'in the shadow' of other women seemed to be present – perhaps of both the daughter-in-law and of her husband's partner. On another level the role of the shadow could be potentially interpreted as a part of Ana's self identity, a part of herself which she feared or suppressed perhaps? In addition the role could also be functioning as a way of enabling Ana to express feelings she feared or had difficulty admitting to.

When Ana had finished the story I asked her if she wanted to say anything more as the shadow. She said no and looked puzzled. I asked her how she was feeling as the shadow. She said lost, rejected, used, left out. I asked her if these feelings were familiar in any way, from anywhere else in her life. After a moment she mentioned the situation with her ex-husband, but said that the shadow wouldn't speak to 'them'.

Still in role as the shadow Ana began to express a great deal of bitterness, anger, rejection, loss and envy towards both her husband and his partner. The daughter-in-law, the son and the representation of herself were present throughout this. The veil, whether deliberately or by accident, had dropped during this time.

When the 'shadow' had finished, Ana said she wanted to leave the role play. I suggested that the shadow might want to say something to those present at the story and her subsequent words, but she said she didn't want to do this, insisting that she wanted to close the role play.

I felt that Ana wanted to get out of role, but was concerned that she should de-role from the shadow persona she had created. In addition, an hour of the session had passed, only thirty minutes remained.

In this way Ana was able to express suppressed feelings and to begin to separate out a set of emotions which had become entwined in a way which was causing her confusion and distress. To me it felt as if there was still much potential for Ana in the material she had created. The levels of feeling she was expressing seemed to indicate this. I have suggested the many possibilities which were in my own mind during the session in terms of what might be present for Ana in the creation of this 'shadow'. However, I did not know what Ana was conscious of, nor yet what meaning she might be able to find in the creation. In the time left it was important that adequate time was left to de-role and complete the session. Ana had also indicated that she wished to leave the role play. I chose to work with her in a way that enabled the completion of the specific enactment but which would leave room for further exploration.

I did not want to push for Ana to begin to analyse the material at a pace which was not her own. In addition, too much conscious analysis of the material at this stage might possibly hinder her creativity and her exploration in further work. Questions in my own mind included why Ana had placed the shadow behind the daughter-in-law. Why had she let the shadow speak in front of herself, the daughter-in-law and the son? In what way could all four of the characters be parts of Ana's own self? I was interested in the shadow character – could this be linked to Jung and von Franz's notions about the shadow – the 'shadow is all that is within you that you do not know about' (von Franz, 1970, 6) – or their discussions of the anima and animus? I was also interested in the choice of red for the veil. The most important element was how Ana responded to and was aware of the material she brought. My reflections were to be taken to supervision – both to explore my own responses to the session, and to consider my task as a therapist in relation to the work. The key to the next stage of the session was to find a way for Ana to leave the enactment and to enable her to begin to make whatever meaning felt right for her at this time.

De-roling and assimilation

Case study 9.6 Ana's Shadow, De-roling and Assimilation

I asked Ana to return to the enrolement/de-roling chairs, to leave the role of the shadow as she had requested, putting the veil aside as an initial way of moving from the role. I suggested that the shadow could be briefly represented through an empty chair. I explained that this was a way of exploring what could be gained from what the shadow had expressed. We put a chair in the performance area, to represent the shadow. Ana could double the chair, giving it the voice of the shadow. Three chairs were presented for the daughter-in-law, the son and herself. The shadow gave a message to each of the people represented and they could give a response.

Ana then came out of the performance area back to the enrolement/ de-roling chairs and spoke to each in turn, giving a message to the daughter-in-law, her son, the shadow and herself. The clients de-roled by leaving the performance area and sitting in the enrolement/de-roling chairs. Here they spoke about how the enactment had felt for the role they had played and how they felt about playing the role. Ana was a part of this and spoke about how the shadow had felt during the playing, and how she felt about playing the role of the shadow. All the players then returned to the audience area, and the group moved to sit in a circle. This was followed by group discussion. Ana, the players and the audience all reflected on the piece. This was followed by a time when group members talked over what they were taking away from the session. Ana said that she felt good about letting her feelings out as she hadn't expressed them before: 'I felt guilty'. In addition she said that it had given her real pleasure to play the shadow, even though it had felt sad and lonely at the same time.

It is usual for a structure used within role activity to have a clear ending. At this point the client or clients will usually leave the roles which have been played. If work has been in a group this involves individuals both leaving the role they have played and acknowledging that others have also left their roles.

Activities often aim to affirm this fact. As noted earlier (see p. 202), the taking on of roles is culturally associated with disturbance. The usual ways in which people consider their own and others' identities have been shifted during the role activity. The notion of disturbance is important to remember in the de-roling process: it is not just a time for people to leave their enacted roles, but also a time for relocating and re-adjusting to people's usual identities. The actors also de-role for the audience. If audience members, those who have witnessed the playing, have strongly identified with roles, emotions or issues, they might need to de-role as audience members, and to witness the return of those involved as players as they move back into their usual selves as group members. For individuals who have been in emotional states, or for people who are vulnerable or who can become confused, or who are not used to dramatic role taking, clear de-roling is seen as important. It is an act of re-orientation. As in enrolement, it is important to understand the individual or group's specific needs in this area. The length, quality and depth of the de-roling will depend upon the specific group and the preceding role activity.

Assimilation involves the establishing of relationship between self and enacted self as represented in the played role. As discussed earlier (see p. 207) there are a variety of opinions concerning this aspect of Dramatherapy practice. Assimilation might take the form of further dramatic activity or verbal discussion within the session. Alternately assimilation might be left to occur outside the session, or might be considered to be happening adequately during the enactment and de-roling and therefore not needing specific attention within the session.

The Dramatherapist's role is to offer a procedure to disengage from the role activity, and to consider and act upon the way of dealing with how the group or individual assimilates the material which has arisen from the role work.

In the session described above the enrolement process helped to establish the de-roling process. The group knew that the chairs present at enrolement were to be used to de-role. This process was aided by the fact that the group were familiar with the procedure. The taking off of the costume was a part of the de-roling process. By asking Ana to give messages to the different roles within the playing, the emphasis is upon her *own* response, not that of the role she played. This helped her to further disengage from being in the role, seeing issues from her own rather than the role's perspective. A further factor was the discussion by all the players of how the parts they played felt in role, and how the players felt about playing the role. I helped the group by insisting that they refer to the played role in the third person – 'When he said . . .' or 'When the shadow cried . . .' – rather than in the first person. This too acts as a way of leaving the role. It does not necessarily mean that the feelings present in the enactment become diminished, but it helps the client to move back to their own identity. This is important both in terms of preparing to return to life outside the session, and in beginning to assimilate the work done in role into their usual identity.

The last part of the session was a verbal reflection, mixed with some silence. This lasted for fifteen minutes in the described session. This was in order to support the process of assimilation as described above.

In later sessions Ana worked further with the material she had brought. Other people worked on their own material, but shortly after Ana returned to the shadow – the persona stayed with her actively in the sessions for a while. Some of the work involved making a mask representing it. She wrote a poem about it and told another story which the group enacted. She later worked directly with her husband and his partner within a role play. She reported to the group that the situation between her daughter-in-law, her son and herself had eased. This was, she felt, in part due to her seeing and understanding the relationship between her feelings for the daughter-in-law and her husband's partner, and in part to acknowledging 'that shadow'. Her subsequent work with the shadow moved more directly to looking at it as a part of herself.

Role work in Dramatherapy enabled Ana to express a number of levels of material simultaneously and to develop and explore this material. Through costume, mask, role enactment, poetry writing and story-telling the role playing was extended – a variety of dramatic means aided the way the client could respond creatively to her problems.

Summary

1 In Dramatherapy a role involves the creation of a dramatic identity. This may be entirely different from the client's usual identity, or may be the dramatic representation of this usual identity. All work with role involves the development of a dramatic identity, the enactment of that identity and the separation from that identity.

2 In certain instances 'role' in Dramatherapy can refer to a focusing upon a particular role function. For example, the Dramatherapy work might focus upon a family role, a social role or a group dynamic role (e.g. daughter, friend or saboteur).

3 Dramatherapy can involve a client in creating a role, but this is only one possible option or element of enactment within the therapy.

4 A role enactment might be connected to other dramatic modes or processes within a session, or over a number of sessions.

5 The length and nature of engagement with role can vary according to the context and to clients' needs. The therapeutic work might involve only the creation of a role with no extended enactment, it might involve a role played within a traditional role play or a role might be taken up over a number of sessions.

6 Within a session the engagement with the created role can involve different degrees of absorption. A client might be highly emotionally involved or highly distanced. There might be a great deal of cognitive analysis and discussion in relation to a role or there may be none at all.

7 Engagement with the role might be momentary or might be prolonged. There is no emphasis put upon catharsis as in Greek tragedy and psychodrama, or the notion of climax as described by Welfare State. Nor is there emphasis upon the completion of a learning process as in the social sciences' use of role play. The dramatic contact is adapted to fit the therapeutic goals and needs of the client in terms of depth of involvement, length of time spent in role and degree of analytic reflection.

Chapter 10
Symbol and metaphor

In order to believe that all these castles, trees and rocks designed
in canvas and unnatural in outline and proportions are real, one
must will them to be real.

Hoffmann, 'Cruel Sufferings of a Stage Director'

Introduction

Symbols and metaphors occur within most aspects of Dramatherapy. The
case studies chosen in this chapter illustrate their variety – from a man
sculpting a group into a barbed wire circle, to a woman enacting a spider
god at the centre of a web, from an autistic young man telling and
enacting the story of a prince locked within a tower to the improvisation
of a hand that is stroked by a telephone.

The formation and expression of a symbol or metaphor within
Dramatherapy involve a particular kind of relationship with the material
presented by the client. This chapter aims to describe this special
relationship to look at how it can assist the therapeutic processes within
Dramatherapy.

The symbol: a nebula of meaning

In certain theatrical traditions, such as Kabuki, the twitch of a mouth or
a gesture of a hand has a deliberate symbolic significance. The bodily
movements and positions function primarily as symbolic signs with deliberate codes of interpretation. So, for example, a movement of the eyes
would symbolise 'the moon'. One way a symbol can function, then, is
as a form which represents something else. It need not have any physical
resemblance to the thing it represents. A symbol can also represent a
complex idea or concept: Christ symbolising compassion or the hammer
and sickle symbolising Communism, for example.

Symbols can also function in a more oblique way. For Jung (1959)
a symbol has many potential clusters of meaning and to try to select
one as final or definitive is to misunderstand the potency of the symbol.
As Eco observes, the content of the symbol is a 'nebula of possible

interpretations'. The symbol says that there is something that it could say, 'but this something cannot be definitely spelled out once and for all; otherwise the symbol would stop saying it' (1984, 161).

For Freud and for Jung the unconscious and dreams are a rich source of symbols which can be used by individuals to gain insight into trauma or distress within analysis. Freud's influential *The Interpretation of Dreams* (1900) centres around processes of symbolic representation. As Jones has said, within Freudian thinking 'A symbol is a manifest expression for an idea that is more or less hidden, secret, kept in reserve' (Jones, 1919). Miller sees the symbol as crucial to the way our unconscious mind relates to the outer world; it represents 'a sort of courier service which passes between the carriers of the internal fantasy life of the mind, and all that goes on out there' (Miller, 1983, 266). So in psychotherapy the symbol is something which is expressed unconsciously – through a dream or free association or through a painting. This is seen as a communication concerning a repressed trauma or problem. The act of psychotherapy involves trying to clarify this communication and by this process the client achieves insight, which leads to therapeutic change.

Dramatherapy acknowledges the wide variety of potentials which the symbol or symbolic ways of relating offer in therapy. The symbol might be used to create and express issues. A dragon seen across a ravine within a session might come to represent a number of important meanings for a client or for clients within a group. The opportunity to develop symbolisation within a therapy group for someone with a learning disability might have important consequences on the way they are able to relate to and understand the world.

The symbolic connection between the world of drama and the real world is crucial to the efficacy of Dramatherapy.

The metaphor: from one object to another

Linguistically the metaphor involves the bringing together of two different objects or subjects which have a particular contact in common. One is spoken of in terms of the other, as if it actually *was* the other. For example,

'My daughter is a butterfly in everything she does'.

Here we are not to believe that the daughter actually is a butterfly. The statement powerfully brings together qualities of the daughter and the butterfly. One thing is spoken of *as if it is* another. The making of a metaphor acknowledges that one thing has important connections with another. The qualities of the daughter and the qualities of a butterfly are brought together so that the butterfly-like aspects of the daughter are highlighted. The reason a metaphor can be made to link these two different subjects is that they have a 'metaphoric connection' – a common quality. This quality in the above example is the state of being unsettled.

A metaphor, then is a statement that brings together two objects and says that they are one. The two objects or subjects are quite different from each other, but are linked through the metaphoric connection. See Figure 10.1.

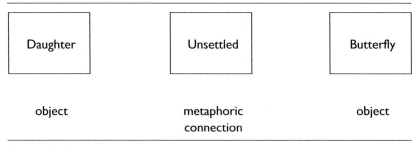

Figure 10.1 The metaphoric connection

Within therapy metaphors are introduced as a way into a closed situation. Often, if a client is blocked in thinking about a situation or problem, a metaphor is introduced. A family might be asked to name their familial roles as if they were kinds of creature. Skynner (1976) gives an example where the relationship between a woman and himself as therapist was illuminated by her use of the metaphor of his being a 'sea anemone'. This enabled her to talk about contradictory experiences of him – firstly as a warm comfortable person 'who made people trust me, but then I suddenly stung them, pulled their insides out and spat them out again' (Skynner, 1976, 343). The use and exploration of the metaphor helped both therapist and client to understand the dynamics of the therapy.

If something cannot be talked about directly then it may be possible to be talk about it through metaphor. The distance from the original object created by the use of metaphor helps the client to talk about something they wouldn't be able to do directly.

Within Dramatherapy the creation of dramatic metaphors performs similar functions. They allow a new perception to be brought into the therapy and can permit access to material which would not usually be allowed.

Two case studies follow which demonstrate the therapeutic potentials of metaphor and symbol in Dramatherapy. The first indicates how the expressive use of the metaphor can create a particular way of relating to problematic material within therapy.

Case study 10.1 The Prince in the Tower

The Dramatherapy group took place at a day centre for young adults who were autistic, over a two-year period. The group met once every week and consisted of one Dramatherapist, an assistant and, initially, three young adults. The clients manifested many of the features often ascribed to autistic people, including hands often being drawn up to cover the face, engagement in forms of ritualistic behaviour and resistance to any form of communication. Eye contact was limited and there was little voluntary verbal communication. Any change in the environment was experienced as extremely distressing and threatening. Having worked with and observed the clients prior to the group, I had noticed an insistence on maintaining an existing state. On one level, if a chair was not in the identical position to the one it was usually in, a client might need to put it back. On another level, if the usual progress of a day or a client's living conditions were disrupted this could result in extreme distress. Clients might self-mutilate or physically attack those around them.

The client I will focus on, Thomas, had many of the above traits. He would, for example, insist verbally on an unchanged situation when change had occurred. He would repeat over and over that a situation had not changed by listing the elements or factors around him which involved the change. When he had come to some level of acceptance in relation to the alteration, then he would list, in a similar fashion, the elements involved in the new situation. He also often withdrew from contact with people. He showed emotional effect from events in his life, such as the changing of some important component, but would not refer directly to his involvement or to any emotion.

Whilst reference to daily occurrences such as eating or day centre activities was allowed, any reference to more immediately personal matters was not permitted. Any question or reference would be met with blocking – no overt recognition that any communication had happened. This took the form of running away, covering eyes, ears or nose whilst humming, rocking, repeatedly jumping high in the air, or self-mutilation, such as biting.

One of the key difficulties experienced by the individuals was that, though they were clearly distressed by events in their lives, there was no apparent way that they could communicate about any experienced problem. In discussion with staff and parents a decision was made to run a Dramatherapy group which aimed to try to find a way to help the expression and exploration of difficult situations.

Two main questions emerged. The first concerned how to establish some sense of relation for individuals who seemed to exist largely in a world where relations were denied, avoided or, when present, were surrounded by difficulties. The second involved how to establish a contact, a method of communication or expression for the clients.

My aim was to see if it was possible to use the metaphoric value of story work. I wanted to see if it would be possible to establish a metaphoric relationship between Thomas's inner experience and the outer expressions of a story.

As has been documented by authors such as Bettelheim (1976), von Franz (1970), Gersie and King (1990), the form of story can provide a useful framework for therapy. Bettelheim sees the child's desire to hear stories repeatedly as due to the fact that in the 'fairytale internal processes are externalised and become comprehensible' (1971, 27). Both von Franz and Gersie and King describe how, for adults and children alike, stories can be used within therapy for their symbolic and metaphoric value. Within this approach the characters, events, scenery and scenarios become charged with symbolic and metaphoric meaning for the client.

The potential of this approach for this particular client group was in two main areas. Firstly, the metaphoric language (characters, story events) would mean that clients could deal with personal material without having to talk about themselves directly. Secondly, by acting the stories the participation would rely on physical and visual expression rather than upon the spoken word alone.

During an assessment period, the story vocabulary to which the individuals already had access was established. Assessment also considered the degree of capability group members had in order to construct and enact stories. In addition it was important to discover the extent to which clients could make connection between the story images and the problems they encountered in their lives.

The work had three stages to it. The first consisted of developing the story vocabulary of the group. It emerged that they knew a few stories, but it was felt that a wider vocabulary would assist the range from which clients could choose to reflect inner emotional states. In addition, due to the lack of verbal skills in the group, we wanted to find a method of storytelling which did not rely on words. To develop the vocabulary and to find a way to tell stories, we devised a series of story cards. These consisted of images of characters, events, scenarios and objects. Clients also made their own images from these stories (see Plates 10.1–10.3).

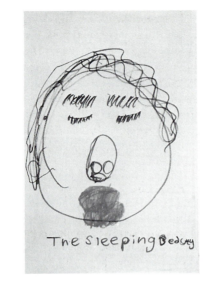

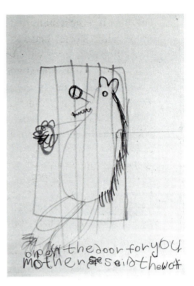

Plate 10.1 Sleeping Beauty

Plate 10.2 Open the Door for You Mother Said the Wolf

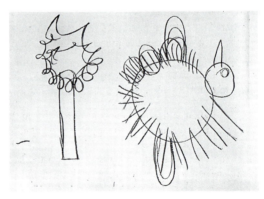

Plate 10.3 The Bird from Tree to Tree

The second stage consisted of group members creating their own images for story cards, creating their own sequences of images into a short story and then acting them out. At first these were simple: a prince who met another prince, for example. Another story was of a bird which flew from a tree to another tree (see Plate 10.3). As the group became more familiar with the approach the stories became more complex, and a move from stereotyped, repeated actions to more individual representations occurred. Images, characters and events from the original stories became transformed into a personal story language. The following story was made by a series of drawn images. The client then made simple statements about what was happening and completed a simple enactment of the story with the group. The story demonstrates this process: it is from the ninth month of the work. The client first created the story cards, then, by answering questions from the Dramatherapist, clarified what was happening. This was followed by a brief enactment of the tale. The story shows traces of *Sleeping Beauty*, *Rapunzel* and the *Three Little Pigs*.

> The story is about a prince. He wants a home. The house and the tower belonged to the witch. The witch was in the house. The prince was in the tower. The prince wanted to find a house outside. The prince in the tower would be happy when he was dead. The prince could get out of the tower if he hit the witch. When the witch came to the tower he hit and killed her and got out. The prince went into the witch's house. He went back to the house and they went for a walk.

It was not possible, for reasons made clear above, to reflect upon personal connections at the end of sessions. At the close clients were taken out of the roles of any characters they'd played, the cards were put away and a simple physical closure exercise was completed. However, in the story related above, it is possible to see that story elements are not only being adapted, but could be expressing feelings, inner dilemmas and anxieties.

The process outlined above is present in the following story from the same period:

> The story is about a hand – it wanted to be stroked. First mother came to it, she stroked it, but she also nipped it. The hand went to father but he was sawing. He stroked the hand but also gave it a nip. The hand went to the telephone. The telephone stroked the hand and didn't nip it. The hand ate an apple. The hand met a dog. The dog ate the hand.

Themes began to emerge as, week after week, images or scenarios would be returned to. This return to situations started to occur from the end of the first year of the work. The stories contained variants or different treatments of the images or scenarios. I would suggest that this marked not only the discovery of the internal resonances of the story work, but also indicated that the clients were returning to areas of conflict or difficulty which needed attention. The story-making and enactment was not only a place to make symbolic and metaphoric representations of unconscious material, but was also becoming a place to develop and explore alternatives, to make attempts to resolve and deal with those

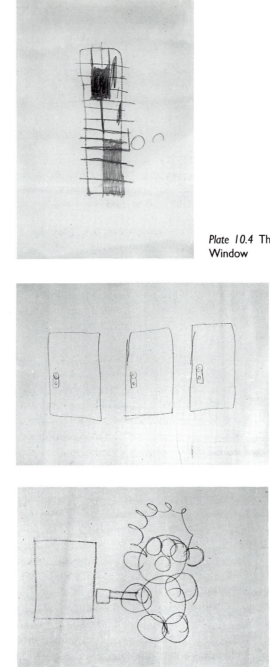

Plate 10.4 The Tower with the Window

Plate 10.5 The Three Doors in the Tower

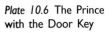

Plate 10.6 The Prince with the Door Key

conflicts. An image and series of stories which were constantly returned to by Thomas came to be called 'The Prince in the Tower'.

For much of the work the story consisted of a prince who stayed in a tower, and narratives usually concerned occurrences within the tower. A long series of stories concerned doors, locks, corridors and rooms within the tower. At first there was no window or door on the outside; gradually, a window shape appeared behind the bricks and a window and door emerged (see Plates 10.4 and 10.5). The tower became populated with images, objects and incidents (see Plate 10.6):

> The Prince is walking in a corridor. He has a key in his hand. He reaches the doors. He looks through the keyholes. The first is a dining room. There's nothing inside except a pile of knives and forks. In the second is a large bed, wardrobe and a table. In the third is a witch.

It became clear that these images were metaphoric. By this I mean that connections were being made by the clients with their lives. However, these were not directly, verbally, acknowledged. Thomas was able to use the stories to look at themes and problems in his life. As the day Centre was in contact with Thomas's parents we knew that themes from the individual's life were present and that the story alternatives seemed to be a way of talking about things which were not usually permitted by Thomas.

One example of this is the story of 'The Two Princes'. We knew that Thomas's brother was going to leave home. As said earlier, any change in the client's life situation was experienced as extremely distressing. His parents had alerted us to this, as on previous occasions when change had occurred Thomas had manifested a great deal of physical distress. At the same time, the prince in the tower was joined by a second prince. For a while the stories involved the princes staying together in the tower. They then went out of the tower together, one prince went on long journeys, returning to the tower. If there were any doubts in our minds about the connections which Thomas was making they were dispelled when, during a Dramatherapy group he, momentarily, referred to the other Prince by his brother's name.

Thomas was not able to discuss the situation or problem concerning his brother directly. However, he seemed to be able to alleviate his anxiety by firstly expressing his desire that his brother should stay, then experimenting with letting his brother go, whilst reassuring himself that his brother would return. The parents reported that the distress they expected did not manifest itself to the extent they had anticipated. This could be taken as some indication that the Dramatherapy group allowed Thomas to explore and express himself through metaphor and that this helped to alleviate some of his distress.

Dramatic metaphor: summary of basic process

A basic process relating to the use of dramatic metaphors in Dramatherapy underpins this work with Thomas. The first stage involves discovering the world of images both verbal and dramatic which the client or clients use or can use. Eco (1984) calls this an 'encyclopedia of reference' which someone draws upon in making a symbol or metaphor.

For the purposes of Dramatherapy it is crucial to discover whether the client can connect the images to themselves, to see whether they can make personal metaphors. In the case study this concerned whether Thomas could make the connection between the tower and himself, for example. One of the central metaphoric connections for Thomas involved the tower and himself – the metaphoric connection was that they were both 'Locked In'. The other involved his brother and the second prince, the metaphoric connection being that they were both 'Leaving'. Figure 10.1, used earlier to illustrate metaphor, is used again below to summarise the metaphoric process as used in the case study:

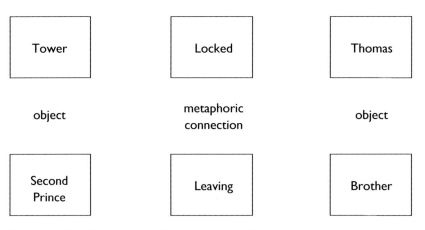

Figure 10.2 The Prince in the Tower: two dramatic metaphors

The next stage involves the use of the connections made within the metaphor to explore a situation. In Thomas's case the exploration took the form of stories. These were drawn and enacted, enabling him to express and look at repressed feelings. The therapeutic effect of the metaphor lay in the way it permitted the release and expression of feelings which were repressed and censored within usual communication. As an alternative mode of relating to and describing an experience, the dramatic metaphor enabled release and change to occur.

The final stage involved the connecting of the metaphoric exploration to the life situation. With Thomas this did not happen through conscious insight expressed within the Dramatherapy session. There is, as described above, some evidence to indicate that this was occurring for him as shown in his verbal 'slip' and in the response to the departure of his brother in real life.

The basic process outlined above consists of three main areas. The first concerns the content and use of the client's vocabulary or encyclopedia relating to dramatic metaphor. The second area involves working with the client's identified problem through dramatic metaphor. The final stage involves the assimilation of the work.

The case study involving Thomas related to dramatic metaphors within Dramatherapy. The next case study illustrates the way a dramatic symbol can be worked with in exploring a problem.

Case study 10.2 Barbed Wire Circle

In a Dramatherapy session within a psychiatric day centre George was making a sculpt concerning his feelings in the group. The Dramatherapy part of an arts therapies programme was running as a closed group and was in its sixth week. Over the previous weeks I had established that the group as a whole was familiar with drama as a medium and was able to use complex dramatic forms. Symbols and metaphors were used naturally by the group in working with individuals' experiences and in looking at the dynamics of the group.

George had sat out of many activities within the first five weeks of the group, but had said that he wanted to show us his feelings soon after the sixth group had started. The group had begun in silence, as was the custom, and people had started to talk about their feelings about working together. George took each group member and sculpted them in a circle. He put himself in the centre of this circle and placed me outside, some distance from the circle. I was placed looking towards the circle and George was looking out towards me. He then doubled each aspect of the sculpt, saying that the circle was made of barbed wire, that I wanted to get in, and that he wanted to get a rifle and shoot at me to keep me away.

I encouraged George to explore this, firstly by free associating with the feelings he had within the circle and then exploring the feelings, briefly taking on the roles of 'the barbed wire' and 'the person on the outside of the circle'. We then looked at whether the symbol and the feelings it contained had any associations or connections for him from other aspects of his life, his past.

He was able to discover a number of meanings in the circle: it brought back memories of his relationships with his father and with his lover, Andrew. He also made connections with the symbol as a representation of different parts of himself in a struggle. One part of himself within the circle wanted to stay isolated, alone. The circle represented the 'ill state', as he called it. The person on the outside represented the part of himself that was well and scared of the ill part of him with the gun.

George selected one area to focus upon. He chose the circle structure as a representation of the internal battle between parts of himself. By becoming the different parts of the sculpt – the ill part inside, the healthy part outside, the circle-barrier and the gun – he was able to develop the exploration of his dilemma. I invited the different parts of the sculpt to enter into dialogue with each other – for the George within the circle to talk to the George outside, for the barrier to have a voice.

Group members also doubled for George when he was playing the different parts. For example, whilst George was playing the 'ill George', saying that he didn't want contact, that he wished to stay inside and would shoot the 'well George', one of the group doubled him in this role saying simply, 'It's safe here, I know what it's like. I don't want to move.' Another immediately doubled, saying, 'I need your help but I don't know how to say this to you.' George accepted both of these doubling statements.

After exploring the different parts of the symbol I asked George to step outside the sculpt and to think of anything he'd like to say to any of the parts of the sculpt. I invited him to address any specific aspects such as the barrier or either 'George' directly. He did so, expressing a wish that the barrier might have a door in it saying, to the gun that it could be put down but not disposed of, and that the 'well' George should extend his arm and hand to the inner George. I asked for a new sculpt to be made reflecting these messages and we explored it as we had done the original sculpt.

At the close I asked George to step outside and, once more, to say anything he wanted to the sculpt. George and the group members in the sculpt de-roled by physically leaving the stage area, stating their identities and discussing what it was like to be in the sculpt. Group members talked about issues the sculpt had raised for them, connections they had made with the symbol. George talked about his experience within the enactment and discussed the connections he had made, both to his relationship to his own illness, his relationship to the Dramatherapy group and to his partner, Andrew. Though the struggle was still there and still difficult for him he explained that it had enabled him to see a little of what was happening inside him and how he might at least begin to feel easier with himself and with the group. At least, he said, the gun was put down. He also said that the sculpt had enabled him to understand that some of his feelings towards me were to do with his own internal struggle and feelings about Andrew.

The symbol of the circle which George brought to the group was used by him to explore a number of significances. When originally creating the sculpt George had a specific attached meaning in mind: it was an image representing his feeling in the group. As the circle was a symbolic expression made by George it was loaded with a number of other possible significances. By identifying other possible meanings and personal connections George was able to have access to the potential of the symbolic nature of the sculpt. By a way of working akin to a dramatic free association, he was able to see parallel or repressed relationships and issues present within the original sculpted circle.

Once these repressed feelings and associations were acknowledged the symbol proved a way of working with the associations. Its specific meaning changed from being a sculpt to represent the group to a sculpt representing an internal struggle within George. The dramatic symbol could contain both situations. As described above, through embodying and playing the part of different aspects of the sculpted symbol George was able to connect with the internal personal struggle. He was also able to consider a way of changing his relationship with the problematic aspects of the struggle. In addition the symbol helped George to try out what it might feel like to make the change. He did this by entering the changed sculpt and experiencing what each part felt like once the change had been made.

The symbolic expression, then, enabled George to express a problematic feeling, to connect it with other repressed feelings, to explore the repressed feelings in the present and to consider and try out change. He was also able to gain insight into the original presenting problem – of how his difficulties in the group reflected an internal struggle of his own. In addition it enabled him to explore some of his transference feelings towards me as therapist. As one group member observed, and as George himself acknowledged, 'the gun was still in the sculpt'. The work described did not aim to achieve immediate change regarding George's situation. Rather, it offered him the opportunity to deal with a part of a problem. The symbol produced many other resonances which George could go on to explore. The symbol itself and the work we did with it in the session marked a part of an ongoing process. The symbol and the themes it raised were worked on by George for the rest of the therapy.

Dramatic symbol: summary of basic process

The basic process beneath this is similar in many respects to that of the metaphor. The first stage consists of discovering the dramatic vocabulary of a group and the way they use this symbolically: the encyclopedia of reference. It also involves discovering whether clients can connect symbols to their own personal feelings. In the case study above, this had been undertaken prior to the sixth session – as stated. I had established the way the group generally related to creating and using dramatic symbols.

The next stage involved exploring George's dramatic symbol. This entailed facilitating the dramatic expression of the symbol and the use of enactment to explore the different parts of the sculpt he created. This led to the development of the work to help to identify key issues around George's connections with the symbol. The form of the symbol was then used to try to help George to resolve some of the problems he identified as being connected to the symbol.

Finally George and the rest of the group were disengaged from the dramatic expression and worked on beginning to assimilate and connect with the exploration that had occurred.

As with the dramatic metaphor work, this area has three main phases: the encyclopedia, working through personal material using symbolic form and the assimilation of this work.

Dramatherapy practice: dramatic symbols and metaphors

Introduction

Some clients or client groups form relationships with dramatic symbols and metaphors quickly and spontaneously. They will be able to create, be aware of and use the richness of the symbol or metaphor. Other clients may create and use symbols within sessions but are developmentally unable to reflect and use them. For others, such as psychotic clients, the emphasis in Dramatherapy would usually be upon concrete and reality-based drama, rather than the exploration of metaphoric or symbolic aspects of enactment. For some clients it is necessary to introduce them to the way in which dramatic symbols and metaphors can be expressed and worked with in Dramatherapy.

Why work with dramatic metaphors or symbols?

As discussed earlier, symbols and metaphors are present in our everyday lives and in much dramatic expression within Dramatherapy. The issue for the Dramatherapist is how to deal with symbols and metaphors present in client work.

In some cases the Dramatherapist would only note the symbolic or metaphoric aspects of clients' expressions and work. In other cases, however, symbol or metaphor would be directly engaged with as a key focus within the work and this would usually be for the following reasons:

• An important symbol or metaphor has arisen in the work – as an individual's expressions such as the barbed wire circle or a group expression, or as something that has arisen for clients outside the actual session, but is presented to the group, such as a symbol in a dream.

• The process of working through symbol or metaphor will introduce a different perspective on the problem being encountered by the client – such as with the 'Prince in the Tower'. The language of metaphor or symbol frees the exploration.

• The process itself, of relating through symbol or metaphor, could be therapeutic. This is less to do with the content of the symbol or metaphor, and more to do with the developmental step or change being made by the client. Someone might only be able to deal with the concrete, the specific. By relating to the world differently through the dramatic symbol this facilitates a new way of relating to the world.

Dramatic metaphors and symbols – main processes in Dramatherapy practice

As briefly described earlier in the summaries of basic processes (see pp. 230 and 234), there are parallels in approaches to working with symbol and metaphor.

The main processes within Dramatherapy practice are:

- The way a client relates to the 'encyclopedia'. This refers to the vocabulary which they draw on for symbols and metaphors in exploring a problem, and the way they use this vocabulary.
- The way dramatic symbols and metaphors are worked with and explored within Dramatherapy.
- The way the symbol or metaphor is assimilated into the clients' awareness of the presenting problem.

The following three sections explore these processes in detail.

The encyclopedia

The Dramatherapist needs to be aware of the kind of terms, issues and objects which a client naturally draws upon in terms of symbol or metaphor, what their vocabulary is and how they use it. A kind of encyclopedia is created, which 'allows both speakers to figure out the "local" dictionary they need in order to ensure the good standing of their communicative interaction' (Eco, 1984, 80).

This may become clear incidentally within enactment and discussion. As the group talk and improvise, the parameters of reference emerge. They might naturally work with certain themes – 'fairy tales', 'the immediate hospital environment' or 'light and dark'. For example, clients might speak of experiencing their lives as 'being lost in the dark'; in drama work a symbol such as a deep well might occur or recur.

The therapist might use exercises to ascertain the language of the group. One example of this is a simple exercise where the therapist invites the group to consider and mime an object that has some quality in common with themselves. A client might mime an armchair, an apple or a discarded paper tissue. A further development of this might be for the client to say something about what they consider the common quality to be. Another exercise involves clients taking on the role of a character or becoming an object which has a quality that is very different from themselves.

To see how a group as a whole relates to symbol and metaphor a similar exercise would be to put a drawn shape such as a circle on the floor. The group are asked what it might be, what group members' associations with the object/image are, or to create brief improvisations based around the shape. The responses give information about the kind of relationships with symbol and metaphor the group form together. There may be a variety of levels of response or one level of response might be expressed. For example, the answers 'hole' and 'plate' would indicate that an imaginative relationship to objects can be made: the group are able to make the circle into imaginative objects. On another level answers that include the circle representing 'completion', 'exclusion' or 'the group' show a capability and willingness to use objects or dramatic material to connect to personal and group themes.

This exploration of the client's encyclopedia of reference also gives information about the levels of connection with the expressed metaphor or symbol. Does the client easily make reference to the implicit levels of meaning or do they work only with the explicit level of meaning? What degree of connection or interpretation is made?

This is ascertained:

- By noting the connections made spontaneously during an exercise or in reflection afterwards
- By simple questions, such as 'Do you think that the creature shared any characteristics with you?' or 'Do you think that there are any things about the circle that are like you or like this group?'

This information begins to reveal the vocabulary the group use to create metaphors and symbols. This, in turn, gives the therapist information about the kinds of concerns or areas present. The way the group or individual use the symbolic or metaphoric expressions also becomes clear. For example, a group may express themselves through a symbol, but might not easily engage in exploring it for personal significance. For example, they might improvise a situation where people were on a journey and came across a chasm. The group might later reflect upon the chasm as a geographical feature only. The therapist may perceive this to be a symbol for clients' experiences of the group or their fears to do with their illnesses. Alternatively, the group might make connections with the chasm as a symbol representing personal processes. In either case the Dramatherapist is given information about the group's current way of relating to symbols present in the work.

The vocabulary, capability to work with symbol or metaphor, and the level of acknowledgement of possible meanings and connections are all part of the 'encyclopedia' which clients work with in creating dramatic metaphors and symbols. Once the therapist has begun to understand the clients' relationships to the encyclopedia, they can begin to develop the relationship and to develop the work which can be undertaken.

Ways of working: exploring the connected world

Most forms of dramatic expression within Dramatherapy can yield symbolic or metaphoric connections or material. All the following can contain dramatic symbols and metaphors.

Story and myth

Stories and myths contain figures, landscapes and objects which can be used as symbols or metaphors by clients. For example, Anansi the spider god at the centre of her web became a metaphor for one woman's self-image. The stealing of the sun in a Native American myth took on symbolic significance for a group, connecting with themes of deprivation, illness, despair, the ending of the group.

Play activity

Objects can take on symbolic or metaphoric value. For example, a small lion toy and its fear of leaving its lair became a metaphor for a small child's fear of leaving the house. An extinct volcano in a group play exercise became a symbol for what was being repressed by the group.

Role/character

A fantasy character or role can become a metaphor for a specific person – for example, a fussing mouse becomes a metaphoric expression of a partner. A role can also take on a symbolic significance. For example, a punishing, blocking character can become a symbol of the different forces that someone has encountered in their life. During enactments the setting or landscape can become metaphoric or symbolic. This can happen overtly, rather like in Bunyan's *Pilgrim's Progress* – a 'Mountain of Joy and Release', a 'Pool of Inertia', a 'Fog of Depression'. More covertly, a slope which clients slip down during an improvisation can take on symbolic significance for 'slipping' in their lives.

Body work

As discussed in Chapter 7, the body can be a rich source of metaphoric and symbolic material.

In Dramatherapy symbols and metaphors are connected to dramatic scenarios – stories, improvisations, object play. It is through the scenarios that the value of the symbol or metaphor is developed.

Case study 10.3 Anansi's Web

The metaphor of Anansi was explored through a series of short improvisations devised by Jan, a client in a Dramatherapy summer school, where different characters representing people in her life became stuck in her web. The client played Anansi, other group members played the characters, and the metaphor was developed as Jan explored the scenario. She improvised a story which told how Anansi wanted the people to stay with her on her web and didn't want to eat them. The characters were frightened by being trapped, and wanted to be freed. They were confused by the fact that they were stuck to a trap for food and yet Anansi was saying she only wanted friendship. Group members improvised these characters, based on brief information given by Jan. Here the client was able to extend her initial metaphoric connection with Anansi. She could deepen the connection, and the metaphor of the spider and web gave her the experience of being present in the living metaphor.

As the enactment developed the ambiguity of the messages Anansi was giving out concerning devouring and friendship became clearer. In addition the client's fear of overwhelming people, along with her own fear of being devoured and need to keep the people in place, to control their distance from her, came out.

The basic metaphor of 'I am Anansi' was connected to a dramatic vehicle which allowed the exploration of the metaphor. The drama allowed the metaphor to deepen and extend in relation to the client's perception of herself and the problem she is encountering. The enactment allowed the client herself to explore her feelings in the Anansi role, and to gain understanding through the actions and relationships of the spider.

In this work it is important for the group to be able to explore the symbolic or metaphoric expressions. If clients are too rational and interpretive then this can block the exploration. The aim should be to find a way for clients to be open to the material which the creation of the symbol or metaphor can yield. In part this is helped by ensuring that the individual or group are adequately warmed up prior to engaging with the metaphor or symbol. This helps in the absorption of the group in the symbols or metaphors created.

Connection and assimilation

Within Dramatherapy there are a number of positions relating to the ways in which clients can connect with and assimilate symbolic and metaphoric material.

Jennings (1987) and Mitchell (1992) state that it is not necessary for the client to reflect verbally or analyse the enactment. Their position is that the unconscious connections are made by the client within the drama. They propose that automatic verbal analysis following the work detracts from the process of assimilation by forcing rational dissection on to the experience. Dokter (1990), however, states that it is crucial to allow the unconscious images to become conscious. She suggests that this can only happen through verbal reflection and acknowledgement of the connections between the conscious self and the unconscious images and scenarios in the drama. Within this approach the connections the clients make verbally and cognitively are crucial to therapeutic change. Some advocate an unstructured time for verbal reflection whilst others advocate structured dramatic and verbal activities to enhance the process of connection (Gersie and King, 1990). The role of verbal interpretation made by the Dramatherapist within the assimilation process also varies within these ways of working (Dokter, 1990, 27; Jennings, 1991, 4, 1992, 41).

Within the approach which stays entirely within the drama the completion of the enactment would be followed by activities designed to de-role participants from roles or characters and to close the session. There would be no emphasis placed on a time to discuss personal connection. The work described in 'The Prince in the Tower' (see pp. 224–229) is a sample of this method.

Within the approach which advocates verbal and dramatic analysis, a time is left to de-role followed by structured or unstructured activity. In an unstructured way of working the Dramatherapist would allow the group members, or individual, to discuss their feelings in character, the responses of group members to the roles they played, and their in-role feelings towards others (see Chapter 9). This would include time to discuss any connections or insights they have in relation to their own life. A structured approach might include specific dramatic exercises and verbal exercises such as symbolic gift giving (Gersie and King, 1990, 57), pair reflection and structured sharing (Blatner and Blatner, 1988b, 112).

In the case study of 'Anansi's Webb' (see p. 239) closure used both these approaches. Each of the characters and Anansi were allocated a chair. The players then gave a short statement in role which summarised their experience during the enactment. The players were asked to leave the chairs and, as they did so, to leave the role behind. They were told that the chairs would represent the characters for a short while. The clients, as themselves, were then invited to give messages or verbally respond to the characters. Any client could give a message or say something to any of the chairs/characters. Following this there was unstructured time for people to reflect upon the enactment.

Closure contains a number of important processes. Firstly the summary enables the player to reflect upon the experience of the character. Leaving the chair helps clients to de-role: physically they leave the role behind. The statement that the role is temporarily represented by the chair reinforces this physical separation: the client can see the chair and they are asked to address the chair as if the chair were the character. In addition they are asked to talk to the character out of role – as themselves. This process reinforces de-roling. It asks the client to think or feel about the role from outside, rather than inside, the skin of the role. The physical changing of position, along with the request for a message, reinforce each other. This also helps the process of assimilation to begin. The clients are being asked to separate from and to relate to the characters they played.

It was at the point of closure that Jan verbally acknowledged her relationship to Anansi; 'I can see that I am like you. I want people too much. I can't let them go.'

The next stage of unstructured feedback allowed her to reflect further, and it allowed group members who had played roles to share with her their own experiences and feelings. It soon became clear that the feelings produced in them by the web scenario were connected to the responses of people in her life. She was able to see the relationship between the spider and the themes mentioned earlier. The initially self-punishing comment, 'I want people too much' was developed into a more balanced, insightful understanding. This change was helped by the verbal reflection of the client, by the responses of other people within the group who had been in role or who had witnessed the enactment, and by the therapist.

Whatever the stance taken on remaining within the drama, or upon the primacy of verbal cognitive reflection, it is clear that the assimilation of the symbolic or metaphoric expressions is crucial to the efficacy of the work. Whether this occurs within the enactment or within a prescribed period of time after the drama, the therapist must engage with the issue of how the client or clients are able to connect their lives with the symbol or metaphor. It is also important to provide space for clients to separate from the dramatic involvement with the material and to re-engage with their usual identity. As this chapter has shown, metaphors and symbols often take fantastic, imaginative forms, and these forms are given powerful emotional investment and involvement by clients. If clients are not offered the space to differentiate at the close of work, then this can feel extremely dislocating and can cause distress and identity confusion.

Summary

Work involving symbol and metaphor in Dramatherapy can help clients to engage with highly problematic material. They serve both to permit expression and to give a form for exploration of the presenting problem. The following summary tries to show how the dramatic symbol and dramatic metaphor operate within Dramatherapy.

In Dramatherapy a *symbol* is a way of encountering unconscious material and a way of negotiating between inner conflict, outer expression and potential resolution.

The symbol in Dramatherapy needs two things: a physical form and particular kind of relationship. It involves the creation of dramatic expression which is symbolic. This expression is an image, action, expression or embodiment which, whilst having a specific form has wider interpretative meaning in its relationship to the client.

Symbols in Dramatherapy can either be created deliberately or can occur spontaneously within an enactment. For example, a group might deliberately use an image such as a forest to explore its symbolic value and connections for individuals. Alternatively an enactment might contain a forest which starts out as an event in an improvisation, but which becomes a symbol as it takes on meaning beyond its original purpose as a functional part of a narrative.

This dramatic symbol may have a specific interpretative value for the client. However, the expressed form of the symbol may be seen as having no one definitive meaning or significance, as a dramatic symbol can take on a wide range of meanings and significances.

The dramatic symbol might be taken from cultural symbols which already exist (e.g. the cross within a Christian framework), it might be a representation of a symbol encountered elsewhere (e.g. in a dream); or it might be created within the therapy session.

The expressed meaning of a symbol in Dramatherapy may be less important than the experience of the making and expressing of the symbolic, dramatic form.

The creation or use of *metaphor* in Dramatherapy involves the bringing together of two separate entities which have a common connection. The two entities are made into a composite dramatic metaphor. For example, a client might experience their father as inaccessible and cold. They might create a castle of ice within an improvisation. Though they are improvising trying to gain entry to an ice castle, through metaphoric connection, the attempted entry is to do with the client trying to gain access to their father. The father and an ice castle are the two entities brought together into the dramatic metaphor.

This metaphor is a dramatic form or image which condenses the two entities into one form or image. The point of contact for this condensation is the common metaphoric connection. The common connection in the example above is 'Cold', 'Unreachable'.

The client is able to deal with one thing by means of another as a result of the metaphoric connection. Hence the client can deal with the father through the dramatic image of the ice castle.

A dramatic metaphor would usually be used in Dramatherapy when the therapist perceives that a new perspective is needed by the client, as they are 'stuck' with the material. The client may spontaneously create a metaphor for a problem during an improvisation.

The therapeutic potential of a dramatic metaphor in Dramatherapy is that:

• The dramatic metaphor creates distance from the actual real-life identity of the problem.
• The distance may enable the client to relate differently to the problem by creating a new perspective.
• The creation of the metaphor brings an altered relationship with the problematic material. By connecting the problem with the dramatic form in making the metaphor the client is opening up the way they see and experience the original.
• The creation of the metaphor enables the problem to be brought into contact with imaginative, dramatic exploration and with the therapeutic potential of the Dramatherapy process.

The process which occurs between the client and the metaphor during the session may help the client to work through the issue and the connecting up of awarenesses made during the exploration of the metaphor and the real-life original problem is important in the efficacy of the metaphor.

Chapter 11
Dramatherapy and ritual

Man must reassume his place between dream and events.

Artaud, *The Theatre and its Double*

Introduction

A relationship between Dramatherapy and ritual has been suggested by a number of theoreticians. Parallels also have been frequently drawn between theatre practice and religious or social ritual. In the twentieth century this connection has ranged from experimental Holy Theatre to the work of Schechner and Boas in the anthropology of performance. The meanings given to the word 'ritual' in these comparisons and relations are extremely varied; in this chapter, I intend to identify a number of these areas of meaning and to look at their relevance to Dramatherapy.

In answering the question 'What is ritual?' it is important to consider the rituals and attitudes towards ritual of different cultures. Themes concerning ritual which are often considered relevant to Dramatherapy cover a range of areas. These include:

- ritual as a means of connecting with a reality or state which is different from the everyday
- the ritual use of artefacts
- behaviours and expressions particular to ritual
- healing and ritual
- the relationship between dramatic enactment and ritual

What is ritual?

Lewis (1980) describes ritual as a fixed procedure bound by rules. Turner has defined ritual as a prescribed formal behaviour 'for occasions not given over to technological routine' (Turner, 1969). Berne refers to ritual as 'a stereotyped series of simple complementary transactions programmed by external social forces ... The form of ritual is ...

determined by tradition . . .' (1964, 36). Haviland defines ritual as a way in which important events are celebrated and in which crises are made less socially disruptive and less difficult for the individual to deal with (1978, 342). Some describe the purpose of ritual as being allied to fundamental processes at work within society: Chapple, for example, says that myth and ritual are forms which mediate between a society's overall social organisation and the biological rhythms of human individuals (Chapple, 1970).

Douglas has described ritual's role in maintaining 'the relation between both individual psychological needs and public social needs, both expressed by symbolic acts' (1975, 61). This mediation includes the rituals of the life cycle and rites of passage at birth, marriage and death. Rituals are also used to create a relationship with the seasons – such as harvest or mid-winter – as part of initiations and in relation to historic events. Others have commented upon the function of rituals to bring together or unify a worshipping community (Ray, 1976, 86), and the ritual's capacity to meet both individual and group needs at the same time (Scheff, 1979, 144).

Myth and ritual are often linked. Harrison, in her researches into early Greek religion, says that myths and rituals are both expressions of collective emotion (Harrison in Perry, 1976, 80). She notes that in some cultures rituals often derive their form from mythic patterns which are considered to be sacred in origin.

Scheff's writings are particularly useful in considering Dramatherapy's relationship to ritual, and describe 'ritual and . . . myth as dramatic forms for coping with universal emotional distress' (Scheff, 1979, 115). He defines ritual as the 'potentially distanced re-enactment of situations' of emotional distress that are 'virtually universal in a given culture' (Scheff, 1979, 118).

The link here between ritual form, enactment and dealing with distress is of interest when considering how ritual and Dramatherapy might relate to each other. It is often argued that ritual and Dramatherapy are connected as they use enactment to deal with experiences of distress.

Attention in Dramatherapy has often focused upon the relationship of healing to ritual. This has involved the consideration of rituals from various cultures. Discussion is mainly in terms of the role of the shaman or healer, along with the nature of the relationship between the activities within the ritual and the way healing occurs.

The following discussion of the 'Wind Babai and the Madusdus Ritual' gives an example of this approach within Dramatherapy.

Case study 11.1　Wind Babai and Madusdus

Connor (1984) describes a ritual connected to the Balinese 'balian' whom she describes as indigenous healers. An individual suffering from a problem is brought to the balian for help. The cultural context of the ritual is described in terms of the way the balian understands the individual's problem. This is seen in terms of possession. Putu, a Balinese woman, is considered to be the victim of witchcraft. She is described as sobbing quietly most of the time, and has been sitting immobile for several weeks. She does not respond. She is vacant-eyed and apparently deaf. The balian feels the body of Putu and locates the problem beneath the jaw and in the armpit; he diagnoses a 'wind babai', *babai angin*, as living there. A babai is described by Connor as a small demon-like creature, which, according to the balian, is the result of witchcraft initiated by a rejected lover of Putu.

An exorcism, a smoking ritual, madusdus, is seen as the solution. This will drive out the babai. Putu's family are asked to be present. Two small human effigies, a male and female, are made out of cooked rice. They are set on the ground to the south of Putu. The babai is driven out of the body by the smoke from a pot between her legs, and is attracted into the effigies. Once the babai is in the two figures it can then be discarded along with the effigies. When this is completed Connor notes behavioural change in Putu – she stays at the house of the balian for a two-week period preparing further purification rituals (Connor, 1984, 253–254).

One way of considering the madusdus is to see it in terms of a ritual of healing which uses an active means to bring about change for Putu. The use of the cooked rice effigies, the physical use of the smoke, the witnessing or presence of the family and the role of the balian in identifying the problem and providing the format are all important aspects of the ritual. Some Dramatherapists would parallel the use of objects here with a client's use of dramatic projection in working with objects such as puppets or dolls in Dramatherapy. Others see this kind of parallel as being problematic, as will be discussed later.

Drama, theatre and ritual

Drama and ritual are connected by both contemporary anthropologists and experimental theatre practitioners. Ritual space is seen by some to be akin to dramatic space. Landy, for example, says, 'Ritual activity . . . is dramatic, as it calls for the subject to create a representational world through symbolic means' (Landy, 1986, 67). Douglas has referred to the way in which a number of rituals rely upon the belief that events can be changed 'by mimetic action' (1975, 23). Authors have analysed part or the whole of ritual forms in terms of dramatic processes or dramatic form. For example, Hope considers the high mass, the role of the celebrant and the Catholic Tridentine in terms of their relation to drama, and sees them as containing 'a degree of role playing' (1988, 79).

Artaud, Brook, Barba and Grotowski have all rooted their theatre in the notion of performance as a form of ritual. They speak of its efficacy as a means of communication, and its power to touch the performer and the audience emotionally and through religious feeling. These different theatre experimenters have linked their theories and their practical work to the concepts and expressive languages of ritual. Grotowski's Theatre of Sources or paratheatrical activities, for example, has been paralleled with ritual. He describes it as 'bringing us back to the sources of life, to direct primaeval experience, to organic primary experience' (Roose-Evans, 1984, 154).

Artaud, in the first manifesto of the Theatre of Cruelty, speaks of theatre as needing to turn away from text and the realistic portrayal of bourgeois life. He argues that the theatre needs to become a place akin to a church, holy place, to 'certain temples in Tibet' (Bentley, 1976, 62). He says that theatre must deal directly with ideas which touch on creation, becoming and chaos. It must provide a 'primary' encounter with these areas in a way which contemporary theatre does not. Theatre becomes, for him, a form which will be able to create 'a kind of passionate equation between Man, Society, Nature and Objects' (1976, 56).

Innes has linked this kind of thinking in theatre to disillusion, to a search for an antidote to an overly rational culture, a desire to turn from Western materialism toward an alternative value scale. Ritual, he argues, becomes linked with a primitivist notion that, in ritual, myth and in non-Western cultures, a pure form of theatre can be discovered which can communicate powerfully (Innes, 1993, 10). He, like others, says that this desire to 'borrow' from other cultures is often 'deeply questionable'. It is often based on nineteenth century imperialist notions of other cultures being simple, basic and pure, or on a 'superficial exoticism', where the work is valued for its surface only.

Brook, speaking about his International Centre of Theatre Research, argues that each person can respond to the cultural forms of races other than their own. He says that 'one can discover in oneself the impulses behind these unfamiliar movements and sounds and so make them one's own' (1988, 129). His route is to find a 'complete human truth' which he sees as global. The task is to bring the 'jigsaw' together, and he sees the theatre as a place to fit the pieces together.

Practitioners such as Schechner (1988) have begun to develop an approach to performance and to ritual which tries to establish a model of intercultural working which is less rooted in racism and colonialism than the work of many of the theatre practitioners mentioned above. This approach stresses the importance of dialogue between cultures, between practitioners and cultural forms rather than the mere appropriation of surface elements of non-Western forms by Western individuals.

Efficacy and ritual

A problem often referred to in relation to ritual concerns its validity and efficacy. For some individuals ritual is felt to be effective: it has meaning for them, it is useful. For others ritual is experienced as alien, meaningless or irrelevant. As Goffman says, 'Ritual is a perfunctory, conventionalised act' (Goffman, 1961, 62). From religion to sport, there is frequently a perception that contemporary rituals are impoverished reflections of their predecessors or those existing in other cultures. This notion is common in Western responses to ritual. Scheff, for example, suggests that in modern Western society the connection between strong emotion and ritual appears to have been severed, and religious rituals are perceived as having decreased emotional meaning (1979, 129).

Some see ritual as a 'negative' force or form which enables society to contain problematic elements. Viewed in this way ritual is seen as essentially conservative and a force against change.

Current studies tend to indicate two possible positions regarding ritual. One viewpoint advocates the power and usefulness of ritual, the other stresses alienation and the lack of efficacy (i.e. negative uses of ritual). One asserts that ritual can function in a number of ways which have beneficial and positive functions for group and individual processes. The other view of rituals includes the notion that they contain and oppress and that contemporary rituals are ineffective.

A research group on ritual was set up with sixteen Dramatherapists, who aimed to explore aspects of the relationship between ritual and Dramatherapy. Each participant filled in a questionnaire concerning their background and their experiences of ritual prior to the start of the work. They completed a form analysing and recording their responses to the active work undertaken within the research. The practical work took the form of a number of activities designed to engage with aspects of ritual using Dramatherapy. Participants came from a variety of different cultural backgrounds and racial groups and were of different religious belief systems. They were asked to identify their experiences or feelings towards ritual. In many ways the findings reflected the two positions described above.

Comments on positive examples of ritual included the following:

- 'Marking significant stages in the development of the individual.'
- 'A strong container to elicit, support and carry through strong feeling.'
- 'Ritual has fulfilled an emotional or physical need which resulted in a shared experience – a coming together.'
- 'Rituals which serve a very personal purpose, where the ritual has grown out of a personal need and where it has structure and rhythm which give their own safety and boundary.'

Negative examples or experiences with ritual included:

- 'Not being initiated into rituals.'
- 'Fears of feeling, participating, being rejected, getting it wrong.'
- 'Feeling of unfinished or unconnected rituals: for example, not closing the curtains at my grandmother's cremation service.'
- 'Incomplete, insensitive, fierce, detached.'
- 'Imposing and controlling . . . imbalance of power . . . no choice.'
- 'A funeral which was cut short because of rain and improper burial equipment. There was no acknowledgement of my family's need (and right) to accompany the deceased, my grandmother, to the graveside.'
- 'Rituals which are shallow or empty because they have become stultified with time.'
- 'Those belonging to something alien to me. For example, religion. These rituals make me feel excluded. I feel as though I'm missing something at a fundamental level that everyone else understands.'

As this chapter will show, this division or ambiguity in relation to ritual's efficacy is at the heart of the way in which Dramatherapy and ritual can usefully connect.

Dramatherapy and ritual

There are two main areas of connection made between Dramatherapy and ritual by theoreticians. One approach says that Dramatherapy is a ritual. The other approach refers to ritual as a mode of healing using enactment. This is then linked to Dramatherapy's use of enactment or becomes a rationale in justifying how and why Dramatherapy uses drama to heal.

Some have argued that the basic assumptions behind Dramatherapy of a fixed structure with active participation can be paralleled with the psychological and emotional functions of ritual. Others have indicated spiritual links between the ways in which ritual can function as an act of worship and the ways in which Dramatherapy can have a spiritual component (Grainger, 1990; McNiff, 1988). They often refer to the spiritual links between health, curing illness and religion which are present in other cultures and which is currently denied in mainstream health provision in the West. Spiritual aspects of the healing which occurs in Dramatherapy are then emphasised, as if Dramatherapy is an equivalent of non-Western rituals.

Landy asserts that one of the key 'reasons' for applying drama to therapy concerns what he calls the 'traditional therapeutic function of theatre' (Landy, 1986, 47). He goes on to connect this with a statement that the ritual and healing aspects of theatre performance have been demonstrated throughout history. This pattern of associations is not uncommon within Dramatherapy: leaps are being made between ritual and healing, theatre performance, history and therapeutic function. This approach tends to take other cultures' phenomena, groups them as a term, 'ritual', and reinterprets them as a pattern for Dramatherapy. Part of this process seeks to create an ancient lineage and cross-cultural significance for Dramatherapy.

Elements of these claims may be of interest when considering and practising Dramatherapy. My concern is that there has been little critical consideration of the ways in which the connection of Dramatherapy with ritual can be of practical use.

I would argue that therapists are often unclear as to what they actually mean by ritual. Vast, vague statements are made about this other world of perceived ancient power.

Dramatherapy has been too quick to claim other cultural practices as its own; too eager to draw parallels between itself and ritual. Dramatherapy is not a ritual. The Dramatherapist is not a shaman. To draw links between the shaman and the Dramatherapist in such a way as to say that the shaman uses role play, or that the contemporary therapist working within a completely different cultural and racial context can 'use' rituals from other cultures and races, is to ignore the complexity of this area.

As Schmais has pointed out, the shaman usually operates in a non-literate tribal society, with roots in a polytheistic, animistic philosophy. Illness is seen as a result of supernatural forces – a loss of soul, an invasion by a spirit power. In the West where most Dramatherapy is practised she says that this would be classified 'as conversion hysteria and simple nuclear forms of schizophrenia' (1988, 281). The primary focus for many shamans is to intervene between spiritual forces and humans. To claim that the Dramatherapist is a shaman presiding over a ritual is inappropriately to 'align ourselves with a mystical religious tradition and declare that our primary mission is to intercede between man and the supernatural' (1988, 301). She stresses the importance of considering the content and form of any process in terms of its cultural and social context. If this is ignored and elements of ritual are simply lifted and transplanted, 'we proceed at our peril'. The Dramatherapist ignores crucial differences when they take techniques rooted in another time and in another social context (1988, 283).

It is important to try to establish a clear framework to describe the relationship between Dramatherapy and ritual. Schmais goes on to say that it is possible to develop a relationship to ritual and shamanic practices but that these must be carefully thought through. Below is an attempt to define a framework and relationship which is based in the practical ways in which ritual and Dramatherapy can usefully connect. The approaches outlined attempt to avoid the problems noted above.

The relationship between Dramatherapy and ritual can be located in three key areas:

- The *reproduction of incomplete or problematic ritual experiences* from the client's past, e.g. a distressing association with a barmitzvah, and *reframing* and reworking the experience.
- The *creation of dramas using ritual forms* to deal with client's material. This might involve the creation of an improvisation using ritual language to acknowledge a life event which has been ignored. Another aspect of this area is the use of ritual form as a way of expressing and dealing with material brought to the therapy: for example, the creation of improvisations using ritual language to mark endings or beginnings.
- Aspects of the Dramatherapy group which can usefully be considered or analysed within a *'ritual' framework* (e.g. rituals which the group create), such as patterns of exercises or ways of relating at the start or close of sessions.

Dramatherapy practice and ritual

The basic relationship between ritual and Dramatherapy for the client and therapist can be summarised as follows.

The client in Dramatherapy:

- can bring material from rituals which have featured in their lives which are experienced as problematic
- can create dramatic representations of these experiences in order to work with and resolve the problem
- can create their own dramatic rituals to deal with personal material

The Dramatherapist:

- can help clients to re-create experiences of ritual which are problematic in order to deal with the difficulty they have encountered
- can work with clients to create their own dramatic rituals using the group or individual's own cultural language of ritual

Re-framing rituals

In Dramatherapy rituals may not only be referred to but can be reworked or worked through using the *language* of ritual. This means that the movements, sounds, words and interactions may be re-created within the expressive language of the therapy. In verbal therapy the ritual can be spoken about, or experiences relived or worked through in recollection or in the transference relationship. In Dramatherapy the recollection or working through can be done in the language of the ritual form itself.

This active use of the language and form of ritual within Dramatherapy is useful, given the area referred to earlier: that some individuals feel disenfranchised or alienated from ritual. Evreinov has pointed out the importance of individuals feeling that they connect to the rituals they experience in society, and says that it is an aspect of the theatrical instinct. Active participation in ritual allows the individual to feel that they are connected with others, have ownership and a sense of power in life. When life becomes actively reflected in the enactment of the ritual, 'it acquires a new meaning, it becomes *his* life, something he has created' (Evreinov, 1927, 27).

In Dramatherapy the ritual is re-created within a framework which allows the individual to explore the ritual and its relationship to them. The enactment of the ritual means that it can be used in improvisation, the individual can explore different ways of responding to the ritual, or can accommodate the ritual to themselves by adapting its form.

So, for example, in 'Hyacinth' below the individual can reframe a funeral. A verbal analysis of the experience would demand some cognitive grasp on what occurred in recollection of the event. Given the individual's age, this would not seem to be the most effective way of dealing with her distress. By using expressive forms of sand play and projective play to reshape and rework the elements, a more effective experience is obtained. A client finds a way of relating to the ritual within a therapeutic framework.

Case describes this work in 'A Search for Meaning: Loss and Transition in Art Therapy with Children' in *Images of Art Therapy* (Daley *et al.*, 1987). Though she is an Art Therapist her use of play in the following example is of interest to reframing in Dramatherapy. She identifies the child's problem in connection with the fact that 'Children often seem to have part knowledge of or part access to the necessary rituals surrounding death' (1987, 59).

Case study 11.2 Hyacinth

A child, Hyacinth, had witnessed and been frightened by the power of her grandmother's cries at the funeral of a close relative. She had cried and screamed as her grandmother had. Case (Daley *et al.*, 1987), however, records that this was problematic for the child; it was an imitation with no working through of her feelings about the death of her younger cousin.

In the art therapy session the child is using sand trays, moving sand from one to another saying, 'I'm clearing up in here, I'm making it clean.' The child makes a mound in the sand. She says 'It's a grave.' Hyacinth uses a box in the art therapy sessions and makes it her home. Case relates how the child remains silent in the box for twenty minutes, then 'an eerie wailing began to emanate from the box, a crying and the words "My son! My son" . . . I saw Hyacinth wailing over the monkey, cradled in her arms, apparently, how her grandmother had wailed over the body of the dead child.'

This wailing continued off and on through the next fortnight, woven into the 'house' play. Case describes the pattern which the child makes in the sessions: house play, work with the monkey and wailing as a 'ritual'. She also describes how the child's participation in these activities gradually reduces in intensity. On the last morning of the therapy she came into the session, leapt into the box, 'announced briefly "My son! My son," and leapt out to begin another activity'. The box is not used again.

This is an example of an almost symbiotic relationship between therapy and ritual. The therapist demonstrates an awareness of the importance of ritual in mourning in terms of emotional development. She also clearly identifies the way it features in the problem offered by the client:

'Children may not be allowed access to rituals surrounding death which provide both a socially accepted expression for grief, and a framework to hold the very basic fears which arise' (Daley *et al.*, 1987, 59).

The practice demonstrates how therapy can provide an environment for the child to work in a way which enables her to create her own images to digest and deal with the ritual. Within the therapy the child creates her own rituals to aid the process of mourning and loss.

A number of people in the research group mentioned above found that the reproduction of elements of ritual involved a powerful re-evaluation of the ritual or the problem attached to the ritual. A participant discovered, for example, just how powerfully the rage was still present with her in terms of an incompleted ritual, 'unhappiness with inadequate . . . incomplete ritual':

> Sculpt of rage. Taking mother's body after long wait for a) dying b) death c) burial service to crematorium. False smile of sympathy on face of flunky bringing flowers unburnt round to the front. Furnace not on that day. Bring to be left like so much rubbish. no guarantee what was in the box of ashes later. Powerless. Frustration.

One set of exercises involved individuals sculpting ritual experiences which had been experienced as problematic. Another involved brief improvisations of difficulties in rituals from people's lives:

> Sculpting my wedding – having talked endlessly and at length about my wedding and marriage I was amazed that the sculpt I used said it all in such a concise and powerful image. (It's a shame I didn't sculpt these feelings prior to the wedding – perhaps I wouldn't have made the mistake of going through with it.)

Opportunities were offered to improvise a different version of the ritual, to rework the ritual experience in order to reframe it. Participants could express feelings through the dramatic representation of the ritual. They could also comment about the ritual and their experience of it during and after the re-enactment. A life experience was identified and described by individuals. They then sculpted others into a depiction of the ritual, and participants were informed of the details of the situation. The individual then directed and watched the improvised version of events: the individuals could then say what they liked to those involved, could talk about the experience and rework it in a way which helped them to deal with the problem.

In this way participants could choose to rework the ritual experience to fit their specific emotional needs. If necessary they could deal with unfinished business left over from the ritual. Individuals could also gain insight into their responses by bringing the event into the here and now of the Dramatherapy work and could discuss the activities and feelings with the group and facilitator. For example, one individual worked with a childhood experience in Africa concerning the pressure put upon him by ritual expectations due to his gender. Another example from a past experience of ritual involved Greek celebrations of Easter.

Case study 11.3 Easter Cake

A chair was put to one side of the performance area and Zanetta sat in it. She described the ritual experience and her problem with it. The focus was the ritual of baking an Easter cake, which in Greek culture is undertaken by the women of the house. The problem was that as an adolescent she had been forbidden to make the family cake one year as she had been menstruating. She had and still felt anger towards the situation and towards her grandmother at her exclusion.

Individuals from the group were invited to play the roles involved in the situation and were sculpted into position by Zanetta who described the kitchen where the activity took place.

The key moment of the grandmother's refusal to let her take part in the ritual was played. Zanetta talked about her feelings at this point and doubled each of the roles. She then re-played it in a way which she would have found satisfying. She chose to make her own cake in the kitchen alongside the grandmother. This, for her, meant both respecting the grandmother's feelings and attitudes toward the ritual, whilst finding a satisfying role for herself. She then addressed her grandmother and the person representing herself in relation to what the experience had revealed to her about the incident, the ritual, her relationship to her grandmother, and what she had discovered to take back to that ritual in the future.

Here the original experience of the ritual is problematic. This is due to the attitude towards women within the ritual and Zanetta's response as an adolescent. Although this experience came from Zanetta's past it is also relevant to her ongoing experience as a woman in relation to this ritual. Additional factors present within the work are Zanetta's relationship with her grandmother, her adolescent self, her own response to cultural attitudes to women, and her own feelings about menstruation.

As so often in working with ritual forms, the chosen image is one which is rich in condensed meanings and issues.

The ritual is reproduced by role playing. Zanetta's relationship to the ritual is explored through enactment and witnessing. She is able to re-experience the ritual, to alter her relationship to the experience and to the ritual itself. She chooses to confront her grandmother with words which were unspoken in the original situation and finds a way of challenging the ritual. She keeps the original ritual of the cake baking and bakes her own cake. As this chapter will later reveal, some of the group felt that this did not fully challenge the attitudes to women and to menstruation, but for Zanetta this was an outcome which satisfied her. She could satisfy her unfinished need to find words and ways to challenge the ritual and yet find a position that felt comfortable in relation to it.

From this, I propose a four-stage process concerning the reframing of ritual in Dramatherapy:

1 The recollection of an issue which is connected with a ritual.

2 The use of ritual 'language' to recollect or to represent the issue. This process begins to adjust and adapt the language and experience to the client's own expressive repertoire.

3 This process of adjustment and adaptation is taken further into the client's work on the issue.

4 A working through of the original stuck or incomplete experience using the new adjusted ritual language OR the client achieving insight into the problems encountered in the ritual experience.

The creation of dramas using ritual forms

Ritual has a specific expressive form and has content which is particular to it. Dramatherapy can enable clients to use their own cultural experiences of ritual form and content to create their own rituals. It is useful to describe these as dramatic rituals as it differentiates them from social and religious rituals present in society at large. Social and religious rituals are the product of large, historic processes and have generally evolved over a period of time. The dramatic ritual is the created product of an individual or group and is created within the space of a Dramatherapy session to deal with the problems brought to therapy.

The dramatic ritual is akin to the rituals created theatrically by practitioners such as Barrault, Grotowski and Barba. Often in this work a group uses ritual language – masking, gesture, posture, chant, repetition.

There is a use of ritual form and patterns. Many work with material from their own culture as well as using the spontaneous creativity of the cast or director to produce their own language of gesture or chant. In the 1980s, the ISTA (International School of Theater Anthropology) attempted to work cross-culturally, exploring the relationship between the languages and forms of Kathakali, Balinese ritual and Noh, for example.

Ritual form is seen to have a specific relationship to the feelings produced whilst it occurs. The production of dramatic rituals often echoes this relationship between form and feeling. This relationship is summarised by Grotowski as a powerful way of creating access to strong feelings and the holding of those feelings:

> There is no contradiction between inner technique and artifice (articulation of a role by signs). We believe that a personal process that is not supported and expressed by a formal articulation and disciplined structuring of the role is not a release and will collapse in shapelessness.
>
> (Grotowski, 1968, 17)

Forms of ritual expression and the production and management of emotion are of relevance to Dramatherapy. The presence of created structure in the context of powerful emotion prevents a collapse into shapelessness; this is true for the shape of sessions and for the way enactment is used as a whole in Dramatherapy. Ritualised expression does, however, have specific aspects of structure. It involves an especially useful relationship between the structure and the expression – the holding and release of strong emotion. It usually involves the creation of a pattern and repetition, with an emphasis upon symbolic and non-narrative expression using chants, gesture or sequences of movement.

Another part of the research work involved utilising the elements of the languages and structures of people's experiences of ritual to create a form to satisfy an emotional need. This could be said to work with the notion that ritual can be seen as suited to deal highly effectively with certain cultural, emotional and psychological areas. These areas are those usually connected to changes in status, position or identity, or to religious contexts.

Small groups of four or five chose areas to work on and then create ritualised dramatic forms. These contained patterns of movements, repetition and chants based on their own cultural experiences of ritual. The form and type of content was seen to evoke particular kinds of responses.

Strong reactions were noted by many members to vocal chants,

- 'Listening to the orchestration of sounds literally made my hair stand on end (on arms and back of neck!)'
- 'It enabled entry into another dimension of experience where voices, intentions and "conversation" became both explicit and symbolic. It was perhaps the closest I came to an "ecstatic" or "altered perception" which I feel is essential to an experience of ritual.'

Patterns of movement to express particular emotions were structured and worked with in the small groups:

- 'I was amazed how just by repeating the movement my emotion of being pulled in all directions became more real and accurately reflected my intense feeling of anger at being in that position.'

Case study 11.4 Menstruation Ritual

One piece of work involved a group of women who all identified a feeling of absence in their lives. This concerned the lack of acknowledgement of women's bodily changes and menstruation. For some of the women the work was triggered by the feelings of anger in Zanetta's exclusion and denial from the Greek Easter ritual. This was seen to be an illustration of the way their bodies and selves had been denied.

In Zanetta's experience of being excluded from the baking ritual because of menstruating I felt so angry on her behalf and I wanted her outcome to be different. I wanted to tell her grandmother that she was continuing a cycle of oppression and to challenge it, not to accept an alternative which still accepted the old way.

The new ritual gave me a chance to work with women who had similar dissatisfactions around the lack of symbolic rites of passage into womanhood; as well as culture's reticence to be explicit about bodily, emotional and psychological changes through the maturation process.

A group of four worked on the creation of a set of repeated movements, vocalisations and the use of objects to achieve a retrogressive acknowledgement:

We were a group of four women – one grandmother, one mother and two women who did not have children. We wanted to make a ritual to celebrate the start of menstruation. This celebration had been absent

> from our lives. We all began by holding a long sheet of material which we threw out in front of us. As we stepped on to it each of us worked with a series of movement patterns.
>
> The use of a symbolic cloth in our new ritual was very effective as it defined a ritual space.

The group had previously worked on anger and had experienced difficulties in working with the feeling, the exercise and with each other, 'not being able to gel as a group and find the same starting point'. In the creation of the ritual they found a way of making contact, uniting in an experience and dealing with an experience that was both individual and collective.

The created ritual involved the following:

• Finding a common need
• Devising a way of working which was effective as an emotional and expressive form
• Dealing with unfinished business

The recollection of an absence, the anger evoked by the experience of an individual and the problem of working together were all used in the new ritual these women had created in the research group. They were able to find a group form which had individual meanings. In one sense the group's work reflected Evreinov's ideas cited in Chapter 3. These described the importance of effective rituals for individuals in owning and taking power in relation to life events. The group's witnessing each other and publicly marking the unacknowledged onset of menstruation was the basis of the therapeutic work.

Many of the group remarked upon the work's effect in validating the experience of menstruation and of being a woman. The importance here was not only in being in the ritual but the therapeutic benefits of *making* the ritual as well.

One woman remarked that the silence around the onset of menstruation was still with her: 'such an important transition in my life but it went almost unnoticed, certainly not celebrated or enhanced'. To create a ritual was a 'wonderful' liberation of this material. 'Something that was always treated as a whispered, frightening, unclean secret into a positive greeting of a life transition'. Another commented of this work 'I was able to find some release and the feeling of having given/received and worked together positively.'

Another participant described the experience of creating a ritual as follows:

These experiences were all planned, meaningful and physical. I found myself very engaged with them and could have repeated them for a great deal of time with the group. I felt the experience worked at a level which was emotional, symbolic, embodied and free of language constraints.

A number commented on how the creation of a planned form using ritualistic theatre form helped to express and contain very powerful emotions:

Amazed at how closely/intimately we related to each other . . . my anger was manageable . . . incredibly powerful and exhausting and safe . . . I was able to get in touch with my feelings of anger quickly and to reach the 'scary' point and go beyond this . . . I felt close to tears but was able to continue until I had released my feelings.

We repeated a movement to work with the emotion . . . when I was reaching a point of frenzy where it might get dangerous my body automatically closed and responded to a movement which the other two in the group were also doing. We had our eyes closed and yet we were doing the same thing. It was as though the body has a memory of a response to a frantic emotion and movement.

Case study 11.5 A Marriage in Reverse

Alan said that he couldn't understand his feelings towards his wife. She had left him for another man and he felt numb: 'I don't feel a thing and I don't know why.' He said that he'd had a dream, but couldn't remember very much about it. One part, however, he could recall. He was standing at the altar with his wife in a church. He said that he couldn't understand why he'd dreamt that, as his situation was 'like a marriage in reverse'.

Initially he presented the dream as a joke, but as the session progressed he decided to explore the image. I suggested that he try to connect the dream with his following phrase concerning the 'reverse' marriage. He described and then improvised his marriage ceremony in reverse. With other group members he improvised the taking off of the ring, its return to the best man. The vows were removed: 'I no longer have you to hold' and 'I am no longer with you in sickness nor in health' were two of the phrases he used.

During the improvised, created ritual he became distressed and started to cry, but wanted to follow it through until they had returned down the aisle and went separately out of the church.

The images created here were experienced by Alan as being very powerful. It enabled him to move from his numbness, both to recognise the actuality of his situation and to release the feelings which were latent in the dream image and 'reverse' phrase he brought to the group. The created ritual acted as a way of releasing and creating access to his feelings which he said had been 'frozen'. In addition, the enactment of the ritual in reverse helped Alan to go on to do further work. The session developed a further role play after the ceremony. In this role work Alan confronted his wife with the things he had kept inside himself, moving on from the 'numbness'. In a later group he said that he had been able to go to his wife and to express his feelings. This was experienced by him as a 'liberation' and enabled him to feel that he could move on in his life.

Summary

Both the 'Menstruation Ritual' and the 'Marriage in Reverse' (see pp. 258 and 260) involved the creation of dramas using ritual forms. The following summarises this process in Dramatherapy:

- In some cases a need is identified concerning the absence of a ritual in the client's life. In others a problem is expressed which might usefully be worked with through ritual, or through ritual forms of expression. Problems or issues most suited to this approach are usually related to areas with which ritual is connected in the client's culture. Examples of these include changes in status, changes in identity or in the life cycle, and religious material.

- The client or clients use ritual forms/patterns and content from their own experience as a basis for the creation of a dramatic ritual. This involves building a dramatic ritual using aspects of form and content such as repetition, chants, patterns of movement, songs, call-and-response.

- The client experiments and improvises with these forms until they arrive at a dramatic ritual which adequately deals with and expresses the problematic feeling or area.

- In some work the expression or creation of the ritual in the therapeutic work results in a change (occurring in the relationship) to the feelings or area to which the dramatic ritual refers. This is due to the use of the form to express material. The experience of the created ritual can also be a means of containing and reaching a different relationship to the problem or issue. Here the emphasis is upon the dramatic ritual as a way of expressing and resolving the material or issue. The creation of the 'Menstruation Ritual' is an example of this way of working.

- For other work the dramatic ritual enables the effective expression of the problematic material or issue. Once expressed, the material can be worked with as in other areas of Dramatherapy as described in Chapter 2. Here the emphasis is upon the created, dramatic ritual as the best way of expressing an issue or problem. Once expressed, the material can be worked with using techniques such as role playing or story work. The 'Marriage in Reverse' is an example of this approach.

Chapter 12
Assessment, recording and evaluation in dramatherapy

> Whatever we see could be other than it is.
> Whatever we describe at all could be other than it is.
> Wittgenstein, *Tractatus Logico-Philosophicus*

Introduction

Vernon, in his survey of assessment in therapy, has pointed out that many dramatists, writers and artists have excelled in the portrayal of character 'but seldom stopped to ask how they, or we, get to know people, or how accurate is our knowledge' (1969, 2). This is debatable – many would argue that the arts and certainly much drama engages with these very questions. However, Vernon does encapsulate the concerns at the heart of assessment, recording and evaluation: how do we know people in Dramatherapy and how accurate is our knowledge? The answer to this must always be 'partially'. There are many routes to apprehending, describing and knowing oneself or another. For Dramatherapy a part of the way the therapist tries to know others is through assessment. Another aspect of this process concerns the way we try to understand what has happened over a period of time within the Dramatherapy – this is evaluation.

Assessment

A basic aim of assessment is to find out as much as possible regarding the client and the difficulties they are encountering. A further aim is to find out how they might proceed to use the Dramatherapy space to work with the material they bring to therapy.

Assessment gathers information. It can do so in a number of ways and from a number of sources. Usually Dramatherapy is practised alongside other therapies and treatments, and a Dramatherapist might use the documented information which has been gathered within these other activities to support their observations. All Dramatherapy, however, uses direct assessment within sessions to gain information. This might include the therapist using a variety of methods to help clients assess themselves.

The Dramatherapist can make use of a variety of formats and approaches to assess the clients they work with.

In some situations the process will be connected to diagnosis. This concerns the identification of the client's problem or condition according to set criteria. The assessment process might also include a consideration of a client's suitability for Dramatherapy.

Assessment is linked to the formation of aims. For some groups the main aims will have been decided beforehand. A setting might decide upon an aim for a Dramatherapy group as a part of its programme. Aims might be advertised in order to help individuals to decide whether they wish to attend the therapy. For example, a women's Dramatherapy group run in a community centre dealing with assertiveness might be advertised locally before its start. For other work the specific aims will be negotiated with the group or individual once the therapy has started. In some work the aims might be very general: 'To bring about personal change'. In other situations aims will be very specific; for example, 'To use role play to enable individuals to become more assertive in their everyday dealings with people in the community'.

Evaluation

Aims are evaluated by the Dramatherapist and by clients within the therapy. Bruscia has defined evaluation as documenting 'whether the client's original status did in fact change as a result of the therapist's interventions' (1988, 5). In some work this might be formal. For example, in a Dramatherapy group whose aim is to develop a particular kind of behaviour or mode of relating to others, the client might be asked to evaluate their own progress. This would entail asking each client to look back at their experiences within the group and within their lives in general. A number of headings or criteria might be used to help to focus this reflection. A group working with assertiveness might look at a series of criteria to evaluate their progress during the group. *Formative evaluation* takes place as the work is in progress and helps to orientate therapist and client. *Summative evaluation* occurs at the close of the work and looks back at the whole process.

Assessment and evaluation: the basic process

The basic process often used in Dramatherapy is as follows:

Referral Referral concerns the way in which clients come to the Dramatherapy group. This might be through self-referral. A setting might refer an individual to Dramatherapy as part of a specific programme for a particular group (e.g. a class in a school for children with emotional or behavioural difficulties). Individuals might be referred by a key worker (e.g. a client is referred to a group by their social worker).

In some settings there might be a referral assessment to establish whether a client's issues or problems are suitable to be worked with through Dramatherapy.

Initial assessment This is a period when the therapist and clients work together to obtain information on the problems to be dealt with, and on the ways in which the Dramatherapy sessions might be used.

Formulation of aims Based on the information gained in the initial assessment, a series of aims are formulated which will guide the Dramatherapy. In some settings main aims might be decided prior to the group. In others they might be formulated once the group has been formed. In either case it is usual that aims reflect the initial assessment. These aims might be very specific or quite general, depending upon the context. Factors such as the Dramatherapist's therapeutic orientation, the length of therapy, and the nature of client group affect the nature of the aims.

Ongoing evaluation (formative) This is an ongoing process during the therapy whereby the work is evaluated. This consists of considering the efficacy of the work according to set criteria. Again, the nature of the criteria varies according to the therapeutic orientation, nature of the client group, etc.

Review of aims From the information gained by the ongoing evaluation, the aims are reviewed to see if they are appropriate and realistic. Following this review aims might need to be adjusted.

Retrospective evaluation (summative) At the close of the work a retrospective evaluation looks back at the process of the Dramatherapy, and considers the nature of the changes which have and have not occurred. This includes a review of the aims in the light of what has occurred in the therapy.

There are ethical considerations to be taken into account in relation to assessment and evaluation. The Dramatherapist must bear in mind the reasons why assessment and evaluation are occurring, how the information to be gained is to be recorded and used, and who will have access to this information. The issue of consent must be engaged with in terms of whether the client has consented to assessment. If the client is severely learning-disabled and cannot understand the concept of assessment, then the therapist must make sure that they deal with the situation with respect.

Ciornai (1983) has emphasised the importance of taking cultural and socio-economic factors into account within diagnosis, assessment and evaluation. She says that it is important for the arts therapist to take into account possible cultural biases and differences. The lack of acknowledgement of these areas can hinder understanding and communication within the therapeutic work. Ciornai gives an example of a therapist unfamiliar with Latino culture who may encounter values which seem to be 'symptoms of dysfunction or immaturity': within Latino culture these values are considered 'signs of health' (1983, 64). She asserts that understanding different cultural values is crucial to the prevention of misdiagnosis.

Approaches to assessment and evaluation in Dramatherapy

A wide number of approaches to assessment and evaluation exist within the fields of psychology, psychotherapy and the arts. As Courtney has said (1981), the form of assessment used within Dramatherapy will be connected to the orientation of the therapy and the therapist. To an extent, the conclusions drawn from assessment and the framework which the assessment uses is also influenced by the orientation of the therapist and setting. Hence analytically orientated therapy will utilise a different approach to work which is being undertaken within a behavioural context. Projective testing using enactment, when conducted to reveal aspects of the client's unconscious world, is more orientated towards a psychotherapeutic way of working with Dramatherapy. A series of drama exercises designed to show the different developmental aspects of the client's way of responding to situations is effective within a developmental framework.

Most assessment approaches, however, can be used within a number of frameworks in Dramatherapy. A projective test which looks at role behaviour through role playing a series of scenarios can be useful to both psychodynamic or behavioural approaches. The way of reading the information gained in the assessment would differ. Within a psychodynamic framework the kinds of themes and content expressed during the role work would be seen as reflecting the client's feelings and unconscious material. The behavioural assessment would be looking at the particular behaviours manifested by the client in the role situations in order to see where work needed to be done in altering behaviour.

Interviews, projective testing, along with structured and unstructured participation, are listed by Bruscia as the main assessment approaches used by Dramatherapists (1988, 8). Dramatherapy often uses profile observation within assessment: the use of a series of observable criteria to describe a state or way of being. In Dramatherapy these usually concern the way in which the client uses drama, the way in which the difficulties they bring to therapy are manifested and how any potential changes might be observed or perceived.

As Read Johnson (1982) has documented, some Dramatherapy work is structured around a developmental paradigm. Here a problem or disorder can be seen as a blockage or halt in development. He identifies a number of developmental processes especially relevant to Dramatherapy (1982, 184):

- the complexity of the media of expression used
- the intensity of affect which an individual can tolerate without overwhelming anxiety
- the degree of interpersonal demand which can be experienced in interactions with others

He connects the assessments of these areas to the way the Dramatherapy's aims are formed: 'Treatment first involves an assessment of where in the developmental sequence the person has stopped him/herself, and then starting the journey again with the therapist as a companion and guide' (1982, 184).

Assessment involves a reciprocal relationship between the therapist and the client. 'New paradigm' approaches to research, as described by Reason (1988) and Rowan (1990), have emphasised this notion. This area has yet to be fully developed within assessment and evaluation approaches in Dramatherapy. However, aspects of new paradigm ways of working are important to consider in relation to assessment. The client becomes a collaborator rather than a subject within assessment, contributing to the planning and operation of any assessment.

The task of the Dramatherapist is to design a form of assessment which is appropriate to a particular individual or group and the setting or context of the work.

Why assess? The problems with assessment and evaluation

Assessment within therapy is a notoriously complex business and its use in the arts is contentious. A number of questions arise concerning the validity and appropriateness of testing, and much debate has taken place in relation to how artistic experiences and products can be assessed. The nature of criteria used and the conclusions drawn from them has been much argued over: there can be no absolute criteria in artistic judgement and assessment, and inevitably criteria are highly value laden and specific. Some schools of therapy have rejected the notion of assessment. In non-directive work the clients bring their own problems and 'effect [their] own re-integration of [their] conflicting perceptions and goals' (Vernon, 1969, 11). The effectiveness of most forms of therapy are difficult to 'prove'.

Why assess at all? The process is intended as a way of helping client and therapist to become as clear as possible about what is needed and what occurs within the therapeutic process. Assessment aims to provide a framework through which the therapist and client can understand what is brought to Dramatherapy and what occurs within the work. As acknowledged earlier this is bound to be a partial process. Many people have asserted that what occurs within an art form is too complex to be fully encompassed by a series of criteria. Others have pointed out the inherent difficulties in trying to reduce the processes of change in therapy to a small area described through assessment and evaluation criteria. However, once these difficulties are acknowledged, it is useful for the therapist and client to find a language to consider what is initially brought to the Dramatherapy and how the potential and actual changes can be described and named. It is important, though, to bear in mind that assessment is a partial process and also to be just as aware of what is not being assessed as what is being assessed.

Questions concerning reliability and validity also arise. Dramatherapy is an emergent discipline: there is not yet a great body of 'tried and tested' assessment methodologies and evaluation processes. However, there are a number of assessment methodologies and approaches utilised within Dramatherapy. Some of the early work in this area was based in the use of dramatic or play based approaches to assess clients for other therapeutic work or areas, but within the past decade an increasing amount of work has been developed which is specifically designed to be undertaken within Dramatherapy.

Historic background to dramatic assessment in therapy

Early forms of assessment using drama are varied in their approach. Moreno utilised a method titled the 'Spontaneity Test' (1953). This aimed to assess the degree of spontaneity manifested by clients. It involved giving clients a basic dramatic scenario and then asking them to respond to instructions without prior warning. He also devised the 'Role Test' in which a subject's role range or repertoire is ascertained. This is achieved by asking the client to enact a series of different roles.

In the 1940s the United States Office of Strategic Services used a test titled 'Improvisation' in the psychological testing of individuals to be recruited into the special missions services in the Second World War. Contained in 'Assessment of men', it describes a technique which was based upon brief improvisations of given situations. A scenario such as a difficulty between a manager and an employee might be given, for example, and testers would attempt to ascertain leadership or interpersonal skills. Rotter and Wickens (1948) developed a system using role play to ascertain the degree of 'social aggression' of an individual. Harrow developed another role playing test which involved the improvising of three different situations between two people. A ratings scale was used to ascertain factors such as 'responsiveness to others' and 'personal security and comfort displayed in role'. Kelly's fixed role therapy used the client's acting out of roles to ascertain their personal constructs (1955); Corsini used role assessment in management within business (1966); social skills were evaluated using role in devices such as the 'Situation Test' (Rehm and Marston, 1948).

Puppetry has featured in assessment for therapeutic purposes, much of it concerning work with children. Lyle and Holly discuss this in 'The Therapeutic Value of Puppets' (1941), and Woltmann has written extensively on the subject in 'The Use of Puppets in Understanding Children' (1940) and 'Diagnostic and Therapeutic Considerations of Non-verbal Projective Activities with Children' (1964). Irwin and Shapiro describe a technique for children which involves the provision of a number of different types of puppet and an analysis of the spontaneous exploration and use of the puppets made by the child. They describe how a therapist deals with the material of a one-hour session: 'The combination of the behavior which the task elicits and the "output" in terms of story material is rich in clinical significance.' The content of the story is used to ascertain 'the child's preoccupation', while the form 'indicates the way he deals with this' (1975, 89). They consider that the hero of the story can be seen to represent a projected perception of the child being assessed.

Early assessment occurred in the field of play and dramatic play; for example, Parten's social participation scale (1932). Piaget developed a series of cognitive play categories, which Rubin, and Serbel combined to assess social-cognitive components of play, looking at areas such as constructive play or dramatic play in terms of solitary, parallel and group interactions (1979). Smilansky produced a sociodramatic play inventory (1968). Murphy developed a miniature toy interview (1956), which aimed to observe free play and involved a series of miniature toys. It was analysed according to a series of criteria such as cognitive, motor and emotional processes. Lowenfeld's World Technique developed an assessment methodology involving sand play with prescribed objects, and Buhler (1951) and Lowenfeld (1970) have developed a series of scoring processes linked to the World Technique.

In the 1970s and 1980s, as Dramatherapy developed a more coherent identity, an increasing number of assessment methodologies based clearly within Dramatherapy emerged. An example of this is David Read Johnson's Diagnostic Role Playing Test (1988).

Until a range of specific thoroughly researched testing devices emerges, the Dramatherapist will usually refer to a variety of sources adapted for the purposes of the particular piece of work. The following section describes some of these and gives examples of their use.

Assessment methodologies

There are two main areas which the Dramatherapist covers in an initial assessment. The assessment:

- identifies the areas or difficulties which might be brought and worked with by clients
- identifies how the client might best find meaning in the dramatic expressive media within Dramatherapy

The first area focuses upon ways of helping to elicit or focus the reasons why the client has come to therapy. The second looks at the different aspects of the dramatic media within Dramatherapy and sees which is most effective for the client to work with in exploring and working with the material to be brought to therapy.

The following two formats aim to assess the way in which a client begins to use the expressive forms or media within Dramatherapy. The first focuses upon the way the client finds meaning in Dramatherapy; the second can be used to consider the way clients involve themselves in the expressive forms used in Dramatherapy.

The following is designed to assess clients' participation in a variety of exercises and activities which clients engage in spontaneously, or which are introduced by the Dramatherapist.

Meaning in Dramatherapy: an expressive inventory

I What expressive means can the clients use?

A = Absent   B = Brief use   C = Sustained involvement

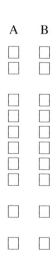

	A	B	C
1 Motor play	☐	☐	☐
2 Concrete play with objects	☐	☐	☐
3 Symbolic play with objects	☐	☐	☐
4 Acting out imaginary situations (as self)	☐	☐	☐
5 Games with rules	☐	☐	☐
6 Character or role for brief period (solitary)	☐	☐	☐
7 Character or role for brief period (with others)	☐	☐	☐
8 Sustained character or role work (solitary)	☐	☐	☐
9 Sustained character or role work (with others)	☐	☐	☐
10 Role from script	☐	☐	☐
11 Imitation of movement	☐	☐	☐
12 Production of movement linked to theme	☐	☐	☐
13 Use of voice to imitate sound	☐	☐	☐
14 Use of voice to represent pretended material (e.g. character or imitation of a sound such as the sea or an explosion)	☐	☐	☐
15 Uninvolved in any of the above	☐	☐	☐

II How does content emerge and develop in the work?

A = Absent   B = Present

	A	B
1 Themes emerge with no therapist intervention	☐	☐
2 Themes emerge with some therapist intervention	☐	☐
3 Themes emerge with high level of therapist intervention	☐	☐
4 Themes do not emerge unless given by therapist	☐	☐
5 Client/s not conscious of themes	☐	☐
6 Themes develop from one another within work	☐	☐
7 Themes develop with little connection	☐	☐
8 Themes develop with no connection	☐	☐
(If group)		
9 Themes mainly common to all group	☐	☐
10 Themes highly divergent with little common ground	☐	☐

III What is the nature of the relationships which clients can use within the work?

A = Not at all   B = With some difficulty   C= With ease

	A	B	C
1 Participation in large group activities	☐	☐	☐
2 Individual work in front of whole group	☐	☐	☐
3 Participation in pair activity	☐	☐	☐
4 Participation in small group activity	☐	☐	☐
5 One-to-one work with the Dramatherapist	☐	☐	☐

IV What is the relationship between the client and their dramatic expression?

A = In none of the activity   B = In some of the activity   C = In all the activity

	A	B	C
1 Shows concentration	☐	☐	☐
2 Shows enjoyment	☐	☐	☐
3 Shows motivation	☐	☐	☐
4 Shows involvement	☐	☐	☐
5 Shows spontaneity	☐	☐	☐
6 Reflection upon own response to activity	☐	☐	☐
7 Reflection upon others' responses to activities	☐	☐	☐
8 Acknowledges connection between personal material and dramatic activities (spontaneously, unsolicited by others/therapist)	☐	☐	☐
9 Acknowledges connection between personal material and dramatic activities (solicited by others/therapist)	☐	☐	☐
10 Evidence that connection may be present but not directly acknowledged to others by client	☐	☐	☐

The above combines elements from developmental play and drama models of assessment, Kott's (1969) semiotic-based assessment and Moreno's models of spontaneity assessment in order to help to ascertain general information about the client's use of drama.

More specific models of assessment are also available and used by Dramatherapists. Some of these are used directly, others are adapted to fits the needs of the context. The adaptation of scales is often necessary as they are designed for drama settings not Dramatherapy, or are aimed at play with children rather than play with adults in therapy. The following scale is an adaptation of the Sutton-Smith, Lazier Scale of Dramatic Involvement (1981). It seeks to give a general impression of involvement for a client's use of drama.

Jones' adaptation of scale of dramatic involvement

I Focus

(a) Within the dramatic activity as a whole

Focused   Occasionally focused   Often distracted   Distracted

☐   ☐   ☐   ☐

(b) in engaging with 'as if' behaviours

Focused   Occasionally focused   Often distracted   Distracted

☐   ☐   ☐   ☐

2 Completion

The degree to which the client completes tasks

Completes all tasks   Completes some tasks   Completes no tasks

☐   ☐   ☐

3 Use of imaginary objects

The capacity for creating and sustaining the use of pretended objects in a manner convincing to self and others

(a) Can create and sustain pretended objects   ☐

(b) Can disengage from object at end of the activity   ☐

(c) Can engage with other's created objects

      Until end   During part   Momentarily   Not at all

    of the activity   of the activity

        ☐   ☐   ☐   ☐

4 Elaboration

Demonstrating the capacity to develop and initiate ideas within improvisation or play

No elaboration   Useful elaboration   Too much elaboration*

☐   ☐   ☐

                                      * (detracts from enactment)

No engagement with   Useful engagement with

others' elaborations   others' elaborations

☐   ☐

5 Use of space

Use of space within dramatic activity: movement in improvisation, games or character-based work

Uses available space easily	Uses space well in relation to others	Confines self to small space
☐	☐	☐

6 Facial expression

Use of face to depict appropriate emotions or responses in pretend or improvised activity

Appropriate and constant use of face	Some attempts to use face	No use of face
☐	☐	☐

7 Body movement

Using body effectively and appropriately to dramatic activity or character, communicating information or messages appropriately

Appropriate and effective use of the body	Some use of the body	No use of the body
☐	☐	☐

Understanding information or messages communicated by others' bodies within dramatic work

Constant	For some of the work	Not at all
☐	☐	☐

8 Vocal expression

Emotional relevance and projection within activities

Constant	For some of the work	Not at all
☐	☐	☐

9 Social relationships

Awareness and response to others within the activities

Constant	For some of the work	Not at all
☐	☐	☐

Projective techniques

Another important area of assessment concerns the use of projective devices in Dramatherapy.

There are two main approaches to projective testing. One approach sees the material as revealing the emotional conflicts, drives and unconscious motivations; the other is object relations orientated. In this approach the material is seen to indicate the patterns and constructs which the individual makes with others. Vernon says that projective techniques are seen as 'revealing covert dynamic forces in the personality through their expression in fantasy, creative activity, play or free associations to verbal or inkblot stimuli' (1969, 13).

The social atom

An early form of assessment which uses the concept of projection is Moreno's social atom, which is a way for the client to express material concerning the relationships and interactions with those around them and acts as a means of eliciting this information. The atom can also be utilised by the client to focus upon the main issues which cause them discomfort within their life. Additionally it can be used as a means of gaining information to evaluate the changes which a client may have experienced in the course of the therapy.

The social atom can be drawn or sculpted. In sculpted form the client uses objects, empty chairs or others in the group to represent other people in their life, and they sculpt a map of their relationships. If the exercise is undertaken on paper then they use simple marks – a circle, for example – to represent the people in their lives. The client also represents themselves within the atom.

The client places the individuals in the room in relation to themselves. The distance and physical position reflects the way the individual feels about them. So, for example, a mother might be placed close to the client, a brother at a distance. The posture and shape of each individual should be used to show something about the nature of the relationship. Hence the mother might be placed with her back to the client, or with her arms stretched between the client and their brother.

The client then explains who is represented in the atom, and describes the nature of the relationships, indicating what they experience as difficult or problematic.

Some therapists use questions to help to elicit information. In some forms the client is invited to double for each of the positions and speak

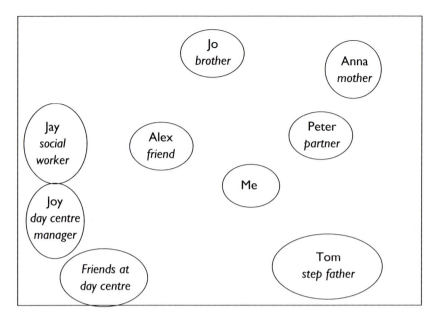

Figure 12.1 Social atom

about the client in role. The client can be asked to rank the people in the sculpt in terms of importance and then to describe the reasons for the choice.

This atom can be recorded through diagrams on paper, or through photographs or video. Later in the therapeutic work the social atom activity can be returned to and the nature of change evaluated through the different representations of the client's atom. Factors to note in any evaluation include the ways in which positioning and posture have changed, the way in which the client's verbal depiction of the different people has changed, and the description of the relationships.

Buchanan gives an example of using the atom in an assessment context and as a means of evaluating change. He describes one patient's use of the social atom over a period of eleven months and another over a period of one month. One client is attending an alcoholism treatment programme. As the therapy proceeds shifts occur in the content of the atom: for example, 'there were three deletions – prison, cousin and an old friend' (1984, 161). These are seen as negative elements by the patient in maintaining his sobriety. Their absence from the atom is seen to indicate a positive change. Buchanan concludes that if therapy is progressing and the patient is changing, 'then there should be a concomitant change in the patient's social atom' (1984, 163). He sees the atom as a barometer of change as well as being an assessment tool.

Role playing tests

A number of assessment and evaluation methodologies have been designed which focus upon role. These vary from Satir's use of sculpting family roles in order to assess family dynamics (1967) to studies based around assessing the effectiveness of dating behaviours. The following describes two ways of framing assessment around role.

Impro-I and Impro-C

Impro-I and Impro-C are two tests devised by McReynolds *et al.* (1976, 1977). They are designed to serve as personality tests and seek to develop a standardised, quantitative approach to the use of improvisation. The tests aim to measure the interpersonal styles of interaction of clients.

Impro-I consists of a series of twelve standardised improvisational role plays and two sets of rating scales. One rating scale concerns the effectiveness of the individual's performance in each role play, the other looks at the overall styles revealed by the client when all the role plays are compared.

Each role play involves the client improvising with one or two members of staff who play prescribed roles. There is an initial scripted dialogue which depicts a specific scenario and leads to a choice which has to be made in terms of the way the individual behaves in relation to the scenario. From this point the client and staff improvise. The dramatic work, including both script and improvisation, usually lasts thirty-five minutes. The scenarios involve the client in dealing with assertiveness, anger, sadness, appreciation. Contexts vary – some occur in work settings, others within intimate relationships. One scenario involves the individual dealing with a friend's experience of the death of a close relative, for example.

Impro-C was devised by two of the team involved in devising Impro-I: Osborne and Pither (1977), and is intended to complement Impro-I and is designed for couples. Like Impro-I it is designed to give information on interactional styles and aims to operate by the construction of a series of lifelike scenarios. The emphasis is upon the interaction and relationship between the two individuals in the couple. There are ten structured role plays, which are undertaken by the couple. Each of the individuals is given a separate brief for the role play scenario, which is a description of the situation described from the point of view of their own role.

The couple begin the role play until the assessor completes the work. Each individual is asked to assess how closely the way their partner and themselves resembled real life. An observer assesses the role plays on two scales: the first is a 'Communication scale' which focuses on the patterns of communications during each role play; the second is an 'Overall style scale' based on the ten role plays together and looks at the interactional styles of the couple. Themes for the role plays include 'conflict, distance, hurt, anger, stress, appreciation of self and appreciation of the partner' (Osborne and Pither, 1977, 262).

Johnson's role playing test

David Read Johnson's role playing test is designed to test and indicate the client's 'internal personality structure'. The individual is asked to enact a short series of roles. This improvisation is undertaken alone, and eleven props are provided (table, wastepaper basket, chair, stick, cloth, paper cup, book, hat, phone, man's coat and woman's dress). Five roles are given to be enacted – grandparent, bum, politician, teacher and lover (1988, 25) – and scenes are usually one minute long. A second test follows this: the props are removed and the individual is asked to improvise three scenes. The scenes involve action between three 'beings'. The individual describes the three beings and then improvises with them, telling the facilitator when they have finished.

The intention is to provide a sample of the client's role playing behaviour. In turn this is seen to give information about the personality structure of the individual, along with information about their concerns bringing them to therapy and about their use of drama in terms of role play.

The material is interpreted according to a series of categories to provide a framework for assessment. These include (1988, 26; 27):

- role repertoire
- patterns in thematic content
- style of role playing
- the way the client structures space, tasks and roles
- the interactions amongst the characters in terms of complexity
- the degree and forms of affect

Categories are divided into criteria to assist assessment. For example, the organisation of the scene is described in Table 12.1.

All of the above role playing tests assume that inferences about personality can be made from dramatised scenarios within the context of therapy. They select an area of behaviour and focus upon it. Each of the

Table 12.1 Diagnostic role playing test – complexity of representations

Item		Description
Organization of scene	1	Developed – characters and their interactions are presented in the context of a story with a plot
	2	Adequate – only characters and their interaction are clearly portrayed
	3	Incomplete – characters and/or plot are incompletely or vaguely portrayed
	4	Incoherent – no discernible plot, characters or interaction

Source: Read Johnson, 1988, 33

tests creates a fixed structure and seeks to assess clients through their individual responses. In all the tests or assessment exercises the emphasis is upon the therapist or professional using information to make conclusions about the client. There is limited opportunity for the client to participate in their own assessment.

Play influenced assessment

Play process and research into the assessment and evaluation of play have influenced the assessment of Dramatherapy. The following present a series of frameworks for assessment which can be useful to work with both adults and children.

Lowenfeld's World Technique

Lowenfeld's World Technique can be used as an assessment technique. As described in Chapter 6, it consists of miniature toys and a tray, usually made of metal or plastic, 75 cm × 52 cm (29 in × 20 in). The toys are divided into a series of basic categories which were listed by her (1970) as:

- human beings
- animals
- countryside objects (trees, fences, etc.)
- buildings such as houses
- transport (cars, ships, ambulances)

The work is divided into two stages: one is called 'The Bridge' the other 'Picture Thinking'. The first stage consists of the therapist informing the child that adults and children live on opposite sides of a river and there is a gap of understanding between the two. The work entails building a kind of bridge across the gap. The sand tray is introduced as a way of forming pictures in the sand: these can be anything the child wants and need not be realistic. The child can use any of the objects along with the contents of the tray.

Whilst the world is being made and after its completion, the therapist tries to find out the meaning the child gives to the different objects in the world and the relationships between the different elements in the world. This is done both through asking questions, and listening and observing what the child does with the created world.

Buhler (1951) has developed this technique for diagnostic purposes. The approach uses 160 set items and uses a square space for children, or a table for adolescents and adults. Some authors, such as Buhler, emphasise quantitative methods of assessing. Bowyer (1970) stresses the importance of qualitative methods, based on observation rather than measurement. This involves looking at the patterns of behaviour which emerge in the sand play and considering the way playing relates to the client's internal constructs.

Bowyer (1970) places assessment using the World Technique within a developmental framework. The therapist looks at the variety of the content of the client's play world, the way the client organises the material and the relationship between the different parts of the play world.

The client is assessed through their work with the created world. A series of areas is used as an assessment framework. A summary of these areas, described by Bowyer (1970) as useful in assessment, are:

- Area of tray used (on a continuum: Empty ⟵⟶ Full)
- Organisation (on a continuum: Chaotic ⟵⟶ Rigid)
- Use of sand: descriptive
- Expressed content: descriptive
- Amount of aggression

The work is recorded by diagram, photograph or video, and by comparing a series of created 'Worlds' conclusions can be made concerning the progress of the client.

As in the role tests the assumption here is that the work with the play world reveals aspects of the client's personality and experiences in a way which can be described and, to some extent, measured. As with the social atom (see p. 275), the use of the 'World' in this fashion can help to focus upon the areas or problems to be worked with as a part of the assessment task.

Sociodramatic Play Inventory

A useful method of assessing play, called the Sociodramatic Play Inventory, has been created by Johnson, Christie and Yawkey (1987) in their adaptation of Smilansky's work (1968). A small number of individuals are focused upon and a decision is made as to which elements of play/drama are present in the work. The designers recommend that two or three individuals are focused upon at a time, and suggest that an observer considers each individual for a one-minute period before moving focus to another individual. The few people focused upon are rotated in terms of the observer's attention. A mark is made in the columns of a Play Inventory Sheet for each element observed in the individual's play. A question mark is placed where a brief or hesitant engagement with a particular kind of activity is observed. This should be undertaken on 'several' occasions.

Summaries are gained by adding the numbers in the different columns of the individual to give a summary of the kinds of play the individual is engaging with. 'A child who shows the full gamut of play components would be judged competent in sociodramatic play' (Johnson, Christie and Yawkey, 1987, 163). This gives information on the kinds of playing an individual engages with and can be used to consider the areas which the facilitator can help the individual to develop. The authors frame the inventory in terms of play development and age, and say that for many children dramatic play would emerge by two years of age and the full elaborate form of sociodramatic play assessed here by three or beyond. However, for Dramatherapy's uses age may not be the chief factor.

Sociodramatic Play Inventory

Name

Role

Make-believe transformation (objects, actions, situations)

Social interaction

Verbal communication – pretend

Verbal communication – metacommunication

Persistence

Pretend metacommunication

Adaptation

Terms Defined

Role – taking on roles as demonstrated by behaviour and/or by declaring a role to be taken

Make-believe transformation – objects are used as if they were other objects, actions are used to represent other actions, imaginary situations are pretended and/or verbally declared

Social interaction – two or more individuals interact within the dramatic play activity

Verbal communication

- *Pretend* describes language used appropriately within a role or character spoken by the individual
- *Metacommunication* describes verbal exchanges which help to set up, structure and maintain play, and are spoken rather like stage directions. They are outside the pretend language spoken 'in role' by the individuals.

Persistence – engagement in sustained dramatic play episodes.

Adaptation – incidents of adapting own ideas or actions in relation to another's ideas or actions.

In Dramatherapy this testing device can be used to ascertain the way in which clients can work with drama. It can also be used to put the work within a developmental paradigm. As described in Chapter 8 the increase in complexity of the client's use of the media would be considered within a therapeutic framework. In this way of working a potential change in the ability to sustain concentration or interaction might be linked to a therapeutic aim. So, for example, in working with an elderly client group who are diagnosed as having senile dementia, an aim in a Dramatherapy group might be to increase concentration, focus and interaction with others. The Play Inventory would be used to establish the level of persistence at the start of the work. Social communication and metacommunication would be used to assess the contact between clients within the group. The Inventory would also help to ascertain whether clients had changed during the therapy.

Adapting assessment methods

Parten's social participation scale

Another example of the adaptation of existing assessment methods is the way that Parten's study of young children and assessment scale was adapted to work with adolescents who had been diagnosed as autistic

(Jones, 1993). The Dramatherapy involved an attempt to enhance clients' social skills through the use of puppetry. Elements of the Parten scale were adapted by Sanctuary (1984) in order to try to ascertain the effect of the Dramatherapy upon the client's interactions outside of the therapy group. A series of criteria based on Parten's scale was used to assess certain behaviours and to evaluate the work.

Eight areas were developed from the Parten scale to produce 'a continuum . . . ranging from withdrawn to active and pro-social behaviours and interactions' (Jones, 1993, 51).

Box 12.1 **Parten's social participation scale**

1 Stereotyped
2 Unoccupied/Withdrawn
3 Solitary
4 Responsive
5 Aggressive
6 Initiated
7 Helping behaviour
8 Parallel activity

Adaptation of Parten (Sanctuary, 1984)

Each area was sub-divided into more specific criteria. So, for example, the fourth area was built of a number of behaviours:

4 Responsive: including

Smiling or laughing in response to another
Answering when addressed
Maintaining conversation
Maintaining eye contact for at least one second
Handing or passing objects in response to another

Clients were assessed for a period two weeks prior to the Dramatherapy group, during the nine-week group, immediately after the closure of the work and finally two weeks after the end of the therapy. The comparison of these assessments was then used to help evaluate the nature of behavioural change in the clients.

Read Johnson (Read Johnson and Quinlan, 1985, 21) describes how an already existing scale for measuring patients' behaviour in a psychiatric hospital was used to measure aspects of patients' responses to being involved in a Dramatherapy group producing plays. Two plays were worked on – one was *A Tendency to Get into Difficult Situations*, the other was *The Future Lies in Eggs*. Virtually all those involved in the plays had been diagnosed as schizophrenic. Two scales were used – one of 'social contact', the other of 'clinical state'. They were assumed to measure social, interpersonal behaviour on the ward ('social contact') and 'more symptomatic, intrapsychic disorder' (1985, 24) in the 'clinical state' assessments. The checklist was used up to fourteen times a week. It was used for (i) four weeks prior to rehearsals, (ii) the four weeks of rehearsal and the performance, and (iii) the four weeks after the performance. The second play had an additional period included from the eighth to twelfth week.

In adapting scales or methods from other areas of study or practice, the Dramatherapist aims to meet the requirements of their own assessment needs. They do so by altering the original criteria to relate more effectively to the dramatic media at the heart of Dramatherapy, or by connecting their work to the assessment strategy of another discipline. As the examples cited in this chapter show, this can be effective. However, there is a danger inherent in this form of adaptation. Payne (1993) has identified this problem in the context of research, saying that, 'A sole reliance on traditional research approaches denies us access to the richness available in the processes and other phenomena intrinsic to practice' (1993, 33).

Recording sessions

Recording Dramatherapy sessions will usually involve the documenting of material for the analysis of the therapist in order to communicate about the work to other colleagues in situations such as case conferences. It is not possible to document and analyse everything that occurs within therapy. However, a good recording format should aid the process of finding a language and structure to describe and consider what has occurred. Recording helps to create a space for reflection, aids the process of considering themes, patterns, key occurrences and interactions within the work. Different modalities of recording sessions are often used. These include video, forms for clients to fill in, the creation of pictoral images, and still photographs of elements of enactments.

The following format, often used by Dramatherapists, seeks to set up a framework for describing, documenting and analysing the session through writing.

This example concerns work in a setting which encouraged clients to engage with a variety of therapy programmes – some were group psychotherapy, others took a more behaviourally orientated approach.

Written Dramatherapy recording sample

Dramatherapy group

Date: 22 May   **Time**: 10.00–11.30am
No. of session 10 out of 20
Present Eva, Janet, Malick, Mark, Miriam, Pete, Jo, Zina
Absent None
Pre-session notes Am informed that community meeting prior to group was argumentative, with some clients expressing anger about an outing which had to be cancelled due to staff shortage. Janet expresses reluctance to come to any sessions at the centre just within my earshot. I feel anxious as group seem quite silent and reticent about entering the room – rather like first sessions.
Overall aims within the Dramatherapy group
　　To increase confidence
　　To improve self-image
　　To increase communication skills
Intended sessional aims
1　To offer the opportunity for clients to present personal issues concerning confidence, self-image and communication skills
2　To enable clients to explore these issues through Dramatherapy
3　Through exploring and working with the problems to enable individuals to look at the way issues from their past relate to their current problems
4　To look at ways of achieving change in order to become more confident, to develop a more accurate relationship to self-image and to develop effective communication
Preparation Last session a heated debate had followed the enactment created by Eva when Zina claimed to have been completely ignored in her role of Eva's mother and said that she felt angry with Eva for ignoring her. She said she felt this was something Eva did to her all the time. Eva had denied this, saying that it was her mother she was ignoring, not Zina herself. The session had ended on this note. It seemed likely that this specific issue might be returned to, along with issues around ignoring, being ignored and parents.
Rationale for sessional aims To give space for unfinished business from last time, given the heated ending. To reflect the group's aims to create opportunities to consider self-image, confidence and communication in working with whatever material group members might choose to bring.

Description Group very silent on entry. All acknowledge me and some acknowledge each other. Eva and Zina do not make any eye contact. As usual at the start of the group there is a silence and people begin to talk about the last session and how they feel now. I suggest a sculpt whereby each person places themselves in a position representing how they felt at the end of the session. In this sculpt they each can say a little about how they felt. This is followed by a partner taking up their position – they then say anything they want to that position from where they are now. The partner then says what it felt like to be in that position.

Several themes emerge.

Eva says she doesn't want to talk about it any more. Zina says that she feels ignored by Eva – that she won't listen to how upset she is. I ask whether she wants to explore this further. She says that she does, and I offer her a number of options – these include telling us a story about the feeling of being ignored, or showing us a situation where she has felt ignored, or exploring the relationship with those in the group by sculpting. She chooses to tell a story. A character is created, 'Jasmin', who shares three qualities with Zina and which relate to being ignored. Zina gives these as shy and unsure, used to being ignored, and feeling unworthy. I suggest that we see a story where her character experiences these feelings in three events. It takes place in a desert in a small bedouin encampment near an oasis. There is a family who live in two tents. The first event involves Jasmin trying to tell someone that she has an aching tooth, but no one will listen. In the second she is sent out to find some wood with her two sisters, but though they come back with damp wood and she returns with dry wood, theirs is chosen for the fire. The third event tells how a stranger arrives. This is someone Jasmin likes but she cannot say to him that she likes him. She is unable to make any contact with him.

Zina chooses Mark for her father, Miriam for her mother, Eva and Janet for her sisters and Malick for the stranger. She sculpts them and describes the desert for us, along with the tents. The boundaries of each tent are set up by chairs. Each character is given two qualities by Zina. The father is preoccupied and works hard, the mother is quiet and loves her two younger daughters best, the middle daughter is hard working and jealous of Jasmin, the youngest daughter is quiet and happy. The stranger is warm and mysterious. Zina chooses to play Jasmin, though she was given the choice to cast one of the group in this role.

The story is kept to by the group. The characters then talk about what it felt like to play these roles. At the end I ask Zina what it is that Jasmin wants and how she might get it. Zina says that Jasmin wants to be appreciated more and to get what she wants more. She should push herself and rely less on others to put her forward and to feel at a loss if they didn't. At this point Zina makes a comparison between herself and Jasmin's position. She talks about the expectations around women and cultural issues concerning her Muslim upbringing and her current rejection of these traditions and her faith.

We re-play the scenario. Zina is to play her role as if she could be more assertive, to rely less on others. As Jasmin, Zina manages to do this in some situations. The enactment is broken into three parts and there is a pause after each to see if Zina wants to try it again differently. At times I invite audience feedback on how Jasmin is doing and, if Zina wants it, to be given some ideas about how to handle things.

When this is completed the players speak to the audience about their experience in role and how they feel in relation to the role. Zina says, though she had needed support, she is astonished to be able to find Jasmin being more forthcoming. She adds that the feelings she experienced as Jasmin reminds her of her family situation.

Some of the group talk about how they could identify with the character and her experience. Eva stays silent during this time.

Analysis The work seemed to be able to reflect the material Zina was becoming aware of in the last session. The underlying relationship between Eva and Zina is still reflected in the content and by the casting of Eva as the 'jealous' sister. The group did not engage with how the casting reflected their actual feelings or relationships between each other.

Personal response I too could recognise the feeling of being ignored. It especially reminded me of the feelings raised in the early days of the group when a number of clients did not participate or participated a little and my interventions were often ignored – I remembered how shut out I felt. I felt warm towards the group as they supported the portrayal of Jasmin.

Evaluation

Sessional aims

1 Zina was able to present personal issues concerning confidence and self-image. She was also able to practise enhancing her communication skills. Others were able to discuss their own issues in relation to the work under-taken by the group through joining in with the enactment, through witnessing and through discussion.

2 The group were able to explore these issues through Dramatherapy. For Zina this was through the story and role she created. Others were able to identify with elements of the content and process. To an extent they were able to engage with their own material by witnessing and in the playing through of fears in the roles they took on.

3 Zina was able to look at issues from her past and how they related to her present situation. A specific example was how her relationship with her mother seemed to reflect the feeling of being ignored by Eva in the last

session. Though this was not verbally acknowledged in the session my opinion is that this was an important aspect of the improvisation.

4 By changing Jasmin's behaviour, Zina was able to identify how change might occur, and experienced effecting that change. She had the skills to work with the family and to work in role with more assertion and with more confidence. Her communication skills were enhanced by the way she talked to the group in putting herself forward as willing to explore the situation. She also communicated to the group the ways she wanted to handle the improvisation. The feedback from the group reinforced this. The group, by identifying, witnessing, by offering support and by playing roles, were able to find some contact and use for themselves within the work.

Other points There were issues around the connecting of the character to reality – 'Jasmin could do it, but could I?' However, Zina seemed pleased that she could manage more assertive behaviour at all. Themes continue within the group of ignoring, lack of communication, isolation, though the ability of the group to support Jasmin was a significant change. The individuals managed to keep roles, though Mark became confused and on two occasions needed help to get back into role.

Evaluation

Earlier in this chapter reference was made to two elements of evaluation within the Dramatherapy process. One referred to 'formative', the other 'summative'. Both concerned the act of trying to establish what had occurred within the Dramatherapy process. There are a number of ways in which this process can occur.

One involves the evaluation of the whole programme. Key questions would include:

What has happened within the group as a whole?
What progress has occurred for individuals?
What has happened in terms of the aims of the work?
Have they been met?
Have other changes or outcomes, not stated in the aims, occurred?

The other involves the evaluation of a particular session. This entails the consideration of what has occurred within the session in terms of the client's responses to the work. In addition any set aims are reviewed in the light of what happened during the session.

Gathering information

The gathering of information is important within any evaluation. Material can be gathered through the kinds of assessment and recording processes described above. A range of choices are available to the Dramatherapist in terms of who takes part in the evaluation. These include:

• information from the client on their experiences concerning the Dramatherapy
• information from the therapist on their perceptions of their own process and those processes observed within the work
• information from observers of the clients (both within the group, e.g. two-way mirror technique or video recordings), and outside the group (information gathered by those involved with clients in other situations)

The evaluation takes the gathered information and attempts to answer questions such as those posed above. Again, the suitability and validity of the instruments used to gather the information must be considered in terms of any claims or conclusions relating to change made in the evaluation.

A number of areas relating to assessment and evaluation need to be as clear as possible prior to the start of the work, or in the negotiations between the Dramatherapist, setting and client. These include:

• the approach to be used in gathering information
• the way in which information will be collated in order to try to understand what has happened and what the effect of the therapy has been
• how any information will be used

If this clarity is not reached then confusion can occur for clients, therapist and setting. Information might be used in such a way as to be unethical or not to be in the interests of the client.

Why evaluate?

Evaluations might be completed for various reasons.

They may be carried out to enable the client to acknowledge or gain insight into changes which have occurred, and into areas where change has not occurred. This might be used by the client to consider further areas to consider in therapy and/or to reinforce changes which have occurred.

An evaluation may help the therapist to give feedback to clients, or to ascertain for themselves the effects of their work. It might be used to give feedback to a staff team or setting in order to assist in the general picture of a client's experiences and progress. It might be necessary as part of a formal requirement, in order to monitor aspects of practice or to justify the continuity of the provision of Dramatherapy.

It might also be completed as a part of a research project or programme considering a specific area of Dramatherapy processes or practice.

Basic forms of evaluation

At its simplest an evaluation might use activities to assist clients to review or look back on their participation. Or it might enable clients to use enactment to reflect and communicate their perceptions of areas where change has and has not occurred. This might involve producing a mime of objects which symbolise the client's perceptions of what they take away from the group, or of something which has changed, something which has stayed the same. Feedback between clients is also used in this way – images of progress or change are used.

A common device is to use a scene which represents a metaphor for the group. Individuals place themselves, or sculpt each other, within the metaphor. A swimming pool or landscape is created within the room to represent the Dramatherapy, and individuals situate themselves within the landscape according to various criteria. These might include 'Where you were at the start of this work', 'Where you feel you are now', 'Where has felt most difficult for you to be?', 'A place that represents change for you'. The individual verbalises why they are in the place, and can reflect upon the process of the Dramatherapy through the image.

Another way of evaluating is for the clients to use a series of criteria to reflect upon their experience or upon those of others. In groups where behavioural change, such as assertiveness or social skills are the focus, this approach is often used. The individual looks at the way they have and have not progressed. Often feedback from others can be a useful way to reinforce change or to help to ground perceptions. This can happen towards the close of a piece of work or at various points during the work.

For some work, the therapist evaluates the individual or group progress by looking back at the recordings and assessments made. This might occur informally – initial aims are considered one by one in the light of the material recorded week by week. It might occur more formally by the use and comparison of material gathered prior to the start of the work, during the work, immediately at the close of the work and at a period of time after the work.

Summary

The development of methods of assessment in Dramatherapy is still an area which needs research. The establishing of clear strategies which are based firmly in the theories, principles and core practices of Dramatherapy are needed. As this chapter has shown, the current approaches toward assessment and evaluation in Dramatherapy are usually adapted from those utilised in related disciplines – dramatic scales, methods from play therapy or psychodrama.

Whilst these approaches and techniques suffice to support the work which the Dramatherapist undertakes, the therapist has to adopt a way of working which must be adapted, rather than working with an approach generated by the field of Dramatherapy itself.

However, the chapter has illustrated the broad range of assessment and evaluation practices available to Dramatherapy. A wide range of processes can be brought to the work in a way which suits the needs and context of the client involved in Dramatherapy.

Conclusion

One of the aims of this book has been to place Dramatherapy within a history of developments in drama, theatre and therapy. In a sense my inspiration was a sentence in Evreinov's short essay about Theatrotherapy, where he says that the use of theatre and drama as a therapy, 'one of the strongest weapons for safeguarding . . health', is 'in its initial stage of development' (1927, 127). He goes on to say that 'Some day I hope to write a book about it' (1927, 127). Though Evreinov's name and writings have been lost, as Chapter 3 of this book has shown, many of his ideas anticipate those of Dramatherapy as it has emerged in the last half of the century. However, he did not succeed in writing a book which developed his ideas on this area fully. In writing *Drama as Therapy* I hope to have created a book which demonstrates how an aspect of theatre and drama can be a way of 'safeguarding health' and of dealing with problems or ill-health.

The centre of this book is Chapter 5 and its description of the core processes. The heart of its ideas lies in asserting that Dramatherapy is based in the healing and affirming potentials within creativity and the art form of drama. One of my aims was to prove, through theoretical exploration and practical example, that Dramatherapy should be approached within its own terms. I hope to have described a form of therapy which can be understood within its own parameters, which does not need to look to models of analytic therapy or to psychodrama for the justification of how change and personal development occur. Too often in the past theorists and practitioners have had to look outside Dramatherapy itself to try to justify its relationship to change; to find clothing which is made up of items from others' wardrobes.

Whilst not ignoring the fact that there are commonalities with other therapies and other arts processes, I hope to have clearly given Dramatherapy its own identity – placing it in history, placing it within a clear set of core processes and showing why and how its approaches and techniques can be used by client and Dramatherapist together.

References

Abrams, M. (1981) *A Dictionary of Literary Terms*, London, Fontana.

Ammar, H. (1954) *Growing Up in an Egyptian Village*, London, Routledge and Kegan Paul.

Anderson, W. (ed.) (1977) *Therapy and the Arts: Tools of Consciousness*, New York, Harper Colophon.

Antinucci-Mark, G. (1986) 'Some Thoughts on the Similarity between Psychotherapy and Theatre Scenarios', *British Journal of Psychotherapy*, vol. 3, no. 1, 14–19.

Argyle, M. (1969) *Social Interaction*, London, Methuen.

Argyle, M. (1972) *The Psychology of Interpreting Behaviour*, London, Penguin.

Aristotle (1961) *Poetics*, tr. Butcher, S.H., New York, Hill and Wang.

Arnheim, R. (1992) 'Why Aesthetics Is Needed', *The Arts in Psychotherapy*, vol. 19, 149–151.

Artaud, A. (1958) *The Theatre and Its Double*, New York, Grove.

Association for the Anthropological Study of Play. Various leaflets. Middle Tennessee State University, Murfreeboro, TN 37132, USA.

Axline, V. (1964) *Dibs: In Search of Self*, New York, Ballantine.

Baker, D. (1981) 'To Play or Not to Play', in McCaslin, N. (ed.) *Children and Drama*, New York, Longman.

Barba, E. and Savarese, N. (1991) *A Dictionary of Theatre Anthropology*, London, Routledge.

Barham, M. (1994) 'Dramatherapy: the Journey to Become a Profession', paper, *ECARTE conference*, Ferrara, Italy.

Barrault, J.L. (1972) 'Best and Worst of Professions', in Hodgson, J. (ed.) *The Uses of Drama*, London, Eyre Methuen.

Barrault, J.L. (1974) *Memories for Tomorrow*, London, Thames and Hudson.

Becker, A.L. (1979) 'Text Building, Epistemology and Aesthetics in Javanese Shadow Theatre', in Becker, A.L. and Yengoyan, A.A. *The Imagination of Reality, Essays in Southeast Asian Coherence Systems*, New Jersey, Ablex.

Becker, A.L. and Yengoyan, A.A. (1979) *The Imagination of Reality, Essays in Southeast Asian Coherence Systems*, New Jersey, Ablex.

Becker, E. (1975) 'The Self As A Locus of Linguistic Causality', in Brissett, D. and Edgeley, C. *Life as Theater: A Dramaturgical Sourcebook*, Chicago, Aldine.

Beckerman, B. (1990) *Theatrical Presentation – Performer, Audience and Act*, London, Routledge.

Beik, J. (1987) *Hausa Theatre in Niger*, New York and London, Garland.

Benjamin, W. (1955) 'Das Kunstwerk im Zeitalter seiner technischen Reproduzierbarkeit', in *Schriften, vol. 1*, Frankfurt, Suhrkamp.

Benjamin, W. (1970) *Illuminations*, London, Penguin.

Benthall, J. and Polhemus, T. (eds) (1975) *The Body as a Medium of Expression*, London, Allen Lane.

Bentley, E. (1976) *The Theory of the Modern Stage*, London, Penguin.

Bentley, E. (1977) 'Theatre and Therapy', in Anderson, W. (ed.) *Therapy and the Arts: Tools of Consciousness*, New York, Harper Colophon.

Berger, P. (1975) *Sociological Perspectives: Society as Drama* in Brissett, D. and Edgeley, C. (eds) *Life as Theater: A Dramaturgical Sourcebook*, Chicago, Aldine.

Berne, E. (1964) *Games People Play*, New York, Grove.

Bettelheim, B. (1976) *The Uses of Enchantment*, London, Thames and Hudson.

Bixler, J. (1949) *Play in Therapy*, New York, John Wiley and Sons.

Blatner, A. (1973) *Acting In*, New York, Springer.

Blatner, A. and A. (1988a) *The Art of Play*, New York, Springer.

Blatner, A. and A. (1988b) *Foundations of Psychodrama*, New York, Springer.

Boal, A. (1974) *Poetics of the Oppressed: Experiments with the People's Theatre in Brazil*, London, Pluto.

Boal, A. (1979) *Theatre of the Oppressed*, London, Pluto.

Boal, A. (1992) *Games for Actors and Non-Actors*, tr. Jackson, A., London, Routledge.

Bolton, G.M. (1981) 'Drama-in-Education – A Re-appraisal', in McCaslin, N. (ed.) *Children and Drama*, New York, Longman.

Bolton, G.M. (1984) *Drama as Education*, Harlow, Longman.

Booth, D. and Martin Smith, A. (eds) (1988) *Recognizing Richard Courtney*, Ontario, Pembroke.

Borges, J.L. (1970) *Labyrinths*, London, Penguin.

Bowyer, R. (ed.) (1970) *The Lowenfeld Technique*, Oxford, Pergamon.

Brecht, B. (1964) *Brecht on Theatre*, (ed.) Willett, J., London, Methuen.

Bretherton, I. (ed.) (1984) *Symbolic Play: The Development of Social Understanding*, Orlando, Florida Academic Press.

Brissett, D. and Edgeley, C. (eds) (1975) *Life as Theater: A Dramaturgical Sourcebook*, Chicago, Aldine.

Brook, P. (1968) *The Empty Space*, London, Penguin.

Brook, P. (1988) *The Shifting Point*, London, Methuen.

Brookes, J.M. (1975) 'Producing Marat/Sade: Theatre in a Psychiatric Hospital', *Hospital and Community Psychiatry*, vol. 26, no. 7, 429–435.

Brown, D. and Pedder, J. (1979) *Introduction to Psychotherapy*, London, Tavistock.

Brown, N.S., Curry, N.E. and Tittnich, E. (1971) 'How Groups of Children Deal with Common Stress Through Play', in Curry, N.E. and Arnaud, S. (eds) *Play: The Child Strives Towards Self Realization*, Washington D.C., National Association for the Education of Young Children.

Brown, R.P. (ed.) (1968) *Actor Training*, Institute for Research in Acting, New York, Drama Book Specialists.

Bruscia, K. (1988) 'Standards for Clinical Assessment in the Arts Therapies', *The Arts in Psychotherapy*, vol. 15, 5–10.

Buchanan, D.R. (1984) 'Moreno's Social Atom: A Diagnostic Treatment Tool for Exploring Interpersonal Relationships', *The Arts in Psychotherapy*, vol. 11, 155–164.

Buhler, N. (1951) *World Technique*, New York, John Wiley and Sons.

Burke, K. (1975) 'On Human Behavior Considered Dramatistically', in Brissett, D. and Edgeley, C. (eds) *Life as Theater: A Dramaturgical Sourcebook*, Chicago, Aldine.

Caldwell Cook, H. (1917) *The Play Way*, London, Heinemann.

Canda, E.R. (1990) 'Therapeutic Use of Writing and Other Media with Southeast Asian Refugees', *Journal of Independent Social Work*, vol. 4, no. 2, 47–60.

Casement, P. (1990) *Further Learning from the Patient*, London, Routledge.

Cassirer, E. (1946) *Language and Myth*, New York, Dover.

Cassirer, E. (1955) *The Philosophy of Symbolic Forms, vol. 1: Language*, New Haven, CT, Yale University Press.

Cattanach, A. (1992) *Play Therapy with Abused Children*, London, Jessica Kingsley.

Cattanach, A. (1994) 'The Developmental Model of Dramatherapy', in Jennings, S., Cattanach, A., Mitchell, S., Chesner, A. and Meldrum, B. (eds) *The Handbook of Dramatherapy*, London, Routledge.

Central Sesame Course Information (1993).

Cerf, K. (1972) 'Drama Therapy for Young People', in Brown, R.P. (ed.) *Actor Training*, Institute for Research in Acting, New York, Drama Book Specialists.

Cervantes, M. (1898) *The History of Don Quixote*, ed. Clark, J.W., London, Cassell Petter and Galpin.

Chapple, E.D. (1970) *Culture and Biological Man: Explorations in Behavioral Anthropology*, New York, Holt, Rinehart and Winston.

Chauncey, H. (ed.) (1969) *Soviet Pre-School Education, vol. 2: Teacher's Commentary*, New York, Holt Rinehart and Winston.

Chesner, A. (1994) 'Dramatherapy and psychodrama: similarities and differences', in Jennings S., Cattanach, A., Mitchell, S., Chesner, A.

and Meldrum, B. (eds) *The Handbook of Dramatherapy*, London, Routledge.

Ciornai, S. (1983) 'Art Therapy with Working Class Women', *The Arts In Psychotherapy*, vol. 10, 63–76.

Clark-Shock, K., Turner, Y. de G. and Boree, T. (1988) 'A Multidisciplinary Psychiatric Assessment, The Introductory Group', *The Arts in Psychotherapy*, vol. 15, 79–82.

Cohen, N. (1944) 'Puppetry with Psychoneurotic Soldiers', *Puppetry Journal*, vol. 4, no. 2, 7–9.

Cohen, R. (1969) 'Play amongst European Kindergarten girls in a Jerusalem Neighborhood' cited in Feitelson, D. (1977) 'Cross-cultural Studies of Representational Play' in Tizard, B. and Harvey, D. (eds) *Biology and Play*, Philadelphia, Lippincott.

Connor, L. (1984) 'The Unbounded Self: Balinese Therapy in Theory and Practice', in Marsella, A.J. and White, G.M. (eds) *Cultural Conceptions of Mental Health and Therapy*, Dordrecht, Reidel.

Corsini, R.T. (1966) *Roleplaying in Psychotherapy*, New York, Aldine.

Coult, T. and Kershaw, B. (1983) *Engineers of the Imagination*, London, Methuen.

Courtney, R. (1974) *Play, Drama and Thought*, New York, Drama Book Specialists.

Courtney, R. (1981) 'Aristotle's Legacy', *Indiana Theater Bulletin*, vol. 2, no. 3, 1–10.

Courtney, R. (1983) 'Human Performance: Meaning and Knowledge', in Booth, D. and Martin Smith, A. (eds) (1988) *Recognizing Richard Courtney*, Ontario, Pembroke.

Courtney, R. (1986a) 'Mirrors: Sociological Theatre/Theatrical Sociology', in Booth, D. and Martin Smith, A. (eds) (1988) *Recognizing Richard Courtney*, Ontario, Pembroke.

Courtney, R. (1986b) 'A Whole Theory for Drama Therapy', in Booth, D. and Martin Smith, A. (eds) (1988) *Recognizing Richard Courtney*, Ontario, Pembroke.

Courtney, R. (1988) *Recognizing Richard Courtney*, eds D. Booth and A. Martin Smith, Ontario, Pembroke.

Cox, M. (1992) *Shakespeare Comes To Broadmoor*, London, Jessica Kingsley.

Curran, F. (1939) 'The Drama As a Therapeutic Measure in Adolescents', *American Journal of Orthopsychiatry*, vol. 9, 215.

Curry, N.E. and Arnaud, S. (eds) (1971) *Play: The Child Strives Towards Self Realization*, Washington, D.C., National Association for the Education of Young Children.

Daley, T., Case, C., Schaverien, J., Weir, F., Nowell Hall, P., Halliday, D. and Waller, D. (1987) *Images of Art Therapy*, London, Tavistock.

Davidoff, E. (1939) 'Reactions of a Juvenile Delinquent Group to Story and Drama Techniques', *Psychiatric Quarterly*, vol. 13, 245–258.

Davies, M.H. (1987) 'Dramatherapy and Psychodrama', in Jennings, S. (ed.) *Dramatherapy, Theory and Practice for Teachers and Clinicians*, London, Routledge.

Davies, M.H. (1992) 'Dramatherapy and Psychodrama' in Jennings, S. (ed.) *Dramatherapy Theory and Practice for Teachers and Clinicians, vol. 2*, London, Routledge.

Dawson, S.W. (1970) *Drama and the Dramatic*, London, Methuen.

Deutsch, N. (1947) 'Analysis of Postural Behaviour', *Psychoanalytic Quarterly*, vol. 16, 195–213.

Deutsch, N. (1952) 'Analytic Posturology', *Psychoanalytic Quarterly*, vol. 21, 196–213.

Dokter, D. (1990) 'Acting In or Acting Out?' *Dramatherapy, Journal of the British Association for Dramatherapists*, vol. 12 no. 2,7–9.

Dokter, D. (1992) 'Dramatherapy A Psychotherapy?' *Dramatherapy, Journal of the British Association for Dramatherapists*, vol. 14, no. 2, 9–11.

Dokter, D. (1993) 'Dramatherapy Across Europe - Cultural Contradictions' in Payne, H. (ed.) *Handbook of Inquiry in the Arts Therapies, One River, Many Currents*, London, Kingsley.

Douglas, M. (1966) *Purity And Danger*, London, Arc/Routledge and Kegan Paul.

Douglas, M. (1970) *Natural Symbols*, New York, Barrie and Rockliff.

Douglas, M. (1975) *Implicit Meaning*, London, Routledge and Kegan Paul.

Dubowski, J. (ed.) (1984) 'Art Therapy as a Psychotherapy with the Mentally Handicapped' Hertfordshire College of Art and Design, Conference Proceedings.

Dunlop, I. (1977) *Edvard Munch*, London, Thames and Hudson.

Dunton, W.R. (ed.) (1950) *Occupational Therapy, Principles and Practice*, Springfield, Charles C. Thomas.

Ebbek, F.N. (1973) 'Learning from Play in Other Cultures', in Forst, K. (ed.) *Revisiting Early Childhood Education*, New York, Holt, Rinehart and Winston.

Eco, U. (1984) *Semiotics and the Philosophy of Language*, London, Macmillan.

Eco, U., Santambrogio, M. and Violi, P. (1983) *Meaning and Mental Representations*, Bloomington, Indiana University Press.

Eifermann, R.R. (1987) 'Children's Games Observed and Experienced', *Psychiatric Study of the Child*, vol. 42.

Ekstein, R. and Friedman, S.W. (1957) 'The Function of Acting Out, Play Action and Play Acting in the Psychotherapeutic Process', *Journal of the American Psychoanalytic Association*, vol. 5, 581–629.

Elam, K. (1991) *The Semiotics of Theatre and Drama*, London, Methuen.

Ellis, G.E. (1954) 'The Use of Dramatic Play for Diagnosis and Therapy', *Journal of Colorado-Wyoming, Academy of Science*, vol. 4, 57–58.

Elsass, P. (1992) 'The Healing Space in Psychotherapy and Theatre', *New Theatre Quarterly*, vol. 8 no. 32.

Emunah, R. and Read Johnson, D. (1983) 'The Impact of Theatrical Performance on the Self Images of Psychiatric Patients', *The Arts in Psychotherapy*, vol. 10, 233–239.

Erikson, E. (1950) *Childhood and Society*, New York, Norton.

Erikson, E. (1963) *Childhood and Society*, Harmondsworth, Penguin.

Esslin, M. (1978) *An Anatomy of Drama*, London, Maurice Temple Smith.

Esslin, M. (1987) *The Field of Drama*, London, Methuen.

Evreinov, N. (1927) *The Theatre in Life*, New York, Harrap.

Fein, G. and Stork, L, (1981) 'Sociodramatic Play: Social Class Effect in Integrated and Pre-school classrooms', *Journal of Applied Developmental Psychology*, vol. 2, 267–279.

Feitelson, D. (1977) 'Cross-cultural Studies of Representational Play', in Tizard, B. and Harvey, D. (eds) *Biology and Play*, Philadelphia, Lippincott.

Feitelson, D. and Landau, M. (1976) *The Home Environment of Two Groups of Pre-Schoolers in Jerusalem*, cited in Feitelson, D. 'Cross-cultural Studies of Representational Play' (1977) in Tizard, B. and Harvey, D. (eds) *Biology and Play*, Philadelphia, Lippincott.

Fenichel, O. (1942) 'On Acting', *Psychoanalytic Quarterly*, vol. 11, 459.

Fenichel, O. (1945) 'Neurotic Acting Out', *Psychoanalytic Review*, vol. 32, 197–206.

Fink, S. (1990) 'Approaches to Emotion in Psychotherapy and Theatre: Implications for Dramatherapy', *The Arts in Psychotherapy*, vol. 17, 5–18.

Florsheim, M. (1946) 'Drama Therapy', paper given at American Occupational Therapy Association Convention.

Fontana, D. and Valente, L. (1993) 'Dramatherapy and the Theory of Psychological Reversals,' *The Arts In Psychotherapy*, vol. 20, 133–42.

Forst, K. (ed.) (1973) *Revisiting Early Childhood Education*, New York, Holt, Rinehart and Winston.

Fortes, M. (1938) 'Social and Psychological Aspects of Education in Taleland', *Africa*, vol. 1 (supplement), 27–42.

Foucault, M. (1986) *The History of Sexuality vol. 2*, New York, Random House.

Freud, S. (1900) *The Interpretation of Dreams*, London, Hogarth.

Freud, S. (1950) *Totem and Taboo*, London, Hogarth.

Frost, A. and Yarrow, R. (1990) *Improvisation In Drama*, London, Macmillan.

Fryrear, J.L. and Fleshman, B. (1981) *The Arts Therapies*, New York, Charles C. Thomas.

Garvey, C. (1974) 'Some Properties of Social Play', *Merrill-Palmer Quarterly*, vol. 20, 163–180.

Garvey, C. (1977) *Play*, Cambridge, MA, Harvard University Press.

Gerould, D. (1985) *Doubles, Demons and Dreamers*, New York, Performing Arts Journal Publications.

Gersie, A. (1987) 'Dramatherapy and Play', in Jennings, S. (ed.) *Dramatherapy, Theory and Practice for Teachers and Clinicians, vol. 1*, London, Routledge.

Gersie, A. (1991) *Storymaking in Bereavement*, London, Jessica Kingsley.

Gersie, A. and King, N. (1990) *Storymaking in Education and Therapy*, London, Jessica Kingsley.

Giffen, H. (1984) 'The Co-ordination of Meaning in the Creation of Shared Make-Believe Reality', in Bretherton, I. (ed.) *Symbolic Play: The Development of Social Understanding*, Orlando, Florida Academic Press.

Gillies, N. and Gunn, T. (1963) 'Live Presentation of Dramatic Scenes', *Group Psychotherapy*, vol. 16, no. 3, 164–72.

Glaser, B. and Strass, A. (1975) 'The Ritual Drama of Mutual Pretense', in Brissett, D. and Edgeley, C. (eds) *Life as Theater: A Dramaturgical Sourcebook*, Chicago, Aldine.

Goffman, E. (1959) *The Presentation of Self In Everyday Life*, New York, Doubleday.

Goffman, E. (1961) *Encounters*, New York, Bobb Merrill.

Goffman, E. (1972) *Relations in Public*, London, Penguin.

Golub, S. (1984) *Evreinov, The Theater of Paradox and Transformation*, Ann Arbor, Michigan, U.M.I. Research Press.

Goodman, J. and Prosperi, M. (1976) 'Drama Therapies in Hospitals', *The Drama Book Review*, vol. 20, no. 1, 20–30.

Goodman, N. (1981) *Languages of Art*, London, Harvester.

Grainger, R. (1990) *Drama and Healing: The Roots of Dramatherapy*, London, Jessica Kingsley.

Green, R. (1966) 'Play Production In A Mental Hospital Setting', *American Journal of Psychiatry*, vol. 122, 1181–1185.

Griffing, P. (1983) 'Encouraging Dramatic Play in Early Childhood', *Young Children*, vol. 38 no. 4, 13–22.

Grolinski, S.A. and Barkin, L. (1978) *Between Fantasy and Reality*, Northvale, NJ, Jason Aronson.

Groos, K. (1901) *The Play of Man*, London, Heinemann.

Gropius, W. (ed.) (1979) *The Theatre of the Bauhaus*, London, Methuen.

Grotowski, J. (1968) *Towards a Poor Theatre*, London, Methuen.

Gunn, G.R.L. (1963) 'The Life Presentation of Dramatic Scenes as a Stimulus to Patient Interaction in Group Psychotherapy', *Group Psychotherapy*, vol. 16, no. 3, 164–172.

Hampson, S. (1988) *The Construction of Personality: An Introduction*, London, Routledge.

Handke, P. (1971) *Offending the Audience and Self-accusation*, London, Holt.

Haviland, W.H. (1978) *Cultural Anthropology*, New York, John Wiley and Sons.

Heathcote, D. (1989) *Collected Writings on Education and Drama*, ed. Johnson, L. and O'Neill, C., London, Hutchinson.

Henry, W.E. (1973) *The Analysis of Fantasy*, New York, Krieger.

Hickling, F.W. (1989) 'Sociodrama in the Rehabilitation of Chronic Mentally Ill Patients', *Hospital and Community Psychiatry*, vol. 40, no. 4, 402–406.

Hodgson, J. (1972) *The Uses of Drama*, London, Methuen.

Hoffman, E.T.A. (1952) 'Cruel Sufferings of a Stage Director', in Nagler, A. M. (ed.) *A Source Book in Theatrical History*, New York, Dover.

Holland, P. (1964) *Self and Social Context*, London, Macmillan.

Hope, M. (1988) *The Psychology of Ritual*, Dorset, Element Books.

Hornbrook, D. (1989) *Education and Dramatic Art*, Oxford, Blackwell.

Horwitz, S. (1945) 'The Spontaneous Drama as a Technic in Group Therapy', *Nervous Child Journal*, vol. 4, 252–273.

Houben, J., Smitskamp, H. and te Velde, J. (eds) (1989) *The Creative Process*, Hogeschool Midden Nederland, Phaedon.

Howes, M. (1980) 'Peer Play Scale', *Developmental Psychology*, vol. 16, 371.

Huizinga, J. (1955) *Homo Ludens*, Boston, Beacon.

Ickes, W. and Knowles, E.S. (eds) (1982) *Personality, Roles, and Social Behavior*, New York, Springer.

Ikegami, Y (1971) 'A Stratificational Analysis of the Hand Gestures in Indian Classical Dancing', *Semiotica*, vol. 4, 365–391.

Innes, C (1993) *Avant Garde Theatre 1892–1992*, London, Routledge.

Irwin, E.C. (1979) 'Drama Therapy with the Handicapped', in Shaw, A.M. and Stevens, C.J. (eds) *Drama, Theater and the Handicapped*, Washington DC, American Theater Association.

Irwin, E.C. (1983) 'The Diagnostic and Therapeutic Use of Pretend Play', in Schaefer, C.E. and O'Connor, K.J. (eds) *The Handbook of Play Therapy*, New York, John Wiley and Sons.

Irwin, E.C. and Shapiro, M.I. (1975) 'Puppetry as A Diagnostic and Therapeutic Technique', in Jakab, T. (ed.) *Transcultural Aspects of Psychiatric Art*, vol. 4, Basel, Karger.

Jakab, T. (ed.) (1975) *Transcultural Aspects of Psychiatric Art*, vol. 4, Basel, Karger.

Jacksons, S. (1988) 'Shadows and Stories: Lessons from the Wayang Kulit for Therapy with an Anglo-Indonesian Family', *Australian and New Zealand Journal of Family Therapy*, vol. 9, no. 2, 71–78.

James, W. (1932) 'A Study of the Expression of Bodily Posture', *Journal of General Psychology*, vol. 7, 405–436.

Jennings, H.H. (1943) *Leadership and Isolation*, New York, Longmans Green.

Jennings, S. (1973) *Remedial Drama*, London, Pitman.

Jennings, S. (ed.) (1975) *Creative Therapy*, London, Kemble.

Jennings, S. (ed.) (1987) *Dramatherapy, Theory and Practice for Teachers and Clinicians vol. 1*, London, Routledge.

Jennings, S. (1991) 'Theatre Art: The Heart of Dramatherapy', *Dramatherapy, Journal of the British Association for Dramatherapists*, vol. 14, no. 1, 4–7.

Jennings, S. (ed.) (1992) *Dramatherapy, Theory and Practice for Teachers and Clinicians vol. 2*, London, Routledge.

Jennings, S., Cattanach, A., Mitchell, S., Chesner, A. and Meldrum, B. (1994) *The Handbook of Dramatherapy*, London, Routledge.

Jernberg, A.M. (1983) 'Therapeutic Uses of Sensory Motor Play', in Schaefer C.E. and O'Connor, K.J. (eds) *The Handbook of Play Therapy*, New York, John Wiley and Sons.

Johnson, D.W. and Johnson, F.P. (1987) *Joining Together, Group Theory and Group Skills*, New York, Prentice Hall.

Johnson, J.E., Christie, J.F. and Yawkey, T.D. (1987) *Play and Early Childhood Development*, Illinois, Scott Foresman and Co.

Jones, E. (1919) 'The Theory of Symbolism', *British Journal of Psychology*, vol. 9.

Jones, P. (1984) 'Therapeutic Storymaking and Autism', in Dubowski, J. (ed.) *Art Therapy as a Psychotherapy with the Mentally Handicapped*, Conference Proceedings, Hertfordshire College of Art and Design.

Jones, P. (1989) 'Dramatherapy – State of the Art' Conference Proceedings, Hertfordshire College of Art and Design.

Jones, P. (1991) 'Dramatherapy, Five Core Processes', *Dramatherapy, Journal of the British Association for Dramatherapists*, vol. 14, no. 1, 5–10.

Jones, P. (1993) 'The Active Witness', in Payne, H. (ed.) *Handbook of Inquiry in the Art Therapies, One River, Many Currents*, London, Jessica Kingsley.

Jung, C.G. (1959) *The Archetypes and the Collective Unconscious, Collected Works*, vol. 9, part 2, London, Routledge and Kegan Paul.

Jung, C.G. (1983) *Selected Works*, ed. A. Storr, London, Fontana.

Kelly, G.A. (1955) *Psychology and Personal Constructs*, New York, Norton.

Kersner, M. (1990) 'The Art of Research', Proceedings of the Second Arts Therapies Research Conference, London City University.

Kipper, D.A. (1986) *Psychotherapy Through Clinical Role Playing*, New York, Brunner/Mazel.

Klaesi, J. (1922) 'Einiges der Schizophrenienbehandlung', in Jakab, I. (ed.)

Transcultural Aspects of Psychiatric Art, Psychiatry and Art, vol. 4, Basel, Karger, 193–200.

Klein, M. (1932) *The Psychoanalysis of Childhood*, London, Hogarth.

Klein, M. (1961) *Narrative of a Child Analysis*, vol. 4, London, Hogarth.

Knowles, E.S. (1982) 'From Individual to Group Members: A Dialectic for the Social Science', in Ickes, W. and Knowles, E.S. (eds) *Personality, Roles, and Social Behavior*, New York, Springer.

Koestler, A. (1977) 'Regression and Integration', in Anderson, W. (ed.) *Therapy and the Arts: Tools of Consciousness*, New York, Harper Colophon.

Kors, S. (1964) 'Unstructured Puppet Shows as Group Procedure in Therapy with Children', *Mental Health*, 7.

Kott, J. (1969) 'The Icon and the Absurd', *The Drama Review*, vol. 14, 17–24.

Kowzan, T. (1968) 'The Sign In Theatre', *Diogenes*, vol. 61, 52–80.

Kreeger, A. (ed.) (1975) *Perspectives and Psychotherapy*, New York, Holt.

Krenger, W.K. (1989) *Body Self and Psychological Self*, New York, Brunner/Mazel.

Lahad, M. (1994) 'What is Dramatherapy?', in Jennings, S., Cattanach, A., Mitchell, S., Chesner, A. and Meldrum, B. (eds) *The Handbook of Dramatherapy*, London, Routledge.

Landy, R. (1982) *Handbook of Educational Drama and Theater*, New York, Greenwood.

Landy, R. (1986) *Drama Therapy*, Springfield, IL, Charles C. Thomas.

Landy, R. (1989) 'One on One', in Jones, P. (ed.) 'Dramatherapy – State of the Art', Conference Proceedings, Hertfordshire College of Art and Design.

Landy, R. (1994) *Persona and Performance*, London, Jessica Kingsley.

Langley, D. (1989) 'The Relationship between Psychodrama and Dramatherapy', in Jones, P. (ed.) 'Dramatherapy: State of the Art', Conference Proceedings, Hertfordshire College of Art and Design.

Langley, D. (1993) 'When Is a Dramatherapist Not A Therapist?', *Dramatherapy*, vol. 15, no. 2, 16–18.

Langley, D. and G. (1983) *Dramatherapy and Psychiatry*, London, Croom Helm.

Laurel, B. (1991) quoted in Rheingold, H., 'Reaching Out To Touch Our Fantasies', *Guardian*, 26 August, 14.

Lassner, R. (1947) 'Playwriting and Acting as Diagnostic Therapeutic Techniques with Delinquents', *Journal of Clinical Psychology*, vol. 3, 349–356.

Lefevre, G. (1948) 'A Theoretical Basis for Dramatic Production as a Technique of Psychotherapy', *Mental Health*, vol. 12.

Leguit, G. and van der Wiel, D. (1989) 'A Family Plays Itself Better', in Houben, J., Smitskamp, H. and te Velde, J. (eds) *The Creative Process*,

Hogeschool Midden Nederland, Phaedon.

Levine, R. and, A. (1963) 'Nyansorgo: A Gusii Community in Kenya', in Whithing, B. (ed.) *Six Cultures: Studies in Childrearing*, New York, John Wiley.

Lewis, G. (1980) *The Day of Shining Red*, Cambridge, Cambridge University Press.

Lindkvist, M. (1966) Radius Document, private collection of Ms Lindkvist.

Lindkvist, M. (1977) BISAT (British Institute for the Study of the Arts in Therapy) leaflet, private collection of Ms Lindkvist.

Lindkvist, M. (1990) The Sesame Institute (UK) Training in Drama and Movement Therapy, Information pamphlet, private collection of Ms Lindkvist.

Lindzey, G. and Aronson, E. (eds) (1968) *Handbook of Social Psychology*, Cambridge, MA, Addison-Wesley.

Loewald, E.L. (1987) 'Therapeutic Play in Space and Time', *Psychiatric Study of the Child*, vol. 47.

Loizos, C. (1969) 'Play Behavior in Higher Primates: A Review', in Morris, D. (ed.) *Primate Ethology*, Garden City, Anchor.

Lomax, A., Bartenieff, I. and Paulay, P. (1968) 'Dance Style and Culture', *American Association for the Advancement of Science*, vol. 88, 222–247.

Lorenz, K. (1966) *Evolution and the Modification of Behavior*, Chicago, University of Chicago Press.

Lowen, A. (1958) *Physical Dynamics of Character Structure: Body Form and Movement in Analytic Therapy*, New York, Grune and Stratton.

Lowenfeld, M. (1970) *The Lowenfeld Technique*, ed. R. Bowyer, Oxford, Pergamon.

Lyle, J. and Holly, S.B. (1941) 'The Therapeutic Value of Puppets', *Bulletin of the Menninger Clinic*, vol. 5, 223–226.

McCaslin, N. (1981) *Children and Drama*, New York, Longman.

McDougal, J. (1989) *Theatres of the Body*, London, Free Association.

McMillen, J. (1956) 'Acting The Activity for Chronic Regressed Patients', *Journal Of Psychiatry*, vol. 7, 56–62.

McNiff, S. (1986) *Educating the Creative Arts Therapist*, Springfield, IL, Charles C. Thomas.

McNiff, S. (1988) 'The Shaman Within', *The Arts in Psychotherapy*, vol. 15, 285–291.

McReynolds, P. (1978) *Advances in Psychological Assessment, vol. 4*, Washington, Jossey-Bass.

McReynolds, P. and DeVoge, S. (1978) 'Use of Improvisational Techniques in Assessment', in McReynolds, P. *Advances in Psychological Assessment, vol.4*, Washington, Jossey-Bass.

McReynolds, P., DeVoge, S., Osborne, S.K., Pither, B. and Nordin, K. (1976) 'Manual for the Impro-I, pamphlet, Department of Psychology, University of Nevada, Reno.

McReynolds, P., DeVoge, S., Osborne, S.K., Pither, B. and Nordin, K. (1977) 'An Improvizational Technique for the Assessment of Individuals', Unpublished Manuscript, Department of Psychology, University of Nevada, Reno.

Magarschack, D. (1950) *Stanislawski – On the Art of the Stage*, London, Faber and Faber.

Maier, N.R.F. (1953) 'An Experimental Test of the Effect of Training on Discussion Leadership', *Human Relations*, vol. 6, 161–173.

Main, G. (1975) 'On Projection', in Kreeger, A. (ed.) *Perspectives in Psychotherapy*, New York, Holt.

Malachie-Mirovich, N. (1927) *Soviet Education*, cited in Chauncey, H. (ed.) (1969) *Soviet Pre-school Education, vol. 2: Teachers' Commentary*, New York, Holt, Rinehart and Winston.

Marcuse, H. (1969) *Eros and Civilisation: A Philosophical Inquiry into Freud*, Harmondsworth, Penguin.

Marineau, R.F. (1989) *Jacob Levy Moreno*, London, Tavistock-Routledge.

Marsella, A.J. and White, G.M. (eds) (1984) *Cultural Conceptions of Mental Health and Therapy*, Dordrecht, Reidel.

Maslow, A (1977) 'The Creative Attitude', in Anderson, W. (ed.) *Therapy and the Art: Tools of Consciousness*, New York, Harper Colophon.

Mast, S. (1986) *Stages of Identity: A Study of Actors*, London, Gower.

Mazor, J. (1966) 'Producing Plays In Psychiatric Settings', *Bulletin of Art Therapy*, vol. 5, 4.

McLoyd, V. (1982) 'Social Class Difference in Sociodramatic Play: A Critical Review', *Developmental Review*, vol. 2, 1–30.

Mead, G.H. (1934) *Mind, Self and Society*, Chicago, Chicago University Press.

Meldrum, B. (1994) 'A Role Model for Dramatherapy and Its Application with Individuals and Groups', in Jennings S., Cattanach, A., Mitchell, S., Chesner, A. and Meldrum, B. (eds) *The Handbook of Dramatherapy*, London, Routledge.

Menninger, K. (1942) *Love Against Hate*, New York, Harcourt, Brace and World.

Messinger, S., Sampson, H. and Towne, R. (1962) 'Life As Theatre: Some Notes on The Dramaturgic Approach to Social Reality', *Sociometry*, vol. 25.

Millar, N. (1973) *The Psychology of Play*, New York, Holt.

Miller, J. (1983) *States of Mind*, London, BBC Publications.

Mitchell, J. and Rose, J. (eds) (1982) *Feminine Sexuality*, New York, Norton and Pantheon.

Mitchell, S. (1990) 'The Theatre of Peter Brook as a Model for Dramatherapy', *Dramatherapy, Journal of the British Association for*

Dramatherapists, vol. 13, 1.

Mitchell, S. (1992) 'Therapeutic Theatre: a Paratheatrical Model for Dramatherapy', in Jennings, S. (ed.) *Dramatherapy, Theory and Practice for Teachers and Clinicians*, vol. 2, London, Routledge.

Mora, G. (1957) 'Dramatic Presentations By Mental Patients in the Middle Nineteenth Century', *Bulletin of the History of Medicine*, vol. 3, no. 3, 260–277.

Moran, G.S. (1987) 'Some Functions of Play and Playfulness', *Psychoanalytic Study of the Child*, vol. 42.

Moreno, J.L. (1946) *Psychodrama, vol. 1*, New York, Beacon House.

Moreno, J.L. (1953) *Who shall Survive? Foundations of Sociometry, Group Psychotherapy and Sociodrama*, New York, Beacon House.

Moreno, J.L. (1983) *The Theatre of Spontaneity*, New York, Beacon House.

Moreno, J.L. (ed.) (1960) *The Sociometry Reader*, New York, Free Press.

Moreno, J.L. and, Z. (1959) *Psychodrama, vol. 2*, New York, Beacon House.

Morris, D. (ed.) (1969) *Primate Ethology*, Garden City, Anchor.

Morton, R.B. (1965) 'The Uses of Laboratory Method in a Psychiatric Hospital', in Schein, E.H. and Bennis, W.G. (eds) *Personal and Organisational Change Through Group Methods*, New York, John Wiley and Sons.

Müller-Thalheim, W.K. (1975) 'Self-Healing Tendencies and Creativity' in Jakab, T. (ed.) *Transcultural Aspects of Psychiatric Art, vol. 4*, Basel, Karger.

Murphy, G. (1944) *Human Potentialities*, New York, Basic Books.

Nagler, A.M. (1952) *A Source Book in Theatrical History*, New York, Dover.

Neubauer, P.B. (1987) 'The Many Meanings of Play', *Psychoanalytic Study of the Child, vol. 42*, New Haven, CT, Yale University Press.

Nietzsche, F. (1967) *The Birth of Tragedy*, New York, Vintage.

Nilli, I. (1984) 'On the Theatre of the Future'('O teatre buduscego'), in Golub, S., *Evreinov, the Theater of Paradox and Transformation*, Michigan, U.M.I Research Press.

Oatley, K. (1984) *Selves In Relation*, London, Methuen.

O'Neill, C. and Lambert, A. (1982) *Drama Structures*, London, Hutchinson.

Parten, M. (1932) 'Social Participation among Pre-School Children', *Journal of Abnormal and Social Psychology*, vol. 27, 3–69.

Pavis, P. (1982) 'Languages of the Stage', *Performing Arts Journal*, New York, Journal Publications.

Pavis, P. (1985) *Voix et images de la scène pour une sémiologie de la réception*, Lille, Presses Universitaires.

Payne, H. (ed.) (1993) *Handbook of Inquiry in the Arts Therapies, One River, Many Currents*, London, Kinglsey.

Pedder, J. (1989) 'Courses In Psychotherapy: Evolution and Current Trends', *British Journal of Psychotherapy*, vol. 6, 2.

Pellegrini, A.D. (1980) 'The Relationship between Kindergartners' Play and Achievement in Prereading, Language and Writing', *Psychology in the Schools*, vol. 17, 530–535.

Pepler, D.J. and Rubin, K.H. (eds) (1982) *The Play of Children: Current Theory and Research*, Basel, Karger.

Perls, S.F., Hefferline, R.F. and Goodmab, P. (1951) *Gestalt Therapy*, Harmondsworth, Penguin.

Perlstein, S. (1988) 'Transformation: Life Review and Communal Theater', *Journal of Gerontological Social Work*, vol. 12, 137–148.

Perry, J.W. (1976) *Roots of Renewal in Myth and Madness*, San Francisco, Jossey-Bass.

Petzold, H. (1973) *Gestalttherapie und Psychodrama*, Nicol, Kassel.

Piaget, J. (1962) *Play, Dreams and Imitation in Childhood*, New York, Norton.

Pickard, K. (1989) 'Shape', in Jones, P. (ed.) 'Dramatherapy – State of the Art' Conference Proceedings, Hertfordshire College of Art and Design.

Polhemus, T. (1975) 'Social Bodies', in Polhemus, T. and Benthall, J. (eds) *The Body as A Medium of Expression*, London, Allen Lane.

Polhemus, T. and Benthall, J. (eds) (1975) *The Body as a Medium of Expression*, London, Allen Lane.

Price, H. and Nagle, L. (1943) 'Recreational Therapy at the Sheppard and Enoch Pratt Hospital', *Occupational Therapy and Rehabilitation*, vol. 30.

Ray, B. (1976) *African Religions*, New York, John Wiley and Sons.

Read Johnson, D. (1980) 'Effects of a Therapeutic Experience on Hospitalized Psychiatric Patients', *The Arts in Psychotherapy*, vol. 7, 265–272.

Read Johnson, D. (1981) 'Some Diagnostic Implications of Dramatherapy', in Schattner, G. and Courtney, R., *Drama in Therapy, vol. 1*, New York, Drama Book Specialists.

Read Johnson, D. (1982) 'Developmental Approaches to Drama Therapy', *The Arts in Psychotherapy*, vol. 9, 183–190.

Read Johnson, D. (1985/6) The Developmental Method in Drama Therapy, *The Arts in Psychotherapy*, vol. 13, 17–33.

Read Johnson, D. (1988) 'The Diagnostic Role Playing Test', *The Arts in Psychotherapy*, vol. 15, 23–36.

Read Johnson, D. (1991) 'The Theory and Technique of Transformations in Drama Therapy', *The Arts in Psychotherapy*, vol. 18, 285–300.

Read Johnson, D. and Munich, R.L. (1975) 'Increasing Hospital Community Contact Through A Theatre Program In A Psychiatric Hospital', *Hospital and Community Psychiatry*, vol. 26, no. 7, 435–438.

Read Johnson, D. and Quinlan, D. (1985) 'Representational Boundaries in

Role Portrayals Among Paranoid and Nonparanoid Schizophrenic Patients', *Journal of Abnormal Psychology*, 94.

Reason, P. (ed.) (1988) *Human Enquiry in Action: Developments in New Paradigm Research*, Chichester, John Wiley and Sons.

Reason, P. and Rowan, J. (eds) (1981) *Human Inquiry*, Chichester, John Wiley and Sons.

Rehm, L.P. and Marston, A.R. (1968) 'Reduction of Social Anxiety Through Modification of Self-reinforcement: An Instigation Therapy Technique', *Journal of Consulting and Clinical Psychology*, 565–574.

Reider, N., Olinger, D., and Lyle, J. (1939) 'Amateur Dramatics as a Therapeutic Agent in the Psychiatric Hospital', *Bulletin of the Menninger Clinic*, vol. 3, no. 1, 20–26.

Reil, J.C. (1803) 'Rhapsodieen über die Anwedung der Psychichen Kurmethode', in Zilboorg, G. (1976), *A History of Medical Psychology, The Age of Reconstruction*, New York, Norton.

Rheingold, H. (1991a) 'Reaching Out to Touch Our Fantasies', *Guardian*, 26 August, 14.

Rheingold, H. (1991b) *Virtual Reality*, London, Secker and Warburg.

Robertson, K. (1990) 'Cultural Differences and Similarities in Dramatherapy Theory and Practice', Conference Paper, Arts Therapies Education – Our European Future, ECARTE.

Roose-Evans, J. (1984) *Experimental Theatre*, London, Routledge.

Rossberg-Gempton, I. and Poole, G.D. (1991) 'The Effect of Open and Closed Postures on Pleasant and Unpleasant Emotions', *Arts in Psychotherapy*, vol. 20, no. 1, 75–82.

Rotter, J.B. and Wickens, D.D. (1948) 'The Consistency and Generality of Ratings of "Social Aggressiveness" Made from Observation of Role Playing Situations', *Journal of Consulting Psychology*, vol. 12, 234–239.

Rowan, J. (1990) 'Recent Work in New Paradigm Research', in Kersner, M., *The Art of Research*, Proceedings of the Second Arts Therapies Research Conference, London, City University.

Rubin, J.A. and Irwin, E.C. (1975) 'Art and Drama: Parts of a Puzzle', in Jakab, T. (ed.) *Transcultural Aspects of Psychiatric Art*, vol. 4, Basel, Karger.

Rubin, K.H. and Seibel, C.C. (1979) 'The Effects of Ecological Setting on the Cognitive and Social Play Behaviors of Preschoolers', Paper to American Educational Research Association, San Francisco.

Sanctuary, R. (1984) 'Role Play with Puppets for Social Training', Unpublished Report, University of London, quoted in Jones, P. (1993) 'The Active Witness', in Payne, H., *Handbook of Inquiry in the Arts Therapies, One River, Many Currents*, London, Jessica Kingsley.

Sandberg, B. (1981) 'A Descriptive Scale for Drama', in Schattner, G. and Courtney, R., *Drama in Therapy, vol. 1 and 2*, New York, Drama Book Specialists.

Sarbin, T. (ed.) (1986) *Narrative Psychology*, New York, Praeger.

Sarbin, T. and Allen, V. (1968) 'Role Theory' in Lindzey, G. and Aronson, E. (eds) *Handbook of Social Psychology*, Cambridge, MA, Addison-Wesley.

Satir, V. (1967) *Conjoint Family Therapy*, Paolo Alto, Science and Behavior Books.

Schaefer, C. (1976) *The Therapeutic Use of Child's Play*, Northvale, NJ, Jason Aronson.

Schaefer, C.E and O'Connor, K.J. (1983) *The Handbook of Play Therapy*, New York, John Wiley and Sons.

Schattner, G. and Courtney, R. (1981) *Drama in Therapy, vols 1 and 2*, New York, Drama Book Specialists.

Schechner, R. (1988) *Performance Theory*, New York, Routledge.

Scheff, T.J. (1979) *Catharsis in Healing, Ritual and Drama*, Berkeley, University of California.

Scheflen, A.E. (1972) *Body Language and Social Order*, Englewood Cliffs, NJ, Prentice Hall.

Schein, E. H. and Bennis, W.G. (eds) (1965) *Personal and Organizational Change Through Group Methods*, New York, John Wiley and Sons.

Schmais, C. (1988) 'Creative Arts Therapies and Shamanism: A Comparison', *Arts in Psychotherapy*, vol. 15, no. 4, 281–284.

Schwartzman, H. (1978) *Transformations: The Anthropology of Children's Play*, New York, Plenum Press.

Shaw, A. (1981) 'Co-respondents: The Child and Drama', in McCaslin, N. (ed.) *Children and Drama*, New York, Longman.

Shaw, A. M. and Stevens, C.J. (eds) (1979) *Drama, Theater and the Handicapped*, Washington, DC, American Theater Association.

Siegal, E. (1984) *Dance Movement Therapy: Mirror of Ourselves*, New York, Human Sciences Press.

Singer, J.L. (1973) *The Child's World of Make Believe*, New York, Academic.

Skynner, A.C.R. (1976) *One Flesh: Separate Persons, Principles of Family and Marital Psychotherapy*, London, Constable.

Slade, P. (1954) *Child Drama*, London, University Press.

Slade, P. (1959) *Dramatherapy as an Aid to Becoming a Person*, Pamphlet, Guild of Pastoral Psychology.

Slade, P. (1981) 'Drama as an Aid to Fuller Experience', in McCaslin, N. (ed.) *Children and Drama*, New York, Longman.

Slade, P., Lafitte, E. and Stanley, R.J. (1975) *Drama With Subnormal Adults*, London, Educational Drama Association.

Smilansky, S. (1968) *The Effects of Sociodramatic Play on Disadvantaged Children*, New York, John Wiley and Sons.

Solomon, A.P. (1950) 'Drama Therapy', in Dunton, W.R. (ed.) *Occupational Therapy, Principles and Practice*, Springfield, IL, Charles C. Thomas.

Solomon, A.P. and Fentress, T.L. (1947) 'A Critical Study of Analytically Orientated Group Psychotherapy Utilizing the Technique of Dramatization of the Psychodynamics', *Occupational Therapy and Rehabilitation*, vol. 26, 42–43.

Sontag, S. (1977) 'Marat/Sade/Artaud', in Anderson, W. (ed.) *Therapy and the Arts: Tools of Consciousness*, New York, Harper Colophon.

Souall, A.T. (1981) *Museums of Madness*, London, Sphere.

Southern, R. (1962) *The Seven Ages of Theatre*, London, Faber.

Stanislavski, C. (1937) *An Actor Prepares*, London, Geoffrey Bles.

Stanislavski, C. (1963) *Creating a Role*, London, Geoffrey Bles.

Stebbins, R. (1969) 'Role Distance, Role Distance Behaviour and Jazz Musicians', *British Journal of Sociology*, vol. 20, no. 4, 406–415.

Steger, S. and Coggins, M. (1960) 'Theatre Therapy', *Hospital Management*, vol. 89, 122–128.

Stock-Whitaker, D. (1985) *Using Groups to Help People*, London, Routledge & Kegan Paul.

Stone, G.P. (1975) 'Appearance and Self', in Brissett, D. and Edgeley, C. (eds) *Life as Theater: A Dramaturgical Sourcebook*, Chicago, Aldine.

Stone, G.P. and Faberman, H. (1970) *Social Psychology Through Symbolic Interaction*, Waltham, Ginn Blaisdell.

Sutton-Smith, B. (1972) *The Folk Games of Children*, Austin, TX, University of Texas Press.

Sutton-Smith, B. (ed.) (1979) *Play and Learning*, New York, Gardner.

Sutton-Smith, B. (1981) 'Sutton Smith-Lazier Scale of Dramatic Involvement', in Schattner, G. and Courtney, R., *Drama in Therapy, Volume I*, New York, Drama Book Specialists.

Tizard, B. and Harvey, D. (eds) (1977) *Biology and Play*, London, Heinemann.

Travisano, R.V. (1975) 'Alternation and Conversion As Qualitatively Different Transformations', in Brissett D. and Edgeley, C. (eds) *Life as Theater: A Dramaturgical Sourcebook*, Chicago, Aldine.

Turner, V. (1969) *The Ritual Process*, Chicago, Aldine.

Turner, V. (1974) *Dramas, Fields and Metaphors*, Ithaca, Cornell University.

Turner, V. (1982) *From Ritual to Theater*, New York, Performing Arts Journal Press.

Valente, L. and Fontana, D. (1993) 'Research into Dramatherapy Theory and Practice', in Payne, H. (ed.) *Handbook of Inquiry in the Arts Therapies, One River, Many Currents*, London, Jessica Kingsley.

Vernon, P.E. (1969) *Personality Assessment, A Critical Survey*, London, Methuen.

Von Franz, M.L. (1970) *The Interpretation of Fairytales*, London, Spring.

Von Franz, M.L. (1974) *Shadow and Evil in Fairytales*, New York, Spring.

Ward, W. (1957) *Playmaking with Children*, New York, Appleton-Century Crofts.

Ward, W. (1981) 'A Retrospect', in McCaslin, N. (ed.) *Children and Drama*, New York, Longman.

Watts, P. (1987) in Jennings, S. (ed.) *Dramatherapy, Theory and Practice, vol. 1*, London, Routledge.

Whithing, B. (ed.) (1963) *Six Cultures: Studies in Childrearing*, New York, John Wiley and Sons.

Williams, A. (1989) *The Passionate Technique*, London, Tavistock, Routledge.

Wilshire, B. (1982) *Role Playing and Identity*, Bloomington, IN, Indiana University Press.

Winnicott, D.W. (1953) 'Transitional Objects and Transitional Phenomena, A Study of the First Not-Me Possession', *International Journal of Psychoanalysis*, vol. 34, Part 2.

Winnicott, D.W. (1966) 'The Location of Cultural Experience', *International Journal of Psychoanalysis*, vol. 48.

Winnicott, D.W. (1974) *Playing and Reality*, London, Pelican.

Witkin, R.W. (1974) *The Intelligence of Feeling*, London, Heinemann.

Wolf, D. and Grollman, S.H. (1982) 'Ways of Playing: Individual Differences in Imaginative Style', in Pepler, D.J. and Rubin, K.H. (eds) *The Play of Children: Current Theory and Research*, Basel, Karger.

Woltmann, G. (1940 'The Use of Puppets In Understanding Children', *Mental Hygiene*, vol. 24, 445.

Woltmann, G. (1964) 'Diagnostic and Therapeutic Considerations of Non-verbal Projective Activities with Children', *Mental Hygiene* vol. 24, 445.

Yalom, I.D. (1985) *The Theory and Practice of Group Psychotherapy*, New York, Basic Books.

Yalom, I.D. (1990) *Existential Psychotherapy*, New York, Basic Books.

Zilboorg, G. (1976) *A History of Medical Psychology, The Age of Reconstruction*, New York, Norton.

Name index

Anderson, W. 120
Antinucci-Mark, G. 9, 63, 64
Argyle, M. 202, 207
Aristotle 44, 46
Artaud, A. 52, 53, 119, 244, 247
Aurelius, C. 45–46
Axline, V. 170

Barba, E. 52, 154, 247, 256
Barrault, J.L. 12, 13, 52, 256
Benjamin, W. 151
Bentley, E. 63–64
Berger, P. 65, 67
Bettelheim, B. 225
Blatner, A. 22, 118, 167, 172–173, 174, 204, 206, 240
Boal, A. 4, 53, 54, 109, 154, 155, 201
Bolton, G. M. 171, 172, 173
Borges, J.L. xv, 50
Boyd, N. 68
Brecht, B. 53, 54, 104, 106, 107, 109, 154, 200, 201
Brissett, D. 66
Brook, P. 3, 4, 52, 109–110, 145, 247–248
Brown, D. 63
Bruscia, K. 264, 266
Burke, K. 65

Caldwell Cook, H. 67
Canda, E.R. 12
Case, C. 253–254
Casement, P. 64
Cassirer, E. 196
Cattanach, A. 116, 181–182

Cerf, K. 78, 79
Cervantes, M. xv
Chesner, A. 63
Ciornai, S. 12, 265–266
Connor, L. 246
Courtney, R. 14, 45, 83, 93, 110, 113, 117, 129, 150, 171, 186, 266
Cox, M. 5, 47
Curran, F. 77

Davies, M. 94
Dokter, D. 11, 240
Douglas, M. 245
Dumas, A. 48

Eco, U. 221–222, 230, 236
Edgeley, C. 66
Elam, K. 113, 152, 153
Elsass, P. 9, 45, 63, 64
Emunah, R. 210
Erikson, E. 170
Esslin, M. 108, 146
Evreinov, N. xvi, 3, 12, 46, 47, 54–57, 119, 167, 204, 252, 292

Fenichel, O. xv
Fleshman, B. 44, 47, 48, 94
Florsheim, M. 44, 79, 80
Fontana, D. 5, 11, 35–36
Fryrear, J.L. 44, 47, 48, 94
Freud, S. 8, 11, 64, 101, 131, 151, 222
Frost, A. 153

Gama, E. 49
Garvey, C. 171, 201
Gersie, A. 146, 225, 240

Techniques index

Subject index

able-bodiedism 33; *see also*
  disability, discrimination
abuse 1–3
acting 5–6, 47–50, 51–54, 55-63, 64,
  78, 132–134, 153–155, 199–203,
  205; *see also* actor/actress,
  performance, theatre
acting out xv–xvi, 133–134
active witness *see* witnessing
Activity Leader Training 93
actor/actress 1–3, 55, 104–107,
  153–155, 199–203, 208; *see also*
  acting, performance, theatre
artistic process 8–9
adolescents 18, 74, 77, 130, 135–138,
  162–163
aesthetics 46, 55, 119; *see also*
  creativity, creativity theory
aims 19, 33, 36, 183, 225, 285, 290;
  overall 16, 264–265, 285; sessional
  20–22, 285; setting and negotiating
  31, 36, 179, 220, 264; *see also*
  assessment, evaluation
anthropology 14, 47, 91, 152, 153,
  245–247; *see also* ritual, body,
  ecstasy
Antony and Cleopatra 129; *see also*
  Hamlet, King Lear, Shakespeare,
  Two Gentlemen of Verona
Apollonian 151–152; *see also*
  Dionysian
applause 27
archetype 8, 217
Art Therapy 32, 88, 91, 121,
  253–253; and Remedial Art
  91

Arts Therapies 7, 14, 48, 91, 95
assessment 60, 107, 157, 168, 225,
  263–291; adaptation of models
  272, 282–284; and aims 264, 265;
  historical background 77, 79,
  268–270; initial 31, 265; and play
  72, 185–194, 269–274; and
  projection 138–140, 266, 275–279
  see also Techniques index
Atari Research 13
audience 9, 27–31, 48–50, 100–101,
  104–107, 109–112, 119, 123, 134,
  148–150, 199–200, 205, 206; *see
  also* applause, interactive audience,
  witness
autism 87, 224–229, 282–284

Babylon 45
basic sessional shape 16–31; *see also*
  structure, completion, closure, need
  identifying, warm up
Bauhaus 148–150, 153
beginning Dramatherapy 32–33,
  263–264, 265, 266
behaviourism 4, 11, 35, 36–37, 56,
  77, 266
black theatre 51, 53–54
body 19, 25, 64, 58, 108, 112-115,
  148–166, 184, 192, 204, 245–246;
  body memory 163–166; and
  communication 112–115, 152,
  153–154, 157–160, 184 (*see also*
  meaning); and dance 148, 151,
  154, 155; and duality 64, 151–152,
  153, 154, 163–164; and feminism
  152; and identity 64, 112–114,